ROXBURGH'S
Common Skin Diseases

17th Edition

Ronald Marks

Emeritus Professor of Dermatology and
Former Head of Department of Dermatology
University of Wales College of Medicine
Cardiff, UK

Clinical Professor
Department of Dermatology and Skin Surgery
University of Miami School of Medicine
Miami, USA

ARNOLD

Hodder Arnold • A member of the Hodder Headline Group • London

First published in Great Britain in 2003 by
Arnold, a member of the Hodder Headline Group,
338 Euston Road, London NW1 3BH

http://www.arnoldpublishers.com

Distributed in the United States of America by
Oxford University Press Inc.,
198 Madison Avenue, New York, NY10016
Oxford is a registered trademark of Oxford University Press

Whilst the advice and information in this book are believed to be true and accurate at the date
of going to press, neither the author nor the publisher can accept any legal responsibility or
liability for any errors or omissions that may be made. In particular (but without limiting the
generality of the preceding disclaimer) every effort has been made to check drug dosages;
however it is still possible that errors have been missed. Furthermore, dosage schedules are
constantly being revised and new side-effects recognized. For these reasons the reader is
strongly urged to consult the drug companies' printed instructions before administering any of
the drugs recommended in this book.

British Library Cataloguing in Publication Data
A catalogue record for this book is available from the British Library

Library of Congress Cataloging-in-Publication Data
A catalog record for this book is available from the Library of Congress

ISBN 0 340 76232 2
ISBN 0 340 76233 0 (International Students' Edition – restricted territorial availability)

1 2 3 4 5 6 7 8 9 10

Commissioning Editor: Joanna Koster
Project Editor: Anke Ueberberg
Production Controller: Deborah Smith
Cover Designer: Terry Griffiths

Typeset in 10.5/12.5 Minion by Charon Tec Pvt. Ltd, Chennai, India
Printed and bound in India

What do you think about this book? Or any other Arnold title?
Please send your comments to feedback.arnold@hodder.co.uk

Contents

Contents

Preface

Recognition and treatment of skin disease is an important part of the practice of medicine. These skills should form an essential part of the undergraduate curriculum because skin disorders are common and often extremely disabling in one way or another. Apart from the fact that all physicians will inevitably have to cope with patients with rashes, itches, skin ulcerations, inflamed papules, nodules and tumours at some point in their careers, skin disorders themselves are intrinsically fascinating. The fact that their progress both in development and in relapse can be closely observed, and their clinical appearance easily correlated with their pathology, should enable the student or young physician to obtain a better overall view of the way disease processes affect tissues.

The division of the material in this book into chapters has been pragmatic, combining both traditional clinical and 'disease process' categorization, and after much thought it seems to the author that no one classification is either universally applicable or completely acceptable.

It is important that malfunction is seen as an extension of normal function rather than as an isolated and rather mysterious event. For this reason, basic structure and function of the skin have been included, both in a separate chapter and where necessary in the descriptions of the various disorders.

It is intended that the book fulfil both the educational needs of medical students and young doctors as well as being of assistance to general practitioners in their everyday professional lives. Hopefully it will also excite some who read it sufficiently to want to know more, so that they consult the appropriate monographs and larger, more specialized works.

In this new edition of *Roxburgh's Common Skin Diseases* account has been taken of recent advances both in the understanding of the pathogenesis of skin disease and in treatments for it. Please forgive any omissions as events move so fast it is really hard to catch up!

An introduction to skin and skin disease

An overview

Skin is an extraordinary structure. We are absolutely dependent on this 1.7 m² of barrier separating the potentially harmful environment from the body's vulnerable interior. It is a composite of several types of tissue that have evolved to work in harmony one with the other, each of which is modified regionally to serve a different function (Fig. 1.1). The large number of cell types (Fig. 1.2) and functions of the skin and its proximity to the numerous potentially damaging stimuli in the environment result in two important considerations. The first is that the skin is frequently damaged because it is right in the 'firing line' and the second is that

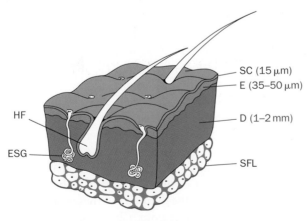

Figure 1.1 Simple three-dimensional plan view of the skin. HF = hair follicle; ESG = eccrine sweat gland; SC = stratum corneum; E = epidermis; D = dermis; SFL = subcutaneous fat layer.

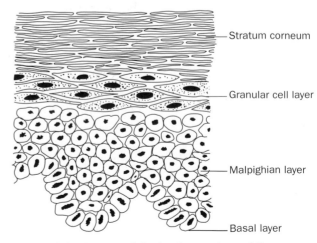

Figure 1.2 Diagram of the basic structure of the epidermis.

1

each of the various cell types that it contains can 'go wrong' and develop its own degenerative and neoplastic disorders. This last point is compounded by the ready visibility of skin, so that minor deviations from normal give rise to a particular set of signs. The net effect is that there seems to be a large number of skin diseases.

Skin disease is very common. However 'healthy' we think our skin is, it is likely that we will have suffered from some degree of acne and maybe one or other of the many common skin disorders. Atopic eczema and the other forms of eczema affect some 15 per cent of the population under the age of 12, psoriasis affects 1–2 per cent, and viral warts, seborrhoeic warts and solar keratoses affect large segments of the population. It should be noted that 10–15 per cent of the general practitioner's work is with skin disorders, and that skin disease is the second commonest cause of loss of work. Although skin disease is not uncommon at any age, it is particularly frequent in the elderly.

Skin disorders are not often dramatic, but cause considerable discomfort and much disability. The disability caused is physical, emotional and socioeconomic, and patients are much helped by an appreciation of this and attempts by their physician to relieve the various problems that arise.

Skin structure and function

It is difficult to understand abnormal skin and its vagaries of behaviour without some appreciation of how normal skin is put together and how it functions in health. Although, at first glance, skin may appear quite complicated to the uninitiated, a slightly deeper look shows that there is a kind of elegant logic about its architecture, which is directed to subserving vital functions.

THE SKIN SURFACE

The skin surface is the delineation between living processes and the potentially injurious outside world and has not only a symbolic importance because of this, but also the important task of preventing and controlling interaction between the outside and the inside. Its $1.7\,\text{m}^2$ area is modified regionally to enable it better to perform particular functions. The limb and trunk skin is much the same from site to site, but the palms and soles, facial skin, scalp skin and genital skin differ somewhat in structure and detail of function. The surface is thrown up into a number of intersecting ridges, which make rhomboidal patterns. At intervals, there are 'pores' opening onto the surface – these are the openings of the eccrine sweat glands (Fig. 1.3). The diameter of these is approximately $25\,\mu\text{m}$ and there are approximately 150–350 duct openings per square centimetre (cm^2). The hair follicle openings can also be seen at the skin surface and the diameter of these orifices and the numbers/cm^2 vary greatly between anatomical regions. Close inspection of the follicular opening reveals a distinctive arrangement of the stratum corneum cells around the orifice.

At magnifications of 500–1000 times, as is possible with the scanning electron microscope (SEM), individual horn cells (corneocytes) can be seen in the process

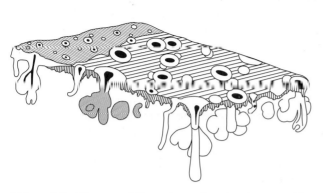

Figure 1.3 Diagram of the skin surface to show sweat pores and hair follicle openings.

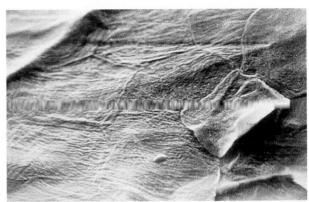

Figure 1.4 Scanning electron micrograph of stratum corneum showing a cell in the process of desquamation.

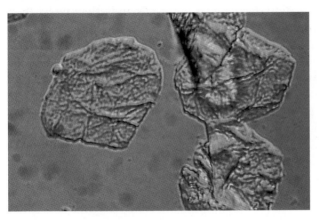

Figure 1.5 Photomicrograph of a corneocyte (×150).

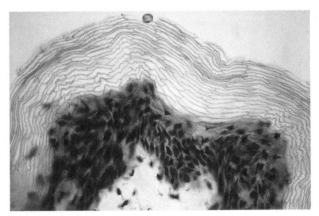

Figure 1.6 Photomicrograph of cryostat section of epidermis to show the delicate structure of the stratum corneum (×90).

of desquamation (Fig. 1.4). Corneocytes are approximately 35 μm in diameter, 1 μm thick and shield like in shape (Fig. 1.5).

THE STRATUM CORNEUM

Also known as the horny layer, this structure is the differentiated end-product of epidermal metabolism (also known as differentiation or keratinization). The final step in differentiation is the dropping off of individual corneocytes in the process of desquamation seen in Figure 1.4. The horny layer is not well seen in routine formalin-fixed and paraffin-embedded sections. It is better observed in cryostat-sectioned skin in which the delicate structure is preserved (Fig. 1.6). It will be noted that at most sites there are some 15 corneocytes stacked one on the other and that the arrangement does not appear haphazard, but is reminiscent of stacked coins.

The corneocytes are joined together by the lipid and glycoprotein of the intercellular cement material and by special connecting structures known as desmosomes.

The orderly release of corneocytes at the surface in the process of desquamation is not completely characterized, but appears to depend on the dissolution of the desmosomes by a chymotryptase protease enzyme near the surface, which is activated by the presence of moisture. On limb and trunk skin, the stratum corneum is some 15–20 cells thick and, as each corneocyte is about 1 µm thick, it is about 15–20 µm thick in absolute terms. The stratum corneum of the palms and soles is about 0.5 mm thick and is, of course, much thicker than that on the trunk and limbs.

The stratum corneum prevents water loss and when it is deranged, as, for example, in psoriasis or eczema, water loss is greatly increased so that severe dehydration can occur if enough skin is affected. It has been estimated that a patient with erythrodermic psoriasis may lose 6 L of water per day through the disordered stratum corneum, as opposed to 0.5 L normally.

The stratum corneum also acts as a barrier to the penetration of chemical agents with which the skin comes into contact. It prevents systemic poisoning from skin contact, although it must be realized that it is not a complete barrier and percutaneous penetration of most agents does occur at a very slow rate. Those responsible for formulating drugs in topical formulations are well aware of this rate-limiting property for percutaneous penetration of the stratum corneum and try to find agents that accelerate the movement of drugs into the skin.

The barrier properties are, of course, also of vital importance in the prevention of microbial life invading the skin – once again the barrier properties are not perfect, as the occasional pathogen gains entry via hair follicles or small cracks and fissures and causes infection.

The mechanical qualities of the stratum corneum are also of great importance. The structure is very extensible and compliant in health, permitting movement of the hands and feet, and is actually quite tough, so that it provides a degree of mechanical protection against minor penetrative injury.

THE EPIDERMIS

The epidermis contains keratinocytes mainly, but also non-keratinocytes – melanocytes and Langerhans cells. This cellular structure is some three to five cell layers thick – on average, 35–50 µm thick in absolute terms (Fig. 1.7a). Not unexpectedly, the epidermis is about two to three times thicker on the hands and feet – particularly the palms and soles. The epidermis is indented by finger-like projections from the dermis known as the dermal papillae (Fig. 1.7b) and rests on a complex junctional zone which consists of a basal lamina and a condensation of dermal connective tissue (Fig. 1.8).

The cells of the epidermis are mainly keratinocytes containing keratin tonofilaments, which are born in the basal generative compartment and ascend through the Malpighian layer to the granular cell layer. They are joined to neighbouring keratinocytes by specialized junctions known as desmosomes. These are visible as 'prickles' in formalin-fixed sections but as alternating light and dark bands on electron microscopy. In the granular layer, they transform from a plump oval or rectangular shape to a more flattened profile and lose their nucleus and cytoplasmic

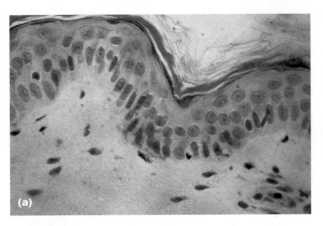
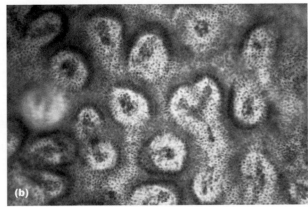

Figure 1.7 (a) Photomicrograph of normal epidermis (H & E, ×90). (b) Photomicrograph of the underside of a sheet of epidermis after removal from dermis showing the indentations made by the finger-like dermal papillae.

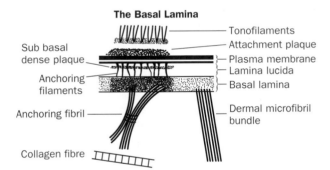

The Basal Lamina

Tonofilaments
Attachment plaque
Sub basal dense plaque
Plasma membrane
Lamina lucida
Anchoring filaments
Basal lamina
Anchoring fibril
Dermal microfibril bundle
Collagen fibre

Figure 1.8 Diagram to show the junctional zone between epidermis and dermis.

organelles. In addition, they develop basophilic granules containing a histidine-rich protein known as filaggrin and minute lipid-containing, membrane-bound structures known as membrane-coating granules or lamellar bodies.

These alterations are part of the process of keratinization during which the keratinocytes differentiate into tough, disc-shaped corneocytes. Other changes include reduction in water content from 70 per cent in the keratinocytes to the stratum corneum's 30 per cent, and the laying down of a chemically resistant, cross-linked protein band at the periphery of the corneocyte.

Of major importance to the barrier function of the stratum corneum is the inter-cellular lipid which, unlike the phospholipid of the epidermis below, is mainly polar ceramide and derives from the minute lamellar bodies of the granular cell layer.

It takes about 28 days for a new keratinocyte to ascend through the epidermis and stratum corneum and desquamate off at the skin surface. This process is greatly accelerated in some inflammatory skin disorders – notably psoriasis.

Pigment-producing cells

Black pigment (melanin) synthesized by melanocytes protects against solar ultra-violet radiation (UVR). Melanocytes, unlike keratinocytes, do not have desmosomes,

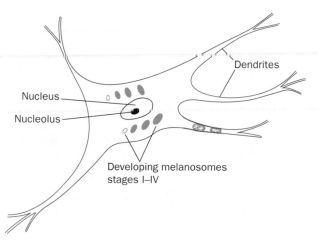

Nucleus

Nucleolus

Dendrites

Developing melanosomes
stages I–IV

Figure 1.9 Diagram to
show a melanocyte with
dendrites injecting
melanin into
keratinocytes.

but have long, branching dendritic projections that transport the melanin they
synthesize to the surrounding cells (Fig. 1.9). They originate from the embryonic
neural crest. Melanocytes account for 5–10 per cent of cells in the basal layer of the
epidermis. Melanin is a polymer, synthesized from the amino acid tyrosine with
the help of a copper-containing enzyme, tyrosinase. Exposure to the sun accelerates
melanin synthesis, which explains suntanning.

Skin colour is mainly due to melanin and blood. Interestingly, the number of
melanocytes in skin is the same regardless of the degree of racial pigmentation –
it is the rate of pigmentation that differs.

Langerhans cells

Langerhans cells are also dendritic cells, but are found within the body of the epidermis in the Malpighian layer rather than in the basal layer. They derive from the
reticuloendothelial system and have the function of picking up 'foreign' material
and presenting it to lymphocytes in the early stages of a delayed hypersensitivity
reaction. They are reduced in number after exposure to solar UVR, accounting for
the depressed delayed hypersensitivity reaction in chronically sun-exposed skin.

THE DERMIS

The tissues of the dermis beneath the epidermis are important in giving mechanical
protection to the underlying body parts and in binding together all the superficial
structures. It is composed primarily of tough, fibrous collagen and a network of
fibres of elastic tissue, as well as containing the vascular channels and nerve fibres
of skin (Fig. 1.10). There are about 20 different types of collagen, but the adult
dermis is made mainly of types I and III, whereas type IV is a major constituent
of the basal lamina of the dermo-epidermal junction. Between the fibres of collagen
is a matrix composed mainly of proteoglycan in which are scattered the fibroblasts that synthesize all the dermal components. Collagen bundles are composed of

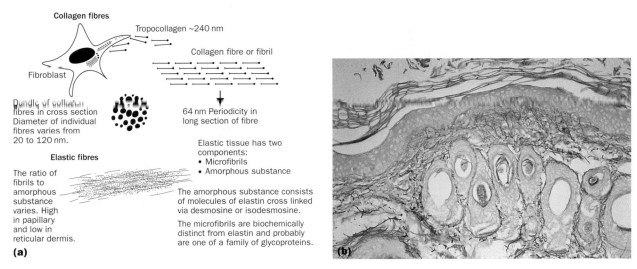

Figure 1.10 (a) Diagram to show components of the dermis. (b) Photomicrograph to show dermal structure.

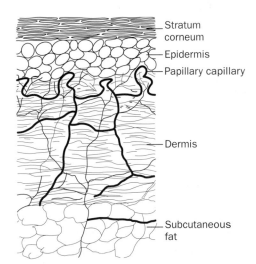

Figure 1.11 Diagram to show the arrangement of the dermal vasculature.

polypeptide chains arranged in a triple helix format in which hydroxyproline forms an important constituent amino acid.

The dermal vasculature

There are no blood vessels in the epidermis and the necessary oxygen and nutrients diffuse from the capillaries in the dermal papillae. These capillaries arise from horizontally arranged plexuses in the dermis (Fig. 1.11).

Nerve structures

Recently, very fine nerve fibres have been identified in the epidermis, but most of the fibres run alongside the blood vessels in the dermal papillae and deeper in the

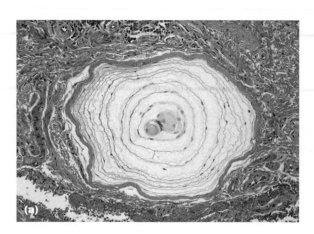
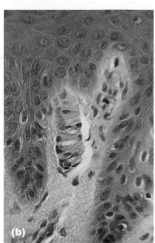

Figure 1.12
Photomicrographs to show (a) Paccinian corpuscle and (b) Meissner corpuscle – specialized neural receptors (H & E, ×150).

dermis. There are several types of specialized sensory receptor in the upper dermis that detect particular sensations (Fig. 1.12).

THE ADNEXAL STRUCTURES

The skin possesses specialized epidermal structures that can be regarded as invaginations of the surface that are embedded in the dermis. These are the hair follicles and the eccrine and apocrine sweat glands.

Hair follicles

Hair follicles are arranged all over the skin surface apart from the palms and soles, the genital mucosa and the vermilion of the lips. Hair growth is asynchronous in humans but synchronous in many lower mammals. The different phases of our asynchronous hair growth occur independently in individual follicles but are timed to occur together in synchronous hair growth, accounting for the phenomenon of moulting in small, furry mammals. The phase of the hair growth is known as anagen and is the longest phase of the hair cycle. Following anagen, a short stage of defervescence is reached known as catagen. This is followed by a resting phase known as telogen, which is again followed by anagen somewhat later (Fig. 1.13).

The hair shaft grows from highly active, modified epidermal tissue known as the hair matrix. The shaft traverses the hair follicle canal, which is made up of a series of investing epidermal sheaths, the most prominent of which is the external root sheath (Fig. 1.14). The whole follicular structure is nourished by a small indenting cellular and vascular connective tissue papilla, which pokes into the base of the matrix. The sebaceous gland secretes into the hair canal a lipid-rich substance known as sebum, whose function is to lubricate the hair (Fig. 1.15). Sebum contains triglycerides, cholesterol esters, wax esters and squalene. Hair

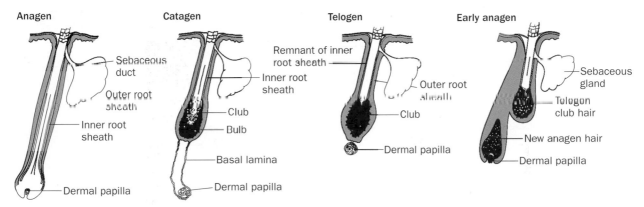

Figure 1.13 Diagram to show hair cycle.

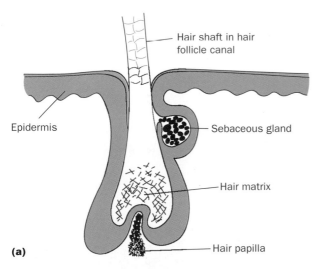

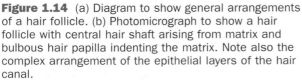

(a)

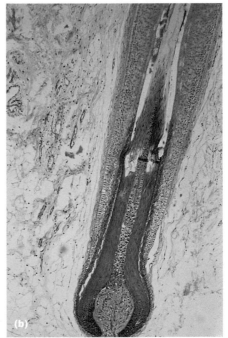

Figure 1.14 (a) Diagram to show general arrangements of a hair follicle. (b) Photomicrograph to show a hair follicle with central hair shaft arising from matrix and bulbous hair papilla indenting the matrix. Note also the complex arrangement of the epithelial layers of the hair canal.

growth and sebum secretion are mainly under the control of androgens, although other physiological variables may also influence these functions.

The eccrine sweat glands are an extremely important part of the body's homeothermic mechanism in that the sweat secretion evaporates from the skin surface to produce a cooling effect. Apart from heat, eccrine sweat secretion may also be stimulated by emotional factors and by fear and anxiety. Certain body sites, such as the palms, soles, forehead, axillae and inguinal regions, secrete sweat selectively during emotional stimulation.

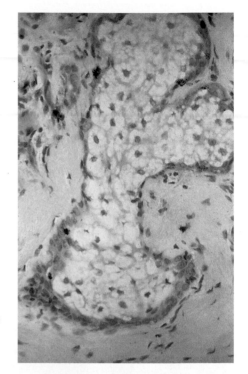

Figure 1.15 Photomicrograph to show sebaceous gland. The 'empty' appearance of the cells is due to the lipid secretion being washed out in the histological preparation (H & E, ×90).

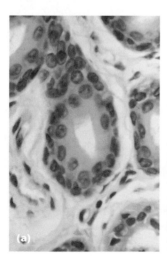

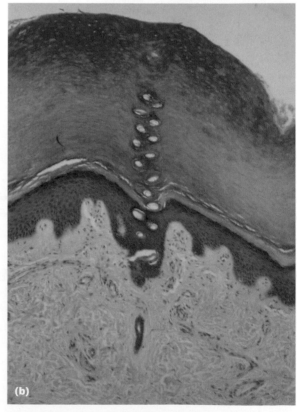

Figure 1.16 (a) Photomicrograph to show tubular structures of a sweat gland deep in the dermis (H & E, ×150). (b) Photomicrograph to show a sweat duct spiralling through the epidermis and stratum corneum of the palm (H & E, ×45).

The eccrine sweat glands consist of a coiled secretory portion deep in the dermis next to the subcutaneous fat and a long, straight, tubular duct whose final portion is coiled and penetrates the epidermis to drain at the sweat pore on the surface (Fig. 1.16). The gland and its duct are lined by a single layer of secretory cells and surrounded by myoepithelial cells.

The apocrine sweat glands drain directly into hair follicles in the axillae and groins. They are larger than eccrine sweat glands and the secretum is completely different, being semi-solid and containing odiferous materials that are thought to have the function of sexual attraction.

Summary

- Skin diseases account for about 15 per cent of a general practitioner's workload.
- Acne, eczema, psoriasis, warts and skin tumours are amongst the commonest of all human disorders.
- Skin is the protective interface between the potentially injurious external environment and the vulnerable organs and tissues of the body.
- The keratinocytes in the epidermis mature into the flattened corneocytes of the stratum corneum. The stratum corneum prevents water loss, penetration by substances in contact with the skin and invasion by micro-organisms.
- Keratinocytes are constantly dividing in the basal layer of the epidermis and corneocytes are shed at the surface.
- Melanocytes are dendritic, pigment-producing cells in the basal layer of the epidermis.
- Langerhans cells are dendritic, bone marrow-derived cells that seize and process foreign substances which manage to penetrate the skin and then present them as antigen to lymphocytes in the first stage of delayed hypersensitivity.
- The dermis is separated from the epidermis by a junctional zone consisting of a basal lamina and a condensation of connective tissue. It contains blood capillaries that reach up near to the epidermis but do not penetrate it. Nerve fibres ending in sensory receptors are also found within the dermis.
- The bulk of the dermis contains fibrous collagen, which gives skin its strength and elasticity, as well as elastic fibres around the collagen fibres and a proteoglycan matrix.
- Adnexal structures – hair follicles and sweat glands – open at the skin surface but reside in the dermis.

Signs and symptoms of skin disease

Skin disorders may be generalized, localized to one or several sites of abnormality known as 'lesions', or eruptive, in which case many lesions appear spottily over the skin. Note that skin that appears normal to the naked eye may have structural abnormalities when inspected microscopically and may also demonstrate functional abnormalities. For example the skin around a psoriatic plaque shows slight epidermal thickening and minor inflammatory changes; similarly, there are alterations in blood flow in the normal-appearing skin near eczematous skin.

Any widespread abnormality of the skin may also affect the scalp, the mucosae of the mouth, nose, eyes and genitalia, and the nail-forming tissues and it is important to inspect these sites whenever possible during examination of the skin.

Alterations in skin colour

The colour of normal skin is dependent on melanin pigment production (see page 5) and the blood supply. Other factors may also influence it, including the optical qualities of the stratum corneum and the presence of other pigments in the skin. One of the most common accompaniments of skin disease is redness or erythema.

ERYTHEMA

The degree of erythema depends on the degree of oxygenation of the blood, its rate of flow and the site, number and size of the skin's blood vessels. Different disorders

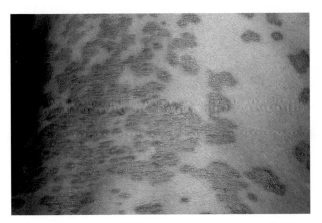

Figure 2.1 Plaques of psoriasis with typical red colour.

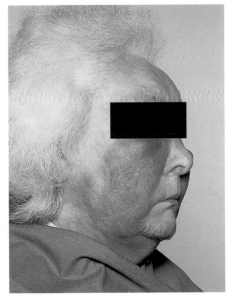

Figure 2.2 Reddened areas on the face in dermatomyositis, showing typical heliotrope discoloration.

tend to be associated with particular shades of red. Psoriatic plaques, for example, tend to be dark red in colour rather than pink, bright red or bluish red (Fig. 2.1). Other diseases associated with specific colours include lichen planus and dermatomyositis. Lichen planus has a well-known mauve hue, which is often helpful in reaching a diagnosis. Dermatomyositis characteristically has the colour of the heliotrope flower associated with the periocular swelling that frequently occurs in this disease (Fig. 2.2).

Measurement of the degree of erythema may be helpful in assessing the effects of treatment on an erythematous skin disease. There are now two types of device that can be used to do this, one is based on the comparator principle and the other uses reflectance spectroscopy. Both employ complex electronics, are available commercially and are easy to use.

BROWN-BLACK PIGMENTATION

The degree of brown-black pigmentation depends on the activity of the pigment-producing cells – the melanocytes – not on the number of cells. It also depends on the size of the granules and the distribution of the pigment particles within the epidermal cells. Shedding of the pigment from keratinocytes into the dermis is known as pigmentary incontinence and causes a kind of tattooing, in which the dusky pigment produced hangs on for many weeks or months.

Brown pigmentation is also caused by a breakdown product of blood – haemosiderin – when this has leaked into the tissues (Fig. 2.3). It is very difficult to tell this apart from melanin pigment, both clinically and histologically, but special stains can help.

A brown-black discoloration of the skin over cartilaginous structures (ears and nose) and, to a lesser extent, at other sites is seen in alcaptonuria, and is due to the

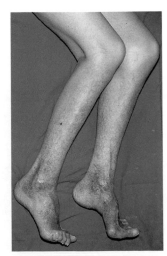

Figure 2.3 Lower legs of a patient with chronic venous hypertension and brown pigmentation due to haemosiderin deposits.

deposition of homogentisic acid. A dark brown pigmentation of acne scars or of areas on the limbs is sometimes observed as an uncommon side effect of the tetracycline-type drug minocycline.

Generalized darkening of the skin, more pronounced in the flexures, is observed in Addison's disease and seems to be due to increased secretion of melanocyte-stimulating hormone and the consequent activation of the melanocytes to produce more pigment. Nelson's syndrome following adrenalectomy is another cause of generalized pigmentation that is also due to the action of melanocyte-stimulating hormone. Darkening of the palmar creases and mucosae may be seen in both these endocrine disorders.

Disorders of pigmentation are also discussed in Chapter 17.

Alterations in the skin surface

The sensation experienced by touching or stroking normal skin is due in part to the normal skin surface markings which vary to some extent in different areas of the body (Figs 2.4 and 2.5). It is also dependent on the presence of hair, sweat and sebum at the skin surface and to the overall mechanical properties of the skin at that site. Horn cells are constantly being shed from the skin surface (desquamation) at a rate that approximates to the rate at which the epidermal cells are being produced. The replacement time (turnover time) of the normal stratum corneum is approximately 14 days, but varies at different body sites and lengthens in old age. Normally, horn cells are shed singly, and the process is imperceptible. When the process of keratinization is disturbed, the horn cells tend to separate in clumps or scales rather than as single cells. Sometimes, the process is so disturbed that shedding of any type is impossible and the horny layer builds up into a thickened, horny patch of hyperkeratosis (Fig. 2.6). When the skin surface is scaly and roughened, it looks dry, and scaling skin disorders are sometimes known colloquially

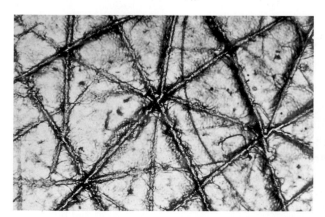

Figure 2.4 Skin surface of the forearm showing typical rhomboidal pattern.

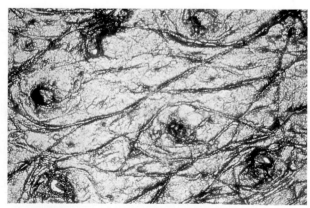

Figure 2.5 Skin surface of the beard area in a man with accentuation of the follicular orifices.

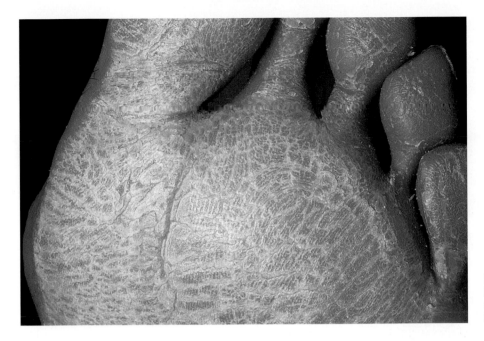

Figure 2.6 Plantar hyperkeratosis in a patient with a congenital disorder of keratinization.

as 'dry skin disorders'. Water placed on scaling skin makes the surface temporarily less scaly, but the scaling is not due to water deficiency.

As mentioned above, scaling is due to disturbances in keratinization, which may be primary or secondary. In primary disorders of keratinization, a metabolic abnormality prevents full and complete differentiation of the stratum corneum, ending in the release of intact single keratinocytes. These disorders are generally congenital in origin – the ichthyoses being the best examples.

Scaling is also seen when keratinization is affected secondary to some other pathological process affecting the epidermis. For example, the scaling seen in psoriasis and eczema is due to the inflammation that affects the epidermis in these disorders. In psoriasis, and probably in some patients with chronic eczema, epidermal cell production is greatly increased and the rapid movement of the epidermal cells upwards results in immature cells within the stratum corneum.

There are no simple ways to quantify scaling, although there are established methods for assessing skin surface contour, in which the contour of skin surface replicas is tracked with a very sensitive stylus and recorded electronically. Skin surface contour may also be recorded optically by measuring the reflection of light from the skin surface.

The size, shape and thickness of skin lesions

When a localized lesion no more than discolours the skin surface, it is known as a macule. If the abnormal area is raised up above the skin surface, it is said to be a plaque. The mild fungal disorder known as pityriasis versicolor (see page 37) causes macules over the chest and back (Fig. 2.7), but the lesions of psoriasis

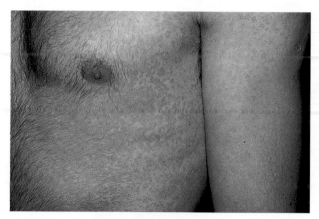

Figure 2.7 Pityriasis versicolor, showing many brownish pink macules on the chest.

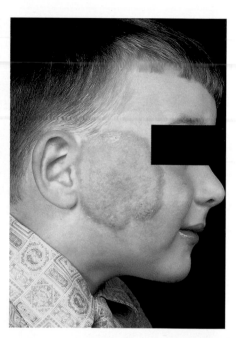

Figure 2.8 Annular lesion of ringworm.

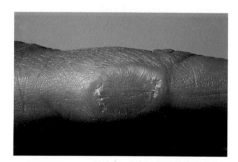

Figure 2.9 Annular lesion of granuloma annulare.

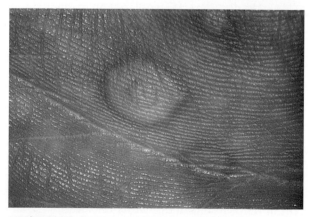

Figure 2.10 Lesion of erythema multiforme showing annular lesion.

(see page 100) are thickened and easily palpable and are called plaques. Sometimes, lesions are very considerably proud of the skin and are known as nodules or tumours. If the tumours are connected with the skin surface by a stalk, they are said to be pedunculated. Nodules and pedunculated tumours are present in the congenital condition called neurofibromatosis (Von Recklinghausen's disease).

The edge of lesions can give some diagnostic help: well-defined edges are especially characteristic of psoriasis and ringworm. Characteristically, it is difficult to discern where the abnormality ends in the eczematous disorders.

The shape of skin lesions can also help in diagnosis. Some skin disorders start off as macular but clear in the centre, making ring-like or annular lesions. Ringworm, granuloma annulare (see page 265) and erythema multiforme (see page 75) are

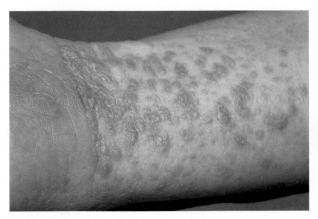

Figure 2.11 Typical lesions of lichen planus on the front of the wrist. The individual papules have a roughly polygonal outline and are mauvish in colour.

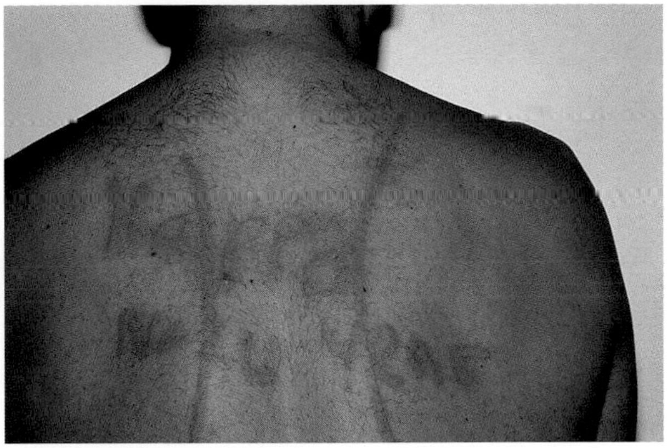

Figure 2.12 Dermographic weals.

three conditions in which the developed lesions tend to be annular (Figs 2.8–2.10). Some skin disorders often produce oval lesions, pityriasis rosea being the best example of this tendency. Occasionally, lesions assume bizarre patterns on the skin surface that almost seem to be representing a particular pattern or symbol. This is termed figurate, and many disorders, including psoriasis, may produce such lesions. For the most part, skin lesions are not usually angular and do not form squares or triangles. However, one condition, lichen planus (see page 144), does produce small lesions that seem to have a roughly polygonal outline (Fig. 2.11).

In some instances, lesions such as plaques or tumours infiltrate into the substance of the skin and, in the case of such malignant lesions as basal cell carcinoma, squamous cell carcinoma or malignant melanoma, it is important to recognize the presence of deep extensions of the lesion in order to plan treatment. Clinically, it is possible for experienced observers to form some impression of the degree of infiltration present by palpation, but this should be validated by histological support before any major surgical decision is made. There is some hope that non-invasive assessment techniques such as ultrasound will be better able to guide the surgeon than clinical examination alone.

Oedema, fluid-filled cavities and ulcers

When a tissue contains excess water both within and between its constituent cells, it is said to be affected by oedema. Oedema fluid may collect because of inflammation, when it is protein rich and known as an exudate, or as a result of haemodynamic abnormalities, when it is known as a transudate. Oedema is a common feature of inflammatory skin disorders, being seen in acute allergic contact dermatitis. Oedema also occurs in urticaria and dermographism (see page 71) in which localized areas of pink, swollen skin (known as weals) occur, lasting for several hours (Fig. 2.12).

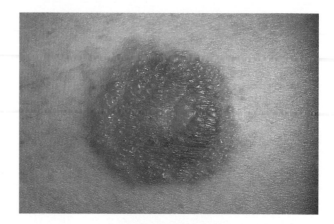

Figure 2.13 Vesicles in eczema from patch test.

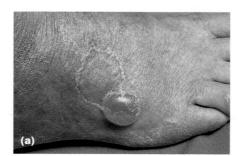

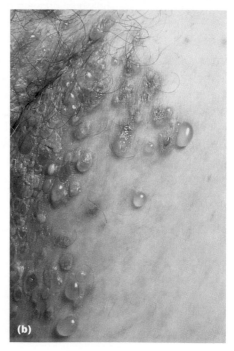

Figure 2.14 (a) Bullous lesion in senile pemphigoid. (b) Numerous bullae in the groin in a patient with pemphigus.

In eczema, oedema fluid collects within tiny cavities less than 1 mm in diameter within the epidermis, known as vesicles (Fig. 2.13). Larger fluid-filled cavities are called bullae (blisters). These may form due to fluid collecting beneath the epidermis (subepidermal), in which case their walls tend to be tough and the captured blister fluid may be blood stained, or they may form by separation or breakdown of epidermal cells (intraepidermal), when the walls tend to be thin, flaccid and fragile. Subepidermal bullae form in bullous pemphigoid, dermatitis herpetiformis and erythema multiforme. Intraepidermal bullae form in the different types of pemphigus (see page 91) and herpes virus infections (see Figs 2.14–2.18).

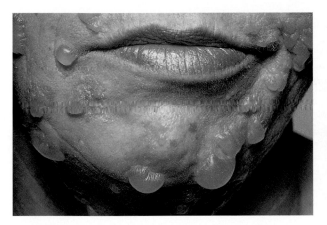

Figure 2.15 Vesicles in dermatitis herpetiformis.

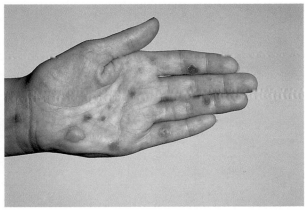

Figure 2.16 Bullae of the palm in erythema multiforme.

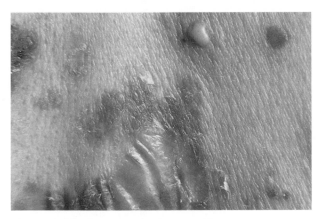

Figure 2.17 Flaccid bullae in pemphigus.

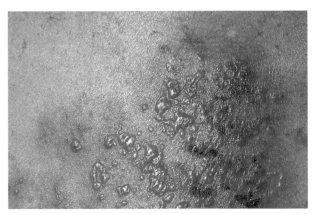

Figure 2.18 Vesicles in herpes zoster.

An erosion is any breach of the epidermis. The term ulcer is used to denote a broad, deep erosion that persists. Erosions may be covered by serous exudates or crust; ulcers tend not to be covered.

Secondary changes

Secondary changes include:

- impetiginization – due to a bacterial infection resulting in exudation and golden-yellow crusting (Fig. 2.19)
- lichenification – the result of constant rubbing and scratching causing thickening, with exaggeration of the skin surface markings (Fig. 2.20)
- prurigo papules – also the result of scratching, but, instead of lichenification, variably sized inflamed papules and even quite large nodules appear (Fig. 2.21).

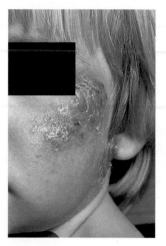

Figure 2.19 Impetigo contagiosa showing exudation and golden-yellow crusting.

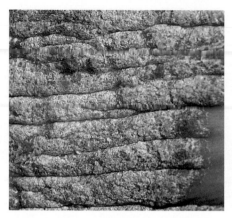

Figure 2.20 Lichenification showing scaling and accentuation of skin markings.

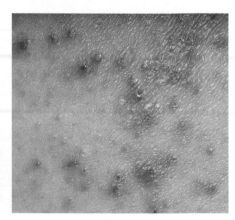

Figure 2.21 Excoriated papules in prurigo.

Case 1

Jack has had severe generalized eczema since the age of 3. It is extremely itchy, and he scratches it vigorously, causing scratch marks or excoriations to appear. In some areas where he scratches and rubs persistently, the skin has become thickened and hypertrophied, with exaggeration of the skin surface markings – a change known as lichenification. In areas that are eczema free, there is xeroderma or drying of the skin with some fine scaling. In places where the eczema is active, the skin is red from the increased blood supply and swollen because of the oedema.

Symptoms of skin disorder

Skin disease causes pruritus (itching), pain, soreness and discomfort, difficulty with movements of the hands and fingers, and cosmetic disability.

PRURITUS

Itching is the classic symptom of skin disorders, but it may occur in the apparent absence of skin disease. Any skin abnormality can give rise to irritation, but some, such as scabies, seem particularly able to cause severe pruritus. Most scabies patients complain that their symptom of itch is much worse at night when they get warm, but this is probably not specific to this disorder. Itching in atopic dermatitis, senile pruritus and senile xerosis is made worse by repeated bathing and vigorous towelling afterwards, as well as by central heating and air conditioning with low relative humidity. If pruritus is made worse by aspirin or food additives such as tartrazine, sodium benzoate or the cinnamates, it is quite likely that urticaria is to blame. Persistent severe pruritus can be the most disabling and distressing symptom, which is quite difficult to relieve. Scratching provides partial and transient relief from the symptom and it is fruitless to request that the patient stop scratching. Scratching itself causes damage to the skin surface, which is visible as scratch marks (excoriations). In some patients, the repeated scratching and rubbing cause lichenification and in others prurigo papules occur. Occasionally, the scratch marks become infected. Uncommonly, the underlying disorder occurs at the site of the injury from the scratch. This phenomenon is found in patients with psoriasis and lichen planus and is known as the isomorphic response or the Koebner phenomenon.

PAINFUL SKIN DISORDERS

Most skin disorders do not give rise to pain. The notable exception to this is shingles (herpes zoster), which may cause pain and distorted sensations in the nerve root involved (see page 52). The pain may be present before the skin lesions appear, while they are there and, occasionally, afterwards. Pain and tenderness are characteristic of acutely inflamed lesions such as boils, acne cysts, cellulitis and erythema nodosum (see page 77). Most skin tumours are not painful, at least until they enlarge and infiltrate nerves. However, there are some uncommon benign tumours that cause pain, including the benign vascular tumour known as the glomus tumour and the benign tumour of plain muscle known as the leiomyoma.

Chronic ulcers are often 'sore' and cause a variety of other discomforts, but they are not often the cause of severe pain. When they do give rise to severe pain, ischaemia is usually the cause. Painful fissures in the palms and soles develop in patches of eczema and psoriasis due to the inelastic, abnormal, horny layer in these conditions.

DISABILITIES FROM SKIN DISEASE

Patients with skin disease may experience a surprising degree of disability. A very major cause of disability is the abnormal appearance of the affected skin. For reasons that are not altogether clear, there is a primitive fear of diseased skin, which even amounts to feelings of disgust and revulsion. The idea of touching skin that is scaling or exudative seems inherently distasteful and it is something that one tries to avoid. These attitudes appear universal and inherent, and it is difficult to prevent them. It is little use pointing out that there is no rational basis for them, and all that can be hoped for is that a mixture of comprehension, compassion and common sense eventually supplants the primitive revulsion felt by all. It has been suggested that the origins of the inherent fear described above are the contagious nature of leprosy and the infestations of scabies and lice. Indeed, the problem is sometimes referred to as the 'leper complex'. Regardless of the origins, it is only too abundantly evident that individuals with obvious skin disease do not do well where the choice of others is concerned. They suffer more unemployment overall, but in addition

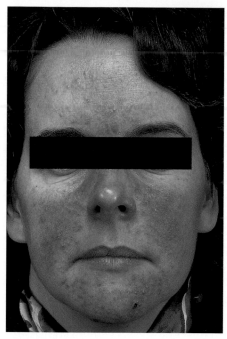

Figure 2.22 Erythema and papules of the cheek in rosacea.

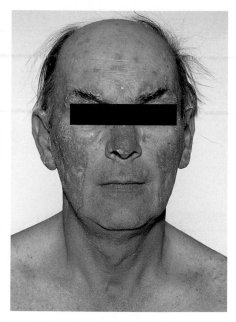

Figure 2.23 Plaques of erythema, scaling and hyperkeratosis in a man with discoid lupus erythematosus.

find great difficulty in obtaining positions that require any kind of interpersonal relationships.

Young patients with acne have particular problems because the disease is only too visible, as it usually affects the face. Psoriasis quite often affects the hands, nails and scalp margin, also causing difficulty for those whose occupations put them into contact with the public.

Numerous other skin disorders put the affected individual at an economic and social disadvantage. Vascular birthmarks and large neurofibromata are disfiguring and tend to isolate the bearers. Chronic inflammatory facial disorders such as rosacea and discoid lupus erythematosus also cause problems (Figs 2.22 and 2.23).

To summarize this point, individuals with visibly disordered skin are disabled because of society's inherent avoidance reaction. One other aspect of this same problem is the sufferers' own perception of the impact they are making on all with whom they come in contact. In most subjects who have persistent, 'unsightly' skin problems, the affected individuals become depressed and isolated. It is especially damaging for those in their late teens and twenties who are desperately trying to make relationships. Self-confidence is, in any case, not at a high point at this time in their emotional development and a disfiguring skin disorder lowers their self-esteem incalculably. Many youngsters with acne and psoriasis find it difficult to conquer their embarrassment sufficiently to have 'girlfriends' or 'boyfriends' and that aspect of their development may become stunted. It was once thought that many skin disorders were caused by neurotic traits, 'stress' and personality disorders. It is

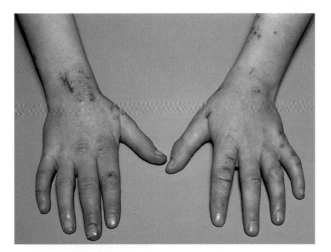

Figure 2.24 Skin fissures in atopic dermatitis.

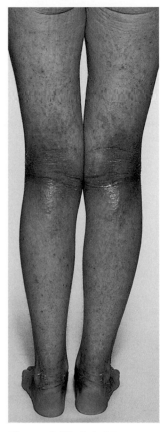

Figure 2.25 Painful fissures in popliteal fossae in atopic dermatitis.

now increasingly appreciated that skin disorders often cause depression, anxiety and stress, so that the wheel has turned full circle.

Skin disease can be enormously disabling when it affects the palms or soles. Although the areas only occupy some 1–2 per cent of the body's skin surface, disease of these sites may prevent walking and use of the hands for anything but simple tasks, i.e. they are virtually completely disabled. Psoriasis and eczema are the usual causes of this form of disablement because of the painful fissures that tend to develop (Fig. 2.24). Patients with a severe atopic dermatitis may develop similar painful fissures around the popliteal and antecubital fossae, so that limb movements become extremely painful (Fig. 2.25). Those with severe congenital disorders of keratinization are often severely troubled by this disordered mobility.

From what has been said so far, it will be appreciated that, contrary to popular belief, patients with skin disorders are often appreciably disabled. They are disabled on account of society's and their own reaction to the disease and because of the physical limitations that the skin disease puts on them.

Skin disease infrequently kills, but often produces unhappiness, usually loss of work and social deprivation as well as considerable physical discomfort.

Summary
- Skin disorders may be generalized or localized to 'lesions'.
- Normal-appearing skin may show structural or functional abnormalities.
- Skin colour is mainly determined by melanin pigmentation and blood content, its oxygenation and distribution. Particular shades of red may indicate particular diseases, e.g. violaceous lichen planus.

- The degree of skin pigment depends on the rate of melanin production and the size of the melanin granules – not the number of melanocytes, which is constant. Pigment shed into the dermis causes persistent darkening.
- The quality of the skin surface depends on hair, sebum and sweat secretion, and desquamation. Scales are aggregates of corneocytes and result from the failure of the usual loss of cohesion

between corneocytes – regardless of the underlying abnormality.

- Erythema, pigmentation and scaling can all be measured objectively.
- Macules are flat; plaques are flat raised patches. Papules, nodules and tumours are progressively larger, localized, raised lesions. Annular lesions occur, for example, in ringworm, erythema multiforme and granuloma annulare.
- Oedema is often a feature of inflammatory disorders of skin, including acute eczema and urticaria.
- Subepidermal blisters (bullae) occur in erythema multiforme, bullous pemphigoid, porphyria cutanea tarda, epidermolysis bullosa and dermatitis herpetiformis.
- Intraepidermal blisters (bullae if large, vesicles if small) occur in pemphigus of various types,

herpes simplex and zoster and sometimes in eczema.

- Pruritus causes scratching and thus scratch marks (excoriations) and skin hypertrophy or lichenification if persistent. Prurigo papules and impetiginization also result from scratching.
- Itching is particularly a problem in atopic dermatitis, scabies, dermatitis herpetiformis and urticaria.
- Pain in skin disorder is a feature of herpes zoster (shingles), some uncommon tumours and fissures in the skin in chronic eczema.
- Disability in skin disorder results from societal rejection and the patient's self-imposed isolation because of fear of the peer response. This results in emotional deprivation, occupational disadvantage and economic loss.

Skin damage from environmental hazards

As already mentioned, a major function of skin is its ability to protect the body from the potentially injurious environment. All parts of the skin contribute to its role in protection. The stratum corneum is a remarkably efficient barrier, protecting against water loss to the environment and against the entry of toxic substances that the skin may encounter. This same, thin structure also helps protect against solar ultraviolet radiation (UVR), thermal injury and, to some extent, mechanical damage.

The vasculature is vital to the maintenance of a constant body temperature. Vasodilatation and vasoconstriction allow loss and conservation of body heat, respectively. The sweat glands, the hair and the subcutaneous fat are other parts of the skin that assist in thermal homeostasis. Evaporation of sweat assists loss of body heat, and the subcutaneous fat and hair help conserve heat because of their insulating functions.

Melanin produced by melanocytes in the basal layer of the epidermis is donated to the epidermal keratinocytes, which become corneocytes, and it is in these that melanin absorbs solar UVR, providing essential protection to the skin against damage from the sun's rays. UVR stimulates melanin production, leading to the well-known 'golden brown' suntan and further protection.

We are subjected to a constant barrage of mechanical stimuli, which vary in intensity, direction, area to which they are delivered and rate of delivery. The dermis contains a network of oriented, tough, collagenous fibres, in the interstices of which there is a viscid proteoglycan ground substance as well as elastic fibres and fibroblasts. Most of the mechanical response to physical stimuli is due to dermal connective tissue. Overall, the mechanical properties can be described as viscoelastic. This means that skin extends in response to a linear force and will tend to regain its original length after release of the force (elastic). It also flows and creeps with some mechanical stimuli (viscous). Skin is also said to be anisotropic, as its mechanical properties vary according to the orientation of the body axis in which the mechanical stimulus is delivered. The anisotropy results from the orientation of the collagen fibres, which vary according to site. Different resting tensions result from the differing orientations and account for the development of broad and ugly scars if incisions are made across the main orientation of the collagen fibres rather than parallel to it. Langer's lines (made by joining the long axes of circular incisions pulled by the internal forces over the skin surface) were an early attempt at revealing the resting tensions in skin. However, they did not take into account important additional local considerations specific to each anatomical region.

The responses to mechanical stimuli vary according to the rate of delivery of the stimulus, i.e. they are time dependent. They are also dependent on the 'stress history' of the anatomical part – recent stress history being more important than distant.

Damage caused by toxic substances

Skin encounters substances with widely ranging toxicities. It must be remembered that many agents used in treatment, such as corticosteroids and salicylic acid, are systemically absorbed when placed on the skin and may cause systemic toxicity.

Detergents, alkaline soaps and lubricating oils are some of the substances that can damage the skin after repeated contact. They damage the horny layer by removing complex lipids and glycoproteins from the intercorneocyte space and then irritate the epidermis, causing a dermatitis characterized by oedema and the presence of inflammatory cells (Fig. 3.1). Although everyone may be injured by irritating substances, susceptibility varies. More heavily pigmented individuals are more resistant, but fair-skinned, blue-eyed people, and especially red-haired individuals, are particularly sensitive. Celtic people are especially vulnerable, though the basis for their vulnerability is not clear. The sensitivity to chemical irritants parallels the sensitivity to UVR (Fig. 3.2).

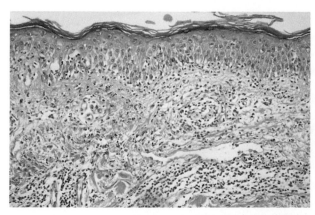

Figure 3.1 Photomicrograph showing inflammation, with inflammatory cells in the dermis and epidermis and oedema (spongiosis) of the epidermis.

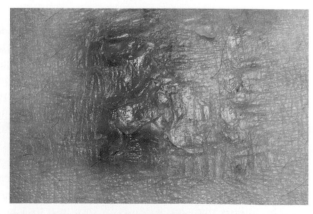

Figure 3.2 Severe irritant dermatitis caused by sodium lauryl sulphate, showing crusting.

LESS COMMON TOXICITIES

Corrosive and blistering injury

Agents that cause blistering are known as vesicants. Blister beetles release vesicants (including cantharidin) when crushed on the skin. Colloquially known as 'Spanish fly', the substance, unjustifiably, had the reputation of being an aphrodisiac. Chemical warfare agents include vesicants known as the mustards, which cross-link DNA, preventing cell division, but also cause severe blistering and erosion on contact with the skin.

Acneiform response

Some materials particularly irritate the hair follicles and stimulate the production of sticky horn, causing comedos and an acneiform folliculitis (Fig. 3.3). Cocoa butter, thick, oily materials including paraffin waxes and substances such as iso-propyl myristate are notorious for doing this in susceptible individuals. Cosmetics were at one time often to blame, but now rarely have this effect because of rigorous safety testing. Lubricating and cutting oils may cause 'oil folliculitis' or 'oil acne' in machine workers at skin sites that come into contact with the oil.

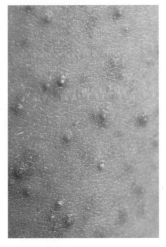

Figure 3.3 Acne lesions induced by cosmetic preparations.

Pigmentary disorders from toxic substances

Some materials can injure melanocytes, causing depigmented patches that may closely resemble vitiligo (see page 297). Substances used in the rubber industry – notably the additive paratertiary butyl phenol – are notorious for causing such a problem. Depigmentation may occur as a temporary phenomenon after irritant dermatitis or other inflammatory dermatoses. Hyperpigmentation can also follow inflammatory skin disease. This can be persistent as it results from the release of melanin particles from injured keratinocytes, which are then engulfed by macrophages, resulting in a 'tattoo'.

Injury from solar ultraviolet irradiation

The sun emits a continuous band of energy over a wide range of wavelengths, but it is only the UVR (250–400 nm) that is of major importance as far as skin is concerned (Fig. 3.4). Three segments of UVR are recognized: UVA (320–400 nm), or long-wave UVR; UVB (280–320 nm), or medium-wave UVR; and UVC (250–280 nm), or short-wave UVR. UVC is mostly filtered out by the ozone layer and would only become biologically important if the ozone layer became seriously depleted.

UVB – especially around 290 nm – is mainly responsible for sunburn, suntan and skin cancer, although other wavelengths contribute to the pathogenesis of these conditions. UVB only penetrates as far as the basal layer of the epidermis, but causes the death of scattered keratinocytes (sunburn cells) and damages others so that they release cytokines and mediators. These produce oedema, vasodilatation and a

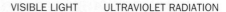

VISIBLE LIGHT ULTRAVIOLET RADIATION

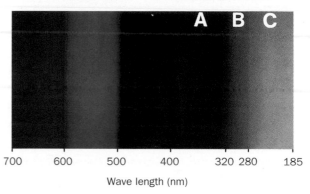

Figure 3.4 Solar spectrum to show visible light and ultraviolet radiation (UVR). The UVR is divided into three portions: (a) long-wave UVR, (b) medium-wave UVR, and (c) short-wave UVR.

subepidermal inflammatory cell infiltrate. Some 2 days after UVR injury, there is an increase in the rate of melanin synthesis. It is probably not possible to stimulate a tan without sustaining UVR-induced epidermal damage. Sunburn is easily recognized by the redness and, when severe, swelling and blistering as well. For some unexplained reason, it is quite sharply restricted to the area of skin exposed. The affected area is very sore and, if blistered and extensive, makes the individual feel unwell and even require in-patient management as for a thermal burn.

An individual's sensitivity to solar UVR depends mostly on the degree of skin pigmentation, but also to some extent on inherent metabolic factors. Sensitivity is conventionally graded as follows in answer to the question 'Do you burn or tan in the sun?'

Type I	Always burns, never tans
Type II	Always burns, sometimes tans
Type III	Sometimes burns, always tans
Type IV	Never burns, always tans
Type V	Brown-skinned individuals of Asian descent
Type VI	Black-skinned individuals of African descent

Although UVA is 1000-fold less effective at causing erythema, there is a lot of it in sunshine and it does penetrate to the dermis. It is thought to play a role in causing the dermal degeneration known as solar elastosis, which is mainly responsible for the appearance of ageing as well as contributing to the cause of skin cancer. UVA is also the part of the spectrum mainly responsible for photosensitivity reactions.

Case 2

Mary and Louise are non-identical twins. Mary has blond hair, blue eyes and pale skin, whereas Louise has brown hair and eyes and slightly darker skin. Mary has found that she becomes red and sunburnt easily and cannot tan, but Louise can stay in the sun longer without burning. At the age of 45, Mary noticed that she had quite a few wrinkles in the crow's feet areas and around the mouth, but Louise still looked quite young.

Chronic photodamage (photoageing)

The wrinkling and other changes in exposed skin commonly believed to be due to ageing are, in fact, mainly due to chronic damage from solar UVR. The changes are more in evidence in those with outdoor occupations, such as farmers, builders or sailors. They are worse in fair-skinned, blue-eyed individuals who are easily sunburnt. However, with the advent of package holidays and cheap air travel, glorification of the great outdoors and the obsession with obtaining a suntan, excess sun exposure is commonplace, resulting in unnecessary photodamage. Persisting sun exposure results in both epidermal and dermal damage.

EPIDERMAL DAMAGE

Minor degrees of epidermal abnormality, with variation in cell and nuclear size, shape, staining and orientation, are known as dysplasia (or photodysplasia). They are common and, although they are not detectable clinically, they may lead on to pre-cancerous solar keratoses or Bowen's disease, frankly invasive squamous or basal cell carcinoma (see Chapter 13) and life-threatening malignant melanoma (see Chapter 13).

DERMAL DAMAGE

Sun-damaged dermal connective tissue loses its fibrous quality and assumes a homogenous, 'blob-like' appearance in some sites and a 'chopped-up', short, stubby fibre appearance in others. When these occur together, they give a 'spaghetti and meatball' appearance. The degenerative change is termed solar elastosis as it stains just like elastic tissue. Solar elastosis starts subepidermally, although separated from the epidermis by a thin layer of normal dermis – the grenz zone. With increasing exposure, elastotic tissue extends deeper and deeper into the dermis.

Solar elastosis imparts a sallow, yellowish tint to affected skin and the altered mechanical properties of the abnormal tissue are responsible for many of the wrinkles and lines around the mouth and eyes on sun-damaged skin (Fig. 3.5). Large telangiectatic blood vessels in the degenerate dermis account for the telangiectasia seen clinically (Fig. 3.6).

Topical retinoids (tretinoin, isotretinoin and tazarotene) used over several months improve the appearance of photodamaged skin by stimulating the synthesis of new dermal connective tissue.

PREVENTION OF PHOTODAMAGE

Complete avoidance of sun exposure is very difficult to achieve and it is better to aim at reducing the UVR dose as much as possible by:

- avoiding exposure between 11.30 am and 2.30 pm
- seeking shade

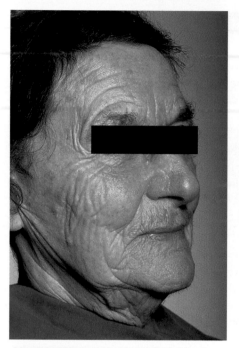

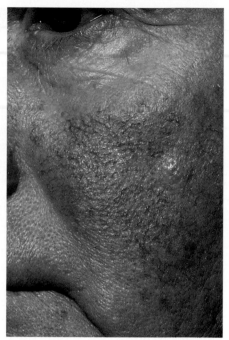

Figure 3.5 Clinical signs of solar elastotic degenerative change, showing marked wrinkling around the mouth and eyes.

Figure 3.6 Solar elastotic degenerative change of the cheek, showing marked telangiectasia.

- using 'opaque' protective clothing, including broad-brimmed hats, trousers and long-sleeved shirts
- using sunscreens.

Sunscreens are creams or lotions that absorb and filter out or reflect off the damaging UVR. Older sunscreens contained substances such as the esters of paraaminosalicylic acid, benzoic acid, the homosalicylates, the benzophenones and the cinnamates, designed primarily to filter out the sunburning 290-nm UVB segment, although some also gave a little protection in the UVA range. Newer sunscreen constituents give protection against UVA as well and may be helpful in protecting against chronic photodamage and skin cancer.

Sunscreen efficacy is usually quoted as a sun protection factor (SPF). The SPF is the ratio of the minimal time of exposure to produce redness of the skin (in minutes) *with* sunscreen protection compared to the minimal exposure time to produce redness without sunscreen protection. For example, if it takes 15 minutes' exposure to a standard UVR source to develop redness and only 1 minute to develop redness without the sunscreen, the SPF of that sunscreen is 15. The test has been carefully standardized so that one can place some confidence in the SPF as an indication of the protection against UVB.

It is more difficult to measure and express protection against UVA. In practice, the protection against UVA provided by sunscreens is often expressed as a ratio of the protection against UVB to that offered to UVA in the 'star system', in which four stars express the best ratio. There are two methods employed. One is the 'pigment-darkening method', in which the time to the production of a transient darkening of the skin is measured. The other method is an *in vitro* spectroscopic method.

Other important points concerning sun exposure include:

- UVR is readily reflected from whitish surfaces such as sand, snow and white walls, and this increases the dose of UVR sustained.
- A significant amount of UVR 'diffuses' through cloudy skies, and it is possible to be burnt even on dull days.
- The nearer the equator, the more direct the UVR and the easier it is to burn. The higher the altitude of exposure, the greater the UVR exposure.
- Lighter-skinned subjects are more at risk, i.e. ginger-haired or flaxen-haired, blue-eyed, pink-skinned individuals 'who never tan and always burn' (type I subjects and, to a lesser extent, type II individuals). A Celtic ancestry, even in comparatively darker-complexioned subjects, usually signifies a marked sensitivity to solar UVR.

DERMATOSES PRECIPITATED AND/OR CAUSED BY SOLAR EXPOSURE

Photosensitivity reactions (see Table 3.1)

Skin can become sensitized to a specific part of the solar spectrum by chemical agents that reach it either via the systemic route or after contacting the skin topically. The molecule damages tissues after absorbing the UVR at a particular wavelength

Table 3.1 Skin diseases precipitated, caused or aggravated by sunlight

Disorder	Wavelengths responsible	Comment
Porphyrias	400 nm	Mostly blistering or erosive disorders, except for EPP, which causes erythema or urticarial patches
Polymorphic light eruption	Mostly the UV part of the spectrum, but visible light may be involved	Papular or eczematous rash on exposed areas
Actinic prurigo	Uncertain	Eczematous rash on exposed areas
Photosensitivities	Mostly the long-wave part of the UV spectrum	Many drugs and chemicals may cause this
Lupus erythematosus	Varies with patients	Acute attack may be precipitated by exposure
Chronic actinic dermatitis (persistent light reaction or actinic reticuloid)	Variable; mostly the long-wave part of the UV spectrum	Patients may be acutely sensitive to light exposure
Eczema/psoriasis	Unknown	Some patients improve, some are aggravated
Rosacea	Unknown	Most are aggravated

EPP = erythropoietic protoprophyria; UV = ultraviolet.

Table 3.2 Examples of common photosensitizing agents

Systemically administered drugs
Tetracyclines
Phenothiazines
Amiodarone
Nalidixic acid
Psoralens

Topically administered drugs
Halogenated salicylanilides
Psoralens
Tars

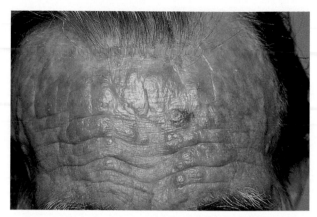

Figure 3.7 Thickening and inflammation of the skin of the forehead in actinic reticuloid.

and becoming activated. This is known as a phototoxic reaction. On occasions, the molecule becomes allergenic after exposure to UVR and a 'photoallergic reaction' develops. Some common photosensitizing agents are given in Table 3.2.

Phytochemical reactions are photosensitivity responses that result from contact with plants or their products on areas exposed to the sun. The psoralens and coumarins are the most common plant sensitizers. Giant hogweed and meadow grass contain coumarins, and psoralens are found in some fruits, such as the bergamot.

Chronic actinic dermatitis (persistent light reaction; actinic reticuloid syndrome)

Patients with this disorder start with severe photoallergic dermatitis and do not respond to routine light avoidance. When photosensitivities are identified to plant extracts or to antimicrobials such as trichlorosalicylanilide, avoidance does not necessarily produce improvement. The skin of a few severely affected individuals may be markedly thickened (Fig. 3.7) and may be involved on all sites – not only light exposed areas. The condition is then known as actinic reticuloid. Severely affected patients need to be nursed in a darkened room to ensure complete protection from irradiation. Some improvement with azathioprine (50–150 mg daily) may be expected, but little else helps.

Polymorphic light eruption

This is a common disorder, occurring in young and middle-aged women and characterized by itchy papules and papulovesicles on exposed sites – particularly the forearms (Fig. 3.8). The rash develops shortly after sun exposure throughout the spring and summer months. Those affected are found to have a marked sensitivity to long-wave UVR.

Patients improve when they avoid sun exposure and use sunscreens blocking UVA. Weak topical corticosteroids may help, but some severely affected patients

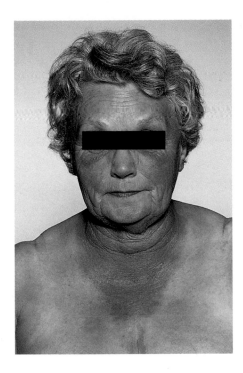

Figure 3.8 Polymorphic light eruption with erythema affecting the face and the light-exposed part of the neck and upper cheek.

may need hydroxychloroquine (200 mg b.d.) or even azathioprine (50 mg b.d.). Desensitizing patients with photochemotherapy with UVA (see Chapter 21) sometimes helps.

Hutchinson's summer prurigo

This occurs in girls and young women and looks somewhat like atopic dermatitis.

Confirmatory tests for the photodermatoses

- *Photopatch tests*. Suspected photosensitizers are placed on the skin and irradiated with broad-spectrum UVR. Controls are run with irradiation alone and with the suspected substances without irradiation. Patches are examined for signs of eczema up to 72 hours after irradiation.
- *Photoprovocation tests*. These specialized tests are only available at a few centres. In one group of tests, the wavelength dependency (action spectrum) of the disorder is determined by shining monochromatic radiation (single wavelength) on the skin using a monochromator.

Sweat rash

The term is quite non-specific and applied by the lay public to any disorder associated with sweating and the hot weather. Dermatoses as diverse as intertrigo and folliculitis are sometimes known as 'sweat rashes'.

A common form of sweat rash is due to blockage of the sweat gland pores or ducts near the surface with swollen over-hydrated horn. The term miliaria crystallina is applied to the tiny, thin walled vesicles that arise from blockage at the pore near the surface. In miliaria rubra, red, inflamed papules occur due to blockage lower in the duct. In miliaria profunda, the blockage is deep down and large inflammatory swellings develop. The most effective treatment is to cool the patient with air conditioning and fans. Systemic antibiotics and anti-inflammatory agents may be required.

Dermatoses aggravated by solar exposure

Lupus erythematosus is very often aggravated by sun exposure, and patients with this disease must not expose themselves to solar UVR. Rosacea is often, and atopic dermatitis occasionally, made worse by the sun. Psoriasis and acne are mostly improved by sun exposure, but some patients are, for some reason, made worse.

COLD INJURY

Frostbite is a form of acute tissue necrosis of fingers, toes, nose or ears due to cold-induced ischaemia.

Chilblains

Chilblains are common in the UK but rare elsewhere. They seem to occur in the 'damp cold' so often experienced in the UK and are also associated with subsequent warming. The lesions occur on the fingers, toes and occasionally elsewhere as raised, dusky red or mauve swellings and are painful and/or itchy. They particularly affect plump young women, for some reason, as well as the elderly. Keeping warm is the only effective treatment.

Raynaud's phenomenon

Table 3.3 Some common causes of Raynaud's phenomenon

| Systemic sclerosis |
| Systemic lupus erythematosus |
| Use of vibratory tools |
| Carpal tunnel syndrome |
| Cervical rib |
| Atherosclerosis |
| Polycythaemia rubra vera |

In the majority of cases, no precipitating cause can be found.

This common, curious response of the digital arteries to the cold is observed in many disorders as well as occurring without any obvious underlying predisposing condition (Table 3.3).

Classically, the fingers suddenly go a deathly white when exposed to the cold. After a variable period, they go pink and then develop a bluish discoloration – the whole sequence lasting approximately 30 minutes. The condition is painful and, during the winter, quite disabling. If severe, it can lead to atrophic changes with loss of tissue and tapering of the fingers. Paronychial infection is a common complication.

If no underlying cause can be found or the cause cannot be removed, symptomatic treatment directed towards keeping the hands warm and producing vasodilatation in them is needed. Electrically heated gloves, oral inositol nicotinate, nifedipine (5–10 mg t.d.s.) and oxypentifylline (400 mg, two to three times daily) may help individual patients.

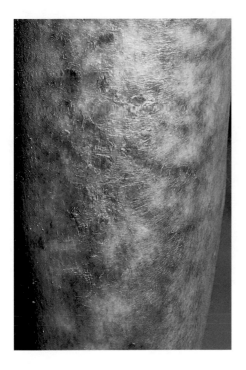

Figure 3.9 Erythema ab igne, showing a brownish reticular network on the leg.

HEAT INJURY

Chronic heating causes injury to the skin, though this is not well characterized. Infra red in the solar spectrum may play a role in chronic photodamage, but it is difficult to determine what that role is. Chronic heat damage to the skin occurs on the shins and elsewhere at sites habitually warmed by focal sources of heat – a condition known as erythema ab igne. Brownish-red reticulate pigmentation is the dominant physical sign (Fig. 3.9), but keratoses and even squamous cell carcinoma can also occur at involved sites.

Summary

- Damage to the skin may be caused by soaps, detergents and oils that remove essential constituents of the stratum corneum, allowing penetration into and irritation of the epidermis.
- Fair-skinned individuals are more susceptible to injury from irritants.
- Some agents, such as cocoa butter, irritate the hair follicles in particular and cause an acne-like response (comedogenic substances).
- Toxic damage to melanocytes by some substances causes areas of depigmentation.
- Solar UVR includes UVB (280–320 nm), which causes sunburn and, over long periods, skin cancer as well as the changes known as photoageing (chronic photodamage). It also contains much UVA (320–400 nm), which is less potent than UVB but can still damage the skin.
- The degree of damage caused by UVR depends on the dose received and the sensitivity of the individual, which mostly depends on the degree of skin pigmentation. Asking whether patients sunburn and can suntan allows categorization into a skin type.

- Persistent sun exposure damages the epidermis and causes pre-cancerous lesions, such as solar keratoses and Bowen's disease, and frankly malignant lesions, including squamous cell carcinoma, basal cell carcinoma and malignant melanoma.
- Sun exposure also damages the dermis, causing the production and deposition of an abnormal elastic tissue. This elastotic degeneration is responsible for many of the appearances of ageing, including wrinkling and telangiectasia.
- Solar damage can be prevented by avoiding exposure at times of maximum irradiation and by the use of sunscreens. The latter should protect against both UVB and UVA.
- UVR also causes certain dermatoses, such as phototoxic and photoallergic reactions when the skin has been exposed to certain chemicals. Some disorders, such as polymorphic light eruptions and actinic prurigo, are caused by exposure to solar UVR alone.
- Exposure to cold can cause frostbite (a type of gangrene) or chilblains or provoke vasospasm of the digital arteries causing Raynaud's phenomenon, in which the fingers go white, pink and blue in sequence. The condition may occur for no obvious reason or be the result of an underlying disorder such as the carpal tunnel syndrome, cervical rib or systemic lupus erythematosus.
- Chronic heating can cause erythema ab igne and skin cancer.

Skin infections

The stratum corneum is an excellent barrier to pathogenic micro-organisms, but is itself sometimes the target of attack. The skin surface and its adnexal structures harbour a stable microflora, which lives in symbiosis with skin and may indeed be beneficial. Gram-positive cocci (*Staphylococcus epidermidis*), Gram-positive lipophilic microaerophilic rods (*Propionibacterium acnes*) and a Gram-positive yeast-like organism (*Pityrosporum ovale* or *Malassezia furfur*) live in the follicular lumina without normally causing much in the way of harm. However, under special conditions, e.g. excess sebum secretion, depressed immunity and compromised stratum corneum barrier protection, they can produce disease. Infection of the skin only occurs when the skin encounters a pathogen that its defences cannot eliminate or control.

Fungal disease of the skin/the superficial mycoses/infections with ringworm fungi (dermatophyte infections)

Dermatophyte infections are restricted to the stratum corneum, the hair and the nails (i.e. horny structures).

PITYRIASIS VERSICOLOR

This disorder is caused by the yeast-like micro-organism *Pityrosporum ovale*. This microaerophilic, lipophilic denizen of the normal follicle only occasionally becomes pathogenic when its growth is encouraged by heightened rates of sebum secretion or there is depressed immunity.

Clinically, pale, scaling macules develop insidiously over the skin of the chest and back in young adults (Fig. 4.1), although, uncommonly, other sites can be affected too (Fig. 4.2). Pale areas are left when the condition resolves. Diagnosis is made by identification microscopically of grape-like clusters of spores and a meshwork of pseudomycelium in skin scrapings made more transparent by soaking the scales for 20 minutes in 20 per cent potassium hydroxide. A more elegant and permanent preparation can be made using cyanoacrylate adhesive (crazy glue) to remove a strip of superficial stratum corneum from the skin surface on a glass slide. The slide is 'rolled off' the skin after 20 seconds and then stained with periodic acid-Schiff reagent (Fig. 4.3). This technique is known as skin surface biopsy. The skin patches often fluoresce an apple green in long-wave UVR (Wood's light).

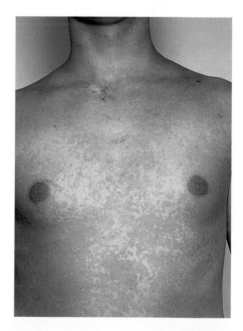

Figure 4.1 Brownish pink macules on the trunk due to infection with *Pityriasis versicolor*.

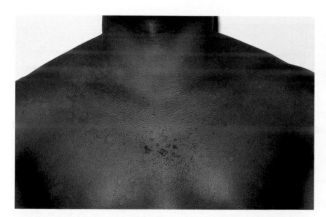

Figure 4.2 Hypopigmented macules on the neck of a black-skinned subject.

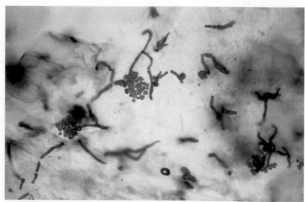

Figure 4.3 Periodic acid-Schiff-positive spores and pseudomycelium of *Pityriasis versicolor* in skin surface biopsy.

Treatment

Topical imidazole creams (e.g. miconazole, clotrimazole, econazole) applied once daily over 6 weeks or use of ketoconazole shampoo to wash the affected areas once daily for 5 days are usually sufficient. Older remedies such as 20 per cent sodium thiosulphate solution and selenium disulphide shampoo are also effective, as is oral itraconazole (1–200 mg/day) for 7–15 days.

TINEA (RINGWORM) INFECTIONS

Trichophyton, *Microsporon* and *Epidermophyton* species are responsible for this group of dermatophyte infections. *Trichophyton rubrum*, *T. mentagrophytes* and *Epidermophyton floccosum* are the most common causes of dermatophyte infection in humans. *Microsporon canis* caught from dogs, cats or children causes tinea capitis in children and, uncommonly, other types of ringworm infection. Occasionally, a quite inflammatory ringworm can be caught from cattle (*T. verrucosum*) and horses (*T. equinum*).

The diagnosis is confirmed by microscopy of skin scrapings, hair or nail clippings treated with 20 per cent potassium hydroxide for 20 minutes and identification of fungal hyphae. Use of the cyanoacrylate 'skin surface biopsy technique' described above makes identification quite easy (Fig. 4.4).

Culture may be positive when direct microscopy is not, but it takes 2–3 weeks or longer before the culture is ready to read.

Clinical features of ringworm infection

Tinea corporis
This is ringworm of the skin of the body or limbs. Pruritic, round or annular, red, scaling, well-marginated patches are typical (Fig. 4.5). It has to be distinguished

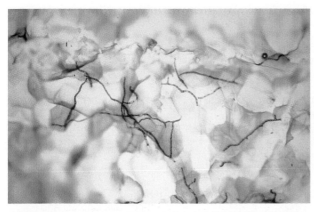

Figure 4.4 Periodic acid-Schiff-positive fungal mycelium hyphae in skin surface biopsy.

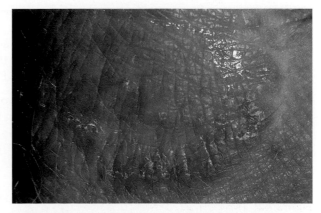

Figure 4.5 Well-demarcated scaling patch due to ringworm.

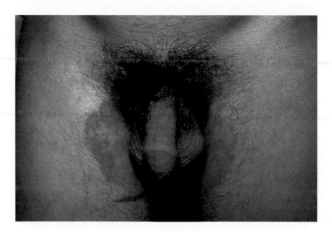

Figure 4.6 Ringworm of the groin (tinea cruris).

from patches of eczema or psoriasis by history and the presence of mycelium in the scales. Any of the species may cause this condition. When an animal species is responsible (e.g. *T. verrucosum*), the affected skin is very inflamed and pustular and heals spontaneously after a few weeks.

Tinea cruris

Tinea cruris or groin ringworm is very itchy and is for the most part a disorder of young men. Well-defined, itchy, red scaling patches occur asymmetrically on the medial aspects of both groins (Fig. 4.6). These gradually extend down the thigh and on to the scrotum unless treated. *T. rubrum* and *E. floccosum* are the causative fungi. Differential diagnosis includes seborrhoeic dermatitis or intertrigo (see page 116) where the rash is symmetrical and does not have a well-defined border, and flexural psoriasis.

Tinea pedis

Ringworm infection of the feet may be:

1 vesicular, with itchy vesicles occurring on the sides of the feet on a background of erythema;
2 plantar, in which the sole is red and scaling; or
3 interdigital, in which the skin between the fourth and fifth toes in particular is scaling and macerated.

Tinea pedis is very common and particularly so in young and middle-aged men, who often contract it from communal changing rooms. It tends to be itchy and persistent. *T. rubrum*, in particular, but also *T. mentagrophytes* and *E. floccosum* cause the infection.

Tinea manuum

This less common, chronic form of ringworm usually involves one palm only, which is usually dull red with silvery scales in the palmar creases. *T. rubrum* is usually to blame.

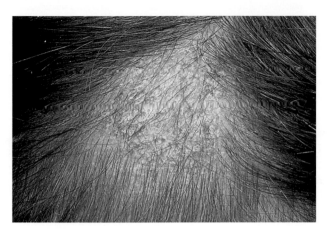

Figure 4.7 Scaling area with hair loss in tinea capitis.

Tinea capitis

Ringworm of the scalp occurs in children exclusively and is mainly due to *M. canis*. It invades the scalp stratum corneum and the hair cuticle (ectothrix infection), causing pink, scaling patches on the scalp skin and areas of hair loss due to the breakage of hair shafts (Fig. 4.7). It is easily spread by, for example, the sharing of hairbrushes. Infected areas sometimes fluoresce a light green under long-wave UVR (the so-called Wood's light).

In another variety of scalp ringworm caused by *T. schoenleini*, the fungus invades the interior of the hair shaft (endothrix) and causes intense inflammation on the scalp, with swelling, pus formation and scalp scarring.

Tinea unguium

This condition is due to ringworm infection of the nail plate and the nail bed. The fungi responsible are *T. rubrum*, *T. metagrophytes* or *E. floccosum*. Infected nail plates are discoloured yellowish or white and thickened (Fig. 4.8). Onycholysis occurs and subungual debris collects (Fig. 4.8). The condition is much more common in the toenails than in the fingernails. Tinea unguium has to be distinguished from psoriasis of the nails (see page 129).

Figure 4.8 (a) and (b) Thickened, yellowish, irregular toenails in tinea unguium.

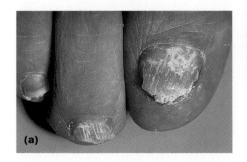

(a)

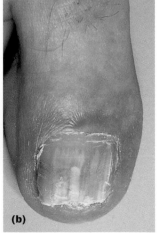

(b)

Case 3

Dai had been a miner for many years and felt that was the reason he had chronic ringworm affecting his toenails and the soles of his feet. He was fed up with having itchy, scaly feet and ugly, thickened toenails and sought treatment. Various creams were prescribed but did not help. Eventually, a 3-month course of oral terbinafine began to clear the problem.

Tinea incognito

This is extensive ringworm with an atypical appearance due to the inappropriate use of topical corticosteroids (Fig. 4.9). The corticosteroids suppress the protective inflammatory response of the skin to the ringworm fungus, allowing it to spread and altering its appearance.

Treatment

For ordinary ringworm of the hairy skin, an imidazole-containing preparation (such as miconazole, econazole and clotrimazole) used twice daily for a 3–4-week period is usually adequate. Topical allylamines such as terbinafine are also effective.

When multiple areas are affected in tinea unguium and tinea capitis and when topical treatment has failed for some reason, one of the following systemic drugs needs to be used.

- Griseofulvin (500 mg b.d.) is only active in ringworm infections and has a low incidence of serious side effects.
- Ketoconazole (200 mg daily) is active in both yeast and dermatophyte infections. This drug should be reserved for patients with severe and resistant

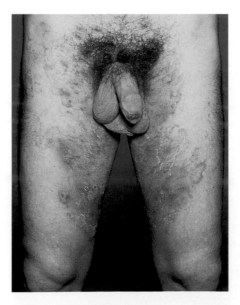

Figure 4.9 Tinea unguium showing extensive and unusual-looking infection due to tinea incognito.

disease because of the possibility of serious hepatotoxicity and the occurrence of other side effects, including rashes, thrombocytopenia and gastrointestinal disturbances.
- Itraconazole (100 mg daily), like ketoconazole, is effective in both yeast and dermatophyte infections. Serious side effects are uncommon.
- Terbinafine (250 mg daily) is indicated for dermatophyte infections only. Serious side effects are uncommon.

These agents are administered for 2–6 weeks except for griseofulvin, which, when given for tinea unguium of the toenails, may need to be given for 6–12 months.

Candidiasis (moniliasis, thrush)

This common infection is due to a yeast pathogen (*Candida albicans*) that resides in the gastrointestinal tract as a commensal. It is a not infrequent cause of vulvo-vaginitis in pregnant women, in women taking oral contraceptives and in those taking broad-spectrum antibiotics for acne. It is also responsible for some cases of stomatitis in infants and the cause of infection of the gastrointestinal tract and elsewhere in immunosuppressed people. It may contribute to the clinical picture in the intertrigo seen in the body folds of the obese and in the napkin area in infancy. Treatment with the imidazole preparations, topical and systemic, is effective. Oral and vaginal moniliasis responds to preparations of nystatin and amiphenazole as well as to the imidazoles. Serious *Candida* infections respond to systemic fluconazole.

DEEP FUNGUS INFECTION

There are several fungal species that cause deep and sometimes life-threatening infection. They are much more common in immunocompromised patients, including those with autoimmune deficiency syndrome (AIDS), transplant patients, those on corticosteroids or immunosuppressive agents and those with congenital immunodeficiencies. Some, such as histoplasmosis, cryptococcosis and coccidioidomycosis, are widespread systemic infections, which only occasionally involve the skin.

Actinomycosis, sporotrichosis and blastomycosis infect the skin and subcutaneous tissues, causing chronically inflamed hyperplastic and sometimes eroded lesions. Sporotrichosis may produce a series of inflamed nodules along the line of lymphatic drainage. Deep fungus infections of this type produce a granulomatous type of inflammation, with many giant cells and histiocytes as well as polymorphs and lymphocytes.

Madura foot is a deep fungus infection of the foot and is seen in various countries of the African continent and India. The affected foot is swollen and infiltrated by inflammatory tissue, with many sinuses. The infection spreads throughout the foot, invades bone and is very destructive and disabling.

Bacterial infection of the skin

ACUTE BACTERIAL INFECTION

Impetigo contagiosa

Impetigo is a contagious, superficial skin infection caused by *Staphylococcus aureus* in most instances and perhaps by the haemolytic *Streptococcus* in a few cases.

Clinical features

Red, sore areas, which may blister, appear on the exposed skin surface (see Fig. 4.10). Yellowish gold crust surmounts the lesions that appear and spread within a few days. It is mostly a disorder of prepubertal children. It is, however, not uncommon for the signs of the lesions to appear over an area of eczema. The condition is then said to be 'impetiginized'.

In tropical and subtropical areas, an impetigo-like disorder is spread by flies and biting arthopods. This disorder is more destructive than ordinary impetigo and produces deeper, oozing and crusted sores and is caused mostly by beta-haemolytic streptococci. It is sometimes known as ecthyma.

There have been several outbreaks of acute glomerulonephritis following episodes of this infective disorder.

Treatment

Local treatment with an antibacterial wash to remove the crust and debris, as well as a topical antimicrobial compound such as betadine or mupirocin are needed in all cases and, unless the area is solitary and very small, a systemic antibiotic such as penicillin V (250 mg 6-hourly for 7 days) is also required. Patients usually respond within a few days.

Erysipelas

Erysipelas is a severe infective disorder of the skin caused by the beta-haemolytic *Streptococcus*.

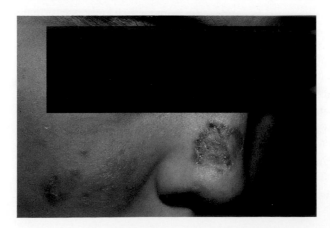

Figure 4.10 Patch of impetigo on the nose.

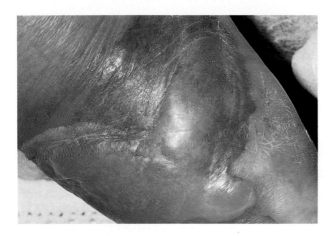

Figure 4.11 Severely inflamed erythematous area on the thigh due to erysipelas.

There is sudden onset of a well-marginated, painful and swollen erythematous area, usually on the face or lower limbs (Fig. 4.11). The inflammation may be very intense and the area may become haemorrhagic and even blister. There is usually an accompanying pyrexia and malaise.

Treatment with antibiotics by mouth (penicillin V, 250 mg 6-hourly) should be rapidly effective.

Cellulitis

This is a diffuse, inflammatory disorder of the subcutis and skin caused by several different micro-organisms and is of variable severity.

It is relatively common, particularly on the limbs, and often occurs on legs affected by venous ulceration or by lymphoedema. There is pain, tenderness, slight swelling and a variable degree of diffuse erythema.

Broad-spectrum antibiotics are indicated, as the micro-organisms may be Gram negative in type (e.g. *Escherichia coli*) or Gram positive. Cephradine and flucloxacillin (250 mg of each 6-hourly) are one suitable combination.

FURUNCLES (BOILS) AND CARBUNCLES

Both these lesions result from *Staphylococcus aureus* infection of hair follicles. They are much less common now than 30 or even 20 years ago, presumably because of improved levels of hygiene. Nonetheless, there are still families and individuals who are troubled by recurrent boils. In many instances, the pathogenic *Staphylococcus* colonizes the external nares, the perineum or other body sites and is difficult to dislodge. The lesions are localized, red, tender and painful swellings; carbuncles may be quite large, perhaps 3 or 4 cm in diameter, and represent the infection of several follicles.

When there is pus centrally, surgical drainage is indicated. Systemic antibiotics are required and, whenever possible, their use should be guided by the pattern of sensitivities found by culture.

ANTHRAX

Anthrax is due to a rare, potentially fatal infection with a Gram-positive bacillus (*Bacillus anthracis*) causing black, scabbed sores and septicaemia. It is spread by farm animals and, because the micro-organism has a resistant spore form, can stay on infected land for years. It has assumed a major importance because of its deliberate spread by terrorists in the USA.

TUBERCULOSIS

Tuberculosis is a multi-system disease caused by varieties of the waxy-enveloped bacterium *Mycobacterium tuberculosis*. Several types of skin tuberculosis were once commonly seen, but are now quite rare in developed countries. However, tuberculosis is, unfortunately, now once again becoming quite common because of the appearance and spread of AIDS. The bacillus can be cultured in special media *in vitro*, but grows very slowly. Special stains are needed to detect it in tissue.

LUPUS VULGARIS

Lupus vulgaris is a rare disorder causing a slowly progressive, granulomatous plaque on the skin caused by the tubercle bacillus. It slowly increases in size, over one, two or three decades. It often has a thickened psoriasiform appearance, but blanching with a glass microscope slide (diascopy) will reveal grey-green foci ('apple jelly nodules') due to the underlying granulomatous inflammation.

Treatment is initially with 'triple therapy' of rifampicin, pyrazinamide and isoniazid over a 2-month period, followed by a 'continuation' treatment phase with isoniazid and pyrazinamide.

Tuberculosis verrucosa cutis (warty tuberculosis)

This is seen on the backs of the hands, knees, elbows and buttocks whenever abrasive contact with the earth and expectorated tubercle bacilli has been made.

Thickened, warty plaques are present, which are sometimes misdiagnosed as viral warts. Diagnosis is confirmed by biopsy showing tuberculoid granulomata and caseation necrosis.

Treatment is as for lupus vulgaris.

Other forms of cutaneous tuberculosis

- A persistent ulcer may arise at the site of inoculation as a 'primary' infection.
- An eroded, weeping area with bluish margins often develops where a tuberculous sinus drains onto the skin from an underlying focus of tuberculosis infection.
- Tuberculides may develop as hypersensitivity to the tubercle bacillus. In papulonecrotic tuberculide, papules arise and develop central necrosis with a black crust. Erythema induratum is an uncommon, odd disorder, which in many cases appears to fulfil the criterion of being a response to tuberculous infection. It is

characterized by the development of plaque-like areas of induration and necrosis on the lower calves and occurs predominantly in young women.

SOME OTHER MYCOBACTERIAL INFECTIONS

Swimming pool granuloma

Mycobacterium marinum, which lives in water, is sometimes caught from swimming pools and fish tanks. It has a 3-week incubation period and causes plaques, abscesses and erosions on the elbows and knees in particular.

The condition responds to minocycline or a trimethoprimsulphamethoxazole combination.

Buruli ulcer

Mycobacterium ulcerans is responsible for this disorder occurring in Uganda and south-east Asia. Large, undermined ulcers form quite rapidly and persist. Surgical removal is currently the best treatment.

SARCOIDOSIS

Recent data suggest that the disorder is, in many patients, an unusual reaction to *M. tuberculosis*. Sarcoidosis is a multi-system disease with manifestations in the respiratory system, the reticuloendothelial system and the skin and occasionally in the bony skeleton and central nervous and cardiovascular systems. In the skin, one of the most common varieties consists of multiple, reddish purple papules (Fig. 4.12). Deeper nodules and plaques are also seen, as are bluish chilblain-like

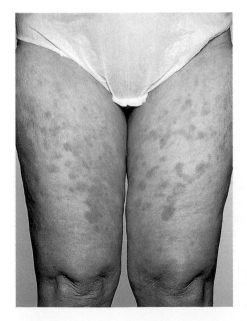

Figure 4.12 Multiple papules and nodules of the skin of the thighs due to cutaneous sarcoidosis.

swellings of the fingers, nose and ears (lupus pernio). These types are infiltrated by typical sarcoid tissue (see below), but another manifestation, erythema nodosum (see page 77), is not.

Histologically, the typical lesion is the 'naked' tubercle, which contains foci of macrophages and giant cells without many surrounding lymphocytes.

Treatment may not be required if the lesions are not troublesome, as they are self-healing, but when large they may leave scarring. For these large lesions, systemic corticosteroids or non-steroidal anti-inflammatory agents may be required.

LEPROSY (HANSEN'S DISEASE)

This is caused by a slow-growing bacillus of the mycobacterial type (*M. leprae*), which cannot be grown *in vitro*, although it can be passaged in armadillos and small rodents. As with the tubercle bacillus, it is detected in tissue by the Ziehl–Nielsen stain or by an immunocytochemical test. The disease is spread by droplet infection and by close contact with an infected individual. It is still a serious problem globally, with 1–2 million people affected, mostly in the poor and underprivileged countries of Africa and Asia.

Clinical features

The pattern of involvement is much dependent on the immune status of the individual. The two extremes are the lepromatous form seen in anergic individuals and the tuberculoid form seen in individuals with a high resistance. Because there are many gradations between these polar types, the range of clinical signs and the corresponding nomenclature have become very complicated. Where the changes are near tuberculoid, the term 'borderline tuberculoid' is used; similarly 'borderline lepromatous' is used for lesions that are close to the other type. 'Dimorphic' refers to both types of lesion being present. In tuberculoid lesions, nerves are infected, which become thickened. The affected areas are well defined, macular and hypopigmented, as well as being anaesthetic because of the nerve involvement. The anaesthesia results in injury, deformity and disability. In lepromatous leprosy, the infection is much more extensive, with thickening of the affected tissue as well as surface changes, with some hypopigmentation. On the face, the thickening gives rise to the characteristic leonine facies, with accentuation of the soft tissues of the nose and supraorbital areas. Where there is resistance, few bacteria can be detected in the lesions (paucibacillary types of leprosy). Types in which many bacteria are found and the patients are anergic are known as 'multibacillary'.

In general, the disease can produce dreadful deformity and disability unless skilfully treated, and it still evokes great fear in primitive communities. Because the disorder causes patchy hypopigmentation, the differential diagnosis includes vitiligo pityriasis versicolor and pityriasis alba.

In tuberculoid types, there is a striking granulomatous inflammation with many giant cells and only a few *M. leprae* to be found. In the lepromatous types, there are many macrophages that are stuffed with *M. leprae* (causing the appearance of foamy macrophages).

Treatment

The treatment of choice is with dapsone (100 mg daily, for periods of a minimum of 6 months) with rifampicin (600 mg monthly) for paucibacillary types of leprosy. During treatment, the patient's condition may flare and deteriorate, causing curious appearances in some, including erythema nodosum-like and ichthyosis-like reactions. Multibacillary types should also be treated with dapsone (100 mg daily) and in addition rifampicin (600 mg once monthly) and clofazimine (50 mg daily). Drug resistance is becoming a major problem.

LYME DISEASE

Lyme disease is caused by the *Borrelia burgdorfii* micro-organism, which is spread by the bite of a tick and has been described in several areas of Europe, including the UK, and in the USA. The disorder is multi-system in that there may be arthropathy, cardiovascular and central nervous components, as well as systemic upset. The skin may be involved in the early stages and show an erythematous ring that expands outwards (erythema chronicum migrans). Later, skin atrophy may be seen (acrodermatitis chronica atrophicans), or fibrosis in a morphoea-like condition. Diagnosis is made by identification of the organism in the tissues or by detection of antibodies in the blood.

Treatment is with antibiotics – preferably penicillin.

LEISHMANIASIS

The term refers to a group of diseases caused by a genus of closely related protozoal parasites with complex life cycles, which include time spent in small rodents. These diseases are spread by biting arthropods (mostly sandflies) in tropical and subtropical areas. Some forms cause severe systemic disease and are prevalent in some areas of Africa and South America and the Indian subcontinent: Others cause predominantly cutaneous or mucocutaneous disease.

Cutaneous forms are found around the Mediterranean littoral and North Africa and in South America. The 'Mediterranean' type is caused by *Leishmania major* and *L. tropica*. After an incubation period of about 2 months, a boil-like lesion appears, usually on an exposed site ('Baghdad boil'). Later, this breaks down to produce a sloughy ulcer ('oriental sore': Fig. 4.13), which persists for some months before healing spontaneously, with scarring and the development of immunity.

Mucocutaneous forms occur mainly in South America (New World leishmaniasis) and are due to *L. mexicana* and *L. brasiliensis*. Small ulcers develop (Chiclero's ulcer) that seem more destructive than the Old World types but also more

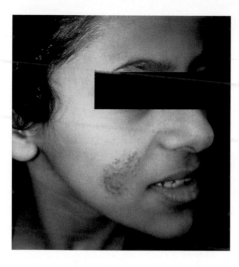

Figure 4.13 Cutaneous leishmaniasis in a boy, showing persistent plaque and papules on the skin of the cheek.

persistent, and later in the disease destructive lesions appear, affecting nasal mucosa in about half of the patients.

A *cutaneous component to visceral forms* is less common, but more extensive, and includes a diffuse cutaneous form with many plaques and nodules resembling lepromatous leprosy, a recidivans form with persistent plaques resembling lupus vulgaris, and post kala-azar (dermal leishmaniasis), occurring after the visceral disease and marked by the appearance of numerous small papules.

Biopsy shows mixed granulomatous inflammation. The parasites can be identified by special stains and can also be cultured in specialized media. There is also an intracutaneous skin test (leishmanin), which becomes inflamed after injection in most patients.

Treatment

The localized small ulcers heal spontaneously, but can be treated by freezing or curettage. Infiltration with sodium stibogluconate has been used. Systemic sodium stibogluconate or pentamidine may also be used for severe and resistant cases.

Viral infection of the skin

HERPES SIMPLEX

This is caused by a small DNA virus of two antigenic types, I and II. Type II herpes simplex infects the genitalia and type I is responsible for the common herpetic infection of the face and oropharynx and, less commonly, elsewhere.

The initial infection may be quite unpleasant, with severe stomatitis, systemic upset and pyrexia mostly in infants. Resolution takes place in about 10 days. Reactivation of the herpes infection occurs in some cases, at varying intervals. Up to 20 per cent of the population suffers from recurrent 'cold sores', so named

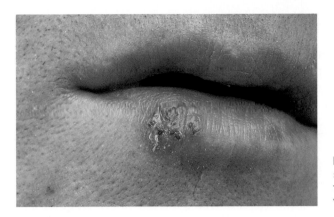

Figure 4.14 Herpes simplex (cold sore) on the lip, with a crust and vesicles.

because the disorder is often precipitated by minor pyrexial disorders. It may also be precipitated by sun exposure. Commonly, the lesions occur around the mouth or on the lip. They start as grouped, tender and/or painful papules or papulovesicles (Fig. 4.14) and then coalesce to form a crusted erosion. The sequence takes some 7–14 days from initial discomfort to the final pink macule marking where lesions have been.

Genital herpes affects the glans penis and the shaft of the penis. In women, the vulval region or labia minora is usually involved, but lesions may occur elsewhere on the buttocks or mons pubis. It may occur cyclically with the menses.

The disorder is caught venereally and has become extremely common. It is painful and inhibits sexual activity.

The vesicle results from epidermal cell degeneration, and smears taken from the lesion showing degenerate cells may help in diagnosis. The diagnosis can also be made by identifying the virus using an immunofluorescent method with antibodies to the herpes virus.

Treatment

Most patients do not require treatment. Idoxuridine is a viral metabolic antagonist, which, as a 5 per cent lotion, can shorten the disorder if started early and used frequently. Aciclovir (5 per cent cream) is the most effective agent for shortening the attack if started early and used five or six times per day. Aciclovir can also be used orally, (200 mg five or six times per day) in severe infections. Famiciclovir has similar properties.

HERPES ZOSTER (SHINGLES) AND CHICKEN POX (VARICELLA)

The same small DNA virus causes both these disorders, which differ only in the extent of the disease, the symptoms caused and the immune status of the individual affected. Most (but not all) cases of chicken pox (varicella) develop during infancy or childhood. Reactivation of the virus occurs in a proportion of those previously affected and causes shingles.

VARICELLA

This common childhood ailment is spread by droplets and debris from the lesions and has an incubation period of 14–21 days. There is accompanying fever and malaise. Lesions are common on the face and trunk, but less common on the limbs. Papules and papulovesicles become crusted, the crust dropping off after some 7–14 days, leaving pock-type scars in many instances.

HERPES ZOSTER (SHINGLES)

This mostly afflicts those past the age of 50 years, but also affects immunosuppressed individuals such as patients with AIDS. It is not 'caught', but is due to the reactivation of a virus that has been 'sitting' latent in a posterior root ganglion of a spinal nerve. Although shingles is not caught from patients with shingles, chicken pox is.

The disorder often starts with paraesthesiae or pain in the distribution of one or more dermatomes. Involvement of one of the branches of the trigeminal ganglion, with lesions in the distribution of the maxillary, mandibular or ophthalmic sensory nerves, is common, as is involvement of dermatomes of the cervical and thoracic regions. Lesions are confined to the skin innervated by the dorsal primary root(s) infected (Fig. 4.15), although there may be a small number of lesions elsewhere. About 25–30 per cent of patients with shingles continue

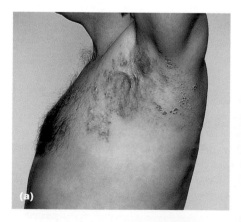

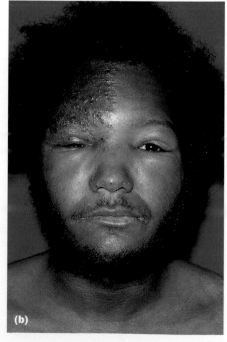

Figure 4.15 (a) Herpes zoster of the axillae and chest wall showing clusters of vesicles and pustules. (b) Herpes zoster affecting the ophthalmic branch of the trigeminal nerve involving the right side of the forehead and eye.

to suffer from pain and paraesthesiae in the area long after the skin lesions have disappeared.

Herpes zoster may occur where there is immunosuppression, as in AIDS or a lymphoma. When this occurs, the disorder is often very severe and may involve several dermatomes.

For most people, no specific treatment is required apart from keeping the lesions clean and, if necessary, the application of antimicrobial preparations to prevent or combat secondary infection. The drug aciclovir, administered by mouth in a dose of 800 mg five times daily (or by infusion) on day 1 of the disorder, shortens the disease and decreases its severity.

VIRAL WARTS

Warts are caused by a member of the human papillomavirus family, of which there are many antigenic types (Table 4.1). Particular clinical types of wart are caused by particular antigenic types. It is likely that they are caught by direct contact of skin with wart virus-containing horny debris. Genital warts are caught mostly (but not exclusively) by venereal contact. Some perianal warts may be transmitted by homosexual contact or by 'child abuse'.

The different varieties are illustrated in Figure 4.16. There are usually little black dots near the surface of the wart, representing thrombosed capillaries in elongated dermal papillae.

Plantar warts are painful, some warts are irritating, and all warts are unsightly and aggravating. They are a particular problem in immunosuppressed patients. In one congenital condition, plane warts spread extensively on the arms, face, trunk

Table 4.1 Human papillomavirus (HPV) types and the common clinical varieties of warts with which they are associated

Clinical type	Most common antigenic type of HPV associated
Common warts of hands and fingers (verruca vulgaris)	2, 4
Deep plantar warts (myrmecia warts)	1
Plane warts	3, 10
Mosaic warts	2
Epidermodysplasia verruciformis	5, 8 (but many others isolated on occasion)
Genital warts (condyloma acuminatum)	6, 11 (NB. Types 16 and 18 are also responsible occasionally, and these are known to be associated with carcinoma of the cervix)
Laryngeal papilloma	6, 11

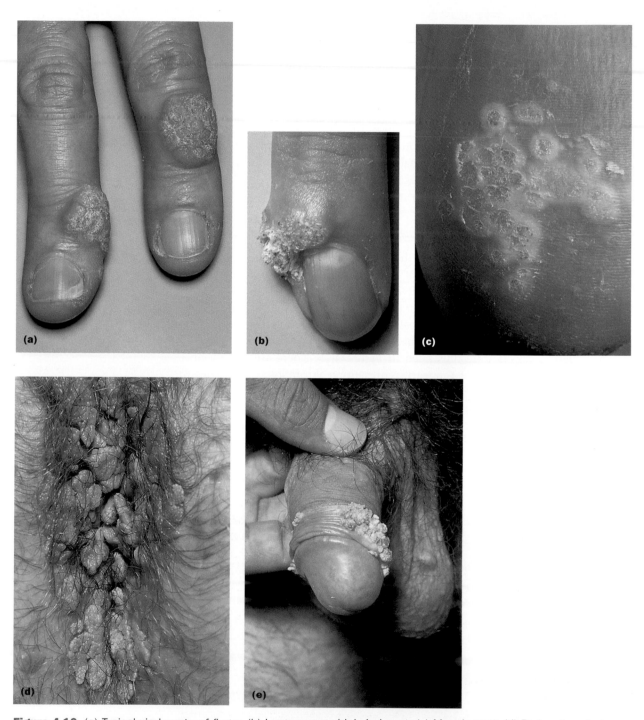

Figure 4.16 (a) Typical viral warts of finger. (b) Large paronychial viral wart. (c) Mosaic wart. (d) Perineal warts in an adult. (e) Multiple penile warts.

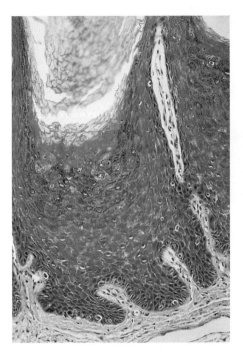

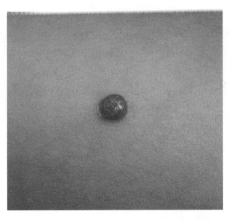

Figure 4.17 Photomicrograph of a viral wart showing marked hypergranulosis and vacuolar change in thickened epidermis.

Figure 4.18 Single lesion of molluscum contagiosum showing central plug.

and limbs and some lesions can transform to squamous cell carcinoma. This rare disorder, known as epidermodysplasia verruciformis, seems to have its basis in a disorder of delayed hypersensitivity.

There is epidermal thickening, with particular increase in the granular cell layer, which also shows a characteristic basophilic stippled appearance (Fig. 4.17).

All warts disappear spontaneously, but may persist for many months or some years. Treatment is, in general, not very satisfactory and relies on some form of local tissue destruction. The techniques mostly used are cryotherapy (tissue freezing with liquid nitrogen or solid carbon dioxide), curettage and cautery or chemical destruction with topical preparations containing salicylic acid, lactic acid, podophyllin or glutaraldehyde. Popular preparations contain high concentrations of salicylic acid (12–20 per cent) and lactic acid (4–20 per cent) or podophyllin (up to 15 per cent). Podophyllin is a plant extract containing potent cytotoxic alkaloids, one of which, podophyllotoxin, is also available as a pure preparation (0.5 per cent). Other methods that have been used include intracutaneous injections of cytotoxics such as bleomycin and injections of recombinant interferon.

MOLLUSCUM CONTAGIOSUM

Molluscum contagiosum is a common infection of the skin caused by a virus of the pox virus group. It is transmitted by skin-to-skin contact.

The typical molluscum lesion is a pink-coloured or skin-coloured, umbilicated papule containing a greyish central plug (Fig. 4.18). There may be one or many lesions. The face and genital regions are commonly involved.

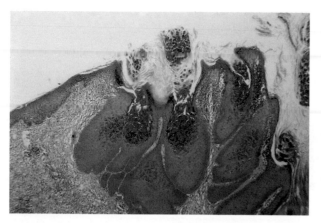

Figure 4.19 Photomicrograph of molluscum contagiosum showing thickened epidermis with central degenerative change and formation of molluscum bodies.

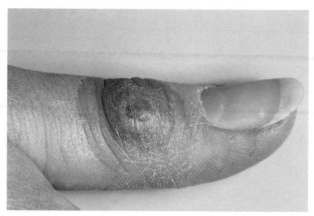

Figure 4.20 Area of orf infection on the thumb.

Pathology

There is cup-shaped epidermal thickening with a characteristic degenerative change in the granular cell layer, in which the cells become converted to globular eosinophilic bodies (molluscum bodies: Fig. 4.19).

Mollusca spontaneously resolve within months of curettage and cautery, strong salicylic acid preparations as for warts or simply squeezing the soft centre out (e.g. with a paper clip).

ORF (CONTAGIOUS PUSTULAR DERMATITIS OF SHEEP)

This disorder is caused by a pox-type virus that mostly affects sheep but also cattle. The lesions are solitary, acute, inflammatory and blistering and are mostly on the fingers (Fig. 4.20). Following the attack, a surprisingly high proportion of patients develop erythema multiforme (see page 75).

Summary

- The normal flora of the skin consists of Gram-positive cocci (*Staphylococcus epidermidis*) Gram-positive rods (*Propionibacterium acnes*) and Gram-positive yeasts (*Pityrosporum ovale*).
- Pityriasis versicolor is caused by *Pityrosporum ovale* when there is depressed immunity or when there is heightened sebum secretion. Fawn, scaling macules occur over the trunk. Treatments with imidazole creams or itraconazole by mouth are effective.

- Tinea infection (ringworm) is caused by *Trichophyton*, *Epidermophyton* and *Microsporum* species of fungus and is restricted to the stratum corneum, the hair and nails. Diagnosis is confirmed by identifying the fungi in the scales by direct microscopy and culture. Tinea pedis, tinea cruris and tinea unguium, affecting the feet, groin and nails, respectively, are the most frequently encountered. Treatments with topical

- imidazoles, topical terbinafine or oral terbinafine are suitable.
- Candidiasis caused by *Candida albicans* causes vaginal and oral thrush and complicates napkin dermatitis and intertrigo.
- Impetigo caused by *Staphylococcus aureus* results in red, sore areas that may blister and later develop a characteristic yellow crust.
- Infection with beta-haemolytic *Streptococcus* is the cause of erysipelas, which is characterized by a sharply marginated, painful, red, swollen area with severe malaise and pyrexia. Cellulitis is a more diffusely swollen area due to bacterial infection.
- Lupus vulgaris and tuberculosis verrucosa cutis are disorders caused by infection with the tubercle bacillus.
- Sarcoidosis is a multi-system disease that may represent a hypersensitivity to the tubercle bacillus and often results in persistent papules and nodules on the skin.
- Leprosy is caused by *Mycobacterium leprae*. The clinical manifestations depend on the immune response. Tuberculoid forms are found in patients with a strong immune response and lepromatous forms where there is a poor immune response.

- The disorder is still a problem for poor communities. Treatment is with dapsone, rifampicin and clofazimine.
- Leishmaniasis is caused by protozoa that reside in rodents and are spread by sandflies. In Europe, the commonest form is a persistent ulcer caused by *Leishmania tropica* or *Leishmania major*.
- Herpes simplex is caused by a small DNA virus that produces intraepidermal vesicles around the mouth and lips (Type I) or on the genitalia (Type II).
- Herpes zoster and varicella are caused by the same virus. Zoster is a painful disorder in which the skin supplied by one (or two) dorsal nerve root is involved in someone who has had varicella previously.
- Viral warts are caused by the human papillomavirus, of which there are many antigenic types. Particular antigenic types cause particular sorts of wart. Treatment is by some form of local destruction – chemical, physical or surgical.
- Molluscum contagiosum causes small, pearly, umbilicated papules and is the result of infection with a member of the pox virus group.

Infestations, insect bites and stings

The way that the skin reacts to the hostile attentions of arthropods and small invertebrates depends partly on the extent and severity of the attack and particularly on the immune status of the individual attacked.

Each geographical region has its own spectrum of skin problems due to the local fauna. Although some disorders, such as scabies, are the same the world over, the pattern and incidence of infestations and bites differ markedly from place to place. In general, the extent of skin problems due to arthropods is directly related to the sophistication and wealth of the society in question, because of the effects of personal hygiene, education, effective waste disposal and prophylaxis.

Scabies

Scabies is due to infestation with the human scabies mite (*Acarus hominis*, *Sarcoptes scabiei*). The mite is an obligate parasite and has no separate existence off the human body.

AETIOLOGY AND EPIDEMIOLOGY

The female mite burrows into the human stratum corneum and lays eggs within the burrow made. The male is smaller than the female and dies shortly after impregnating the female. The symptom of itch and the characteristic eczematous rash caused by invasion of the scabies mite are the result of the affected individual becoming sensitive to the waste products of the mites within the intracorneal

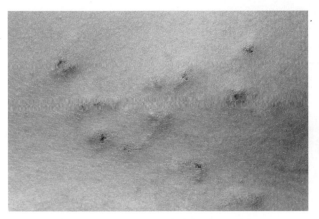

Figure 5.1 Papules and excoriations in scabies.

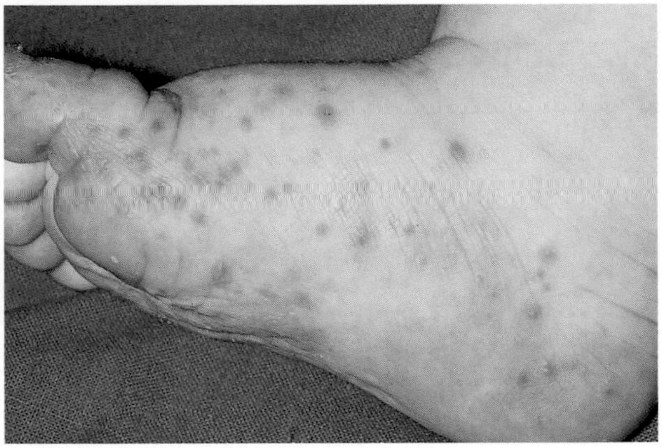

Figure 5.2 Multiple papules and vesicles due to scabies.

burrows. This generally does not happen before 1 month after the initial invasion of the mite; subsequent infestations cause symptoms and signs within a few days as the individual is already sensitized.

Infestation occurs after close skin-to-skin contact with an infested individual, sexual contact being the most frequent but not the only cause of infestation.

There have been several notable pandemics of scabies in recent history. The most recent of these started in the mid-1960s and ended in the early 1970s, although between peaks of incidence the disorder continues to appear sporadically and in localized mini-epidemics – such as within families or in nursing homes.

CLINICAL FEATURES

The disorder is notorious for the intensity of itch that it causes, even in the presence of relatively minor physical signs. The physical signs are essentially those of eczema and the effects of scratching. Vesicles are seen, but excoriations and prurigo-like papules are more common (Figs 5.1 and 5.2). Scaling, oozing and crusting can also be present in some sites due to secondary infection. However, the primary lesion is that of the scabies 'burrow' or run, which is a tiny, raised, linear or serpiginous white mark (Fig. 5.3).

The favourite sites for lesions are portrayed in Figure 5.4. It is odd that they should be symmetrical and concentrated in certain sites consistently. The best sites on which to find scabies burrows are the palms and the interdigital areas of the fingers, the flexural creases and over the elbows. Scabies lesions also commonly occur around the anterior axillary fold, the areolae of the breast, the buttock folds, lower abdomen, genitalia, knees, ankles and soles. Lesions are observed on the head and neck in infants only.

The severity of the eruption depends on the number of mites present and this is mostly dependent on the immune status of the individual. In severely immunosuppressed individuals, such as those with human immunodeficiency virus (HIV)

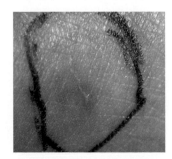

Figure 5.3 Scabies burrow on the foot.

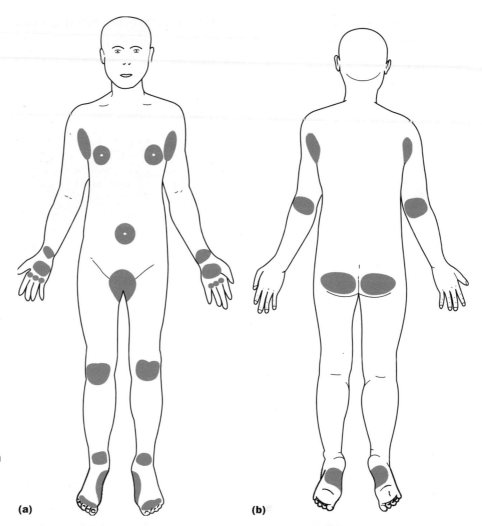

Figure 5.4 Diagrams showing sites of predilection for scabies infestation on (a) the front of the trunk and limbs, and (b) the back of the trunk and limbs.

(a)   **(b)**

infection or patients receiving immunosuppressive drugs for renal transplants, the infestation is very heavy and the resulting eruption correspondingly severe. Norwegian scabies is the term used to describe a very severe and extensively crusted version of the infestation seen in the frail elderly and congenitally immuno-deficient population (Fig. 5.5).

DIAGNOSIS

The diagnosis of scabies is not always easy, but is much helped by finding the burrows of the female scabies mite, which are pathognomonic of the disease and their recognition is important. The burrows are grey-white, linear, slightly raised marks, some 1–4 mm long, and are present on the favoured sites. The number of burrows present is variable – myriads in severe infestations in the elderly, but few in the fastidiously hygienic young.

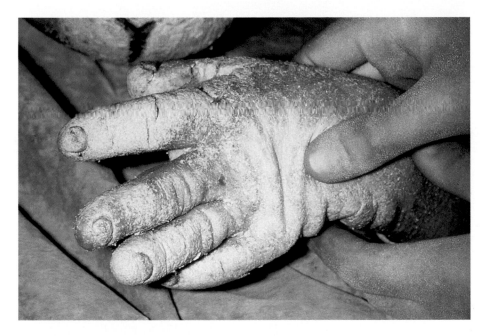

Figure 5.5 Severely crusted eruption due to scabies in an immunosuppressed child.

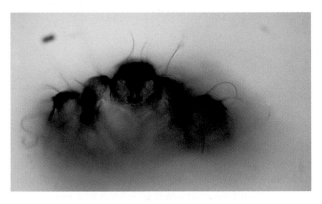

Figure 5.6 Scabies mite seen by microscopy in skin scrapings treated with potassium hydroxide.

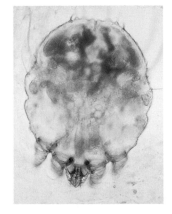

Figure 5.7 Scabies mite seen on microscopic examination of skin surface biopsy.

Finding the mite (or its eggs) by using a pin or by examining skin scrapings (Fig. 5.6) or a skin surface biopsy taken with cyanoacrylate glue confirms the diagnosis (Fig. 5.7).

Identification of the telltale burrows or mite is not always easy, even for the experienced! For the 20 per cent of scabies patients in the UK in whom burrows cannot be identified, a positive family or social history with itching contacts is helpful evidence and, in the presence of a compatible clinical picture, treatment should be instituted. Differential diagnosis is set out in Table 5.1.

TREATMENT

Treatment should be instituted as soon as the diagnosis has been made to prevent the infestation spreading. It should also be offered to everyone who lives with the

Table 5.1 Differential diagnosis of scabies

Disorder	Comment
Canine scabies	Different distribution – not transmitted between humans
Eczematous diseases	Particularly atopic dermatitis – usually a history of eczema is present for the patient or family
Dermatitis herpetiformis	Similar distribution; vesicles and urticarial lesions more prominent – biopsy discriminates
Mechanical irritation by fibreglass	The glass fibres can be found microscopically in clothes
Pediculosis	Presence of lice and nits

Table 5.2 Treatments used for scabies

Agent	Percentage	Comment
Malathion	0.5	Second line treatment
Permethrin	1.0	New effective agent
Crotamiton	10.0	Claimed to be antipruritic as well
Monosulfiram	25.0	May cause Antabuse (disulfiram)-like alcohol reaction

patient and to all other sexual contacts, who should use the treatment at the same time as the patient.

The treatments employed are applied to the whole skin surface apart from the head and neck, and are for this reason usually lotions, although creams are also sometimes used. The patient should be instructed to have a hot bath before applying the treatment, after which no further application or bathing is permitted for 24 hours. The particular agents used are set out in Table 5.2.

Case 4

Sydney was 35 and began to itch all over two weeks ago. Now his girlfriend was also itching, as were her mother and brother. Close inspection of the skin showed many excoriations. Over the buttocks and genitalia there were papules and tiny, whitish lines, at the end of which there were minute black specks. Microscopy of these showed them to be scabies mites. Sydney was given permethrin lotion and told to use it all over from the neck down after a hot bath. His girlfriend and her family were also given the treatment. Improvement in the itching started some 2 weeks later.

DOG SCABIES

The mite causing dog scabies is similar to that causing human scabies, but the dog scabies mite does *not* cause the same clinical picture as human scabies. The rash only occurs at the site on the skin with which the dog has been in contact and does not spread to other areas. Scabies burrows are not found. The correct treatment is to treat the dog and to give any topical anti-itch preparation to the patient for the affected site.

Pediculosis

Pediculosis is the result of infestation with one of the varieties of the human louse. The different varieties cause different patterns of infestation.

PEDICULOSIS CAPITIS (HEAD LICE)

Infestation with *Pediculus capitis* is extremely common and seems to be becoming even more so. Although once more often seen in the poorer sections of society, the head louse is now seen in long-haired schoolchildren regardless of social background. It is more common during times of social upheaval, such as war. The louse is passed amongst children by casual contact and by sharing combs and brushes.

Clinical features

Itching is the predominant complaint. The scratching that results can cause secondary infection with exudation and crusting, but if this does not occur, all that may be seen are excoriation and red papules on the skin surface.

Examination of the hair will reveal the louse eggs (nits) stuck to the hair shaft (Fig. 5.8). Careful inspection will also detect the adult louse itself, which is less than 1 mm long and greyish or, after feeding, reddish in hue. When it moves it deserves the description of 'mobile dandruff'.

Confirmation of the diagnosis is the microscopic identification of the louse (Fig. 5.9) or the nits stuck to the hair shafts.

Treatment

The pediculicides used are set out in Table 5.3. The recommended regimen is application to the scalp of malathion or carbaryl lotion for a 12-hour period, followed by shampooing with shampoo containing the same pediculicide. Care must be taken to ensure that all close friends and family are also treated. A further treatment 1 month later is also necessary to kill off all the young lice that may have hatched from nits that remained alive after the initial treatment.

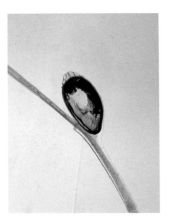

Figure 5.8 Louse egg (nit) on hair.

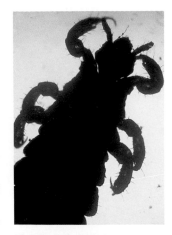

Figure 5.9 Hair louse seen microscopically.

Table 5.3 Treatments for pediculosis capitis

Agent	Percentage	Comment
Malathion	0.5	Both lotion and shampoo
Carbaryl	0.5	Both lotion and shampoo
Phenothrin	0.2	Lotion

PEDICULOSIS CORPORIS (BODY LICE)

Infestation with body lice is uncommon in modern developed societies, but may reach epidemic proportions in times of war or natural disaster. It also occurs sporadically in poor, socially deprived communities where there is poor hygiene. Transmission is via infested clothes or bedding or by close contact with the infested subject. The body louse is responsible for transmission of epidemic typhus, which is due to *Ricketessia prowazeki*, as well as trench fever and relapsing fever due to *Borrelia recurrentis*.

The body louse spends most of its time attached to the fibres of clothing, where it and its eggs should be sought if the disorder is suspected.

Clinical features

Itching without a great deal to see to account for the symptom is usual in the early stages. Some excoriations, blood crusts and bluish marks on the skin where the louse has fed may also be seen. Later in the disease, lichenification and eczema complete the picture of 'vagabond's disease'.

Treatment

Destruction and/or disinfestations of all clothes and bedding of the infested individual, the individual's family, friends and close contacts are necessary. In many countries, there are 'disinfestation centres' where this essential task is performed. Treatment with one of the pediculicides in Table 5.3 is mandatory. A further treatment after 1 month is advised.

PEDICULOSIS PUBIS (PUBIC LICE, CRAB LICE)

The pubic louse (*Phthirus pubis*) looks different from the head and body lice as it is broader, with crab-like rear legs (Fig. 5.10). It is mostly spread by sexual contact. The crab lice cling tenaciously to pubic hair, nipping down to skin level every so often to have a blood meal. In heavy infestations, the lice spread to body hair and even to the eyebrows and eyelashes! Diagnosis is confirmed by finding the louse and/or its nits.

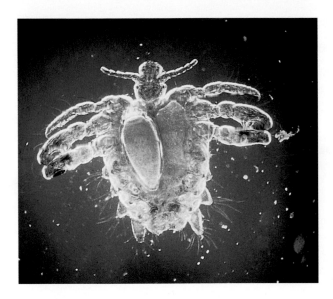

Figure 5.10 Pubic louse.

Treatment

One of the pediculicides in Table 5.3 should be used, with a repeat treatment after 1 month. Shaving of pubic hair is sometimes advised, but is not really necessary. All sexual contacts should be treated.

Insect bites and stings

A vast number of flying, jumping and crawling arthropods are capable of causing injury in a variety of ways to human skin. Some are capable of transmitting disease and some important examples of this are given in Table 5.4 (see also Table 5.5).

MOSQUITOES

Mosquito bites tend to be on exposed areas. Some varieties of mosquito (e.g. the culicine mosquitoes) can cause blisters when they bite. The bites may be extremely itchy and prominent (Fig. 5.11) and may become infected after being scratched.

FLEAS

Flea bites are mainly sustained from cat and dog fleas, which occasionally temporarily 'visit' a human host. They drop off their original hosts and live on carpets and rugs, as do their young, and jump up when they feel the vibration of footsteps. The bites, which are small and itchy, are often, but not exclusively, on the legs.

Table 5.4 Examples of important arthropod-spread diseases

Disease	Arthropod	Micro-organism
Malaria	Mosquitoes (*Anopheles* species)	Malaria parasite[a] (*Plasmodium* species)
Trypanosomiasis (sleeping sickness)	Tsetse fly	*Trypanosoma brucei*[a]
Leishmaniasis Visceral Cutaneous Mucocutaneous	Sandfly (*Phlebotomus* species)	*Leishmania donovani*[a] *Leishmania tropica*[a] *Leishmania braziliensis*[a]
Onchocerciasis	Blackfly (*Similium* species)	*Onchocerca volvulus*[b]
Bubonic plague	Rat flea	*Pasteurella pestis*[c]

[a] Protozoon.
[b] Thread-like nematode worm.
[c] Bacterium.

Table 5.5 Examples of methods of injury to the skin by arthropods

Mechanism	Arthropod
Bites from piercing and cutting mouthpieces – injection of saliva	Mosquitoes, ticks, sandflies, blackflies
Stings from 'purpose-built' structures with injection of toxic materials	Wasps, bees, scorpions, jellyfish
Release of toxic body fluids after being crushed on the skin surface, causing blistering	'Blister beetles' – cantharidin

Figure 5.11 Mosquito bites on the leg.

TICKS

Ticks stay stuck to the skin for some time after biting and are found mainly in agricultural communities, as the principal host is mostly sheep.

MITES

A large variety of mites may occasionally bite humans. Most of these, such as bird mites or *Cheyletellia* mites living on cats, dogs and rabbits (amongst others), cause small, red, itchy papules and are quite difficult to identify (Fig. 5.12).

BEDBUGS (*CIMEX LECTULARIUS*)

This primitive creature lives in the woodwork of old houses and comes out at night to bite its sleeping victims. The bites are often quite large and inflamed and arranged in straight lines where the creature has taken a 'stroll' over the skin surface.

WASPS AND BEES

The stings of wasps and bees are usually quite painful. The stung part may become very swollen a short time after the sting and, when hypersensitivity is present, the individual may develop a widespread reaction. Rarely, such a reaction can cause anaphylactic shock and even death.

PAPULAR URTICARIA

Papular urticaria is a term used to describe a recurrent, disseminated, itchy papular eruption due to either insect bites or hypersensitivity to them.

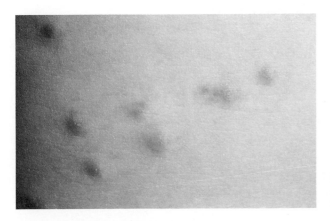

Figure 5.12 Multiple small papules due to mite bites.

Diagnosis

The lesions themselves should be compatible, i.e. they should be papules or, less commonly, blisters, and it helps if puncture marks can be found in the lesion. It is commonplace for the patients (or their parents) to deny the possibility of insect bites being responsible for the lesions, as there seems to be a social stigma attached to being the recipient of them. A detailed history is necessary, with particular attention being given to the presence of domestic animals, proximity to farms, the occurrence of similar lesions in other family members, and the periodicity of lesions.

Biopsy may occasionally be helpful in that it may well rule out other disorders. The presence of a mixed inflammatory cell infiltrate in the upper and mid dermis is typical, but the pattern and density of cellular infiltrate are variable (Fig. 5.13).

Searching for the biting arthropod in the home may be fruitless unless the assistance of trained personnel is sought. Examination of 'brushings' from the coats of dogs by veterinarians may be successful in identifying the culprit – cheyletellia, for example.

Treatment

Identification of the creature responsible and prevention of further attack are important. Uncommonly, when there is evidence of hypersensitivity (as in a bee or wasp sting), systemic antihistamines may be required and, when there is a severe systemic reaction, systemic steroids and even adrenalin may be needed.

A major problem with insect bites is their intense itchiness. Occasionally, this may result in infection in the excoriated skin, when treatment is required for this complication. Topical antihistamines (e.g. diphenhydramine, promethazine, dimentidine) are often prescribed and may have a slight antipruritic effect, but all that is usually required is a calamine or mentholated calamine preparation.

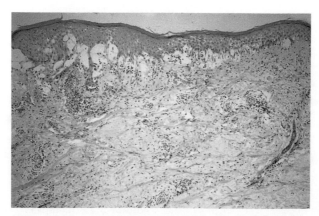

Figure 5.13 Pathology of inspect bite showing marked inflammation and subepidermal oedema.

Helminthic infestations of the skin

ONCHOCERCIASIS

This is caused by the parasite *Onchocerca volvulus* and is found in equatorial West Africa. The disorder is spread by the bite of the blackfly *Simulium damnosum*, which is found around rivers. The larval forms, known as microfilariae, are injected into the skin by the blackfly and develop after some years into adult onchocercal worms. These are extremely long (up to 1 m) but very thin (1–2 mm in diameter) creatures that live curled up in the subcutis surrounded by a palpable, host-supplied fibrous capsule. The adult worm procreates by producing enormous numbers of microfilariae, which invade the subcutis of large areas of truncal skin.

Clinical features

The disorder is characterized by severe and persistent irritation of affected skin. Affected areas become thickened, lichenified (see page 119), slightly scaly and often hyperpigmented (Fig. 5.14). The microfilariae may also invade the superficial tissues of the eye and cause blindness ('river blindness').

Diagnosis

Biopsies show non-specific inflammation, but occasionally demonstrate portions of the microfilariae. A more successful way of identifying the larval forms is by taking a series of skin 'snips' with a needle and scalpel. The tiny portions of skin are then immersed in saline and observed microscopically to watch for the emergence of microfilariae. There is usually a marked eosinophilia and there is also a complement fixing test for antibodies that is available in some centres.

Treatment

The pruritus is much improved by Hetrazan (diethyl carbamazine). The drug must be given cautiously because of the possibility of a severe systemic reaction

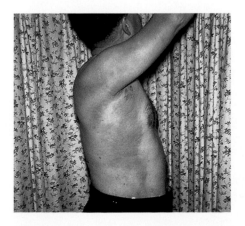

Figure 5.14 Skin changes of onchocerciasis, with marked thickening and discoloration.

due to the liberation of toxic products from the dying microfilariae. Hetrazan has no effect on the adult worm and it is necessary to treat with the potentially toxic drug Suramin to kill off the worm and prevent further production of microfilariae. Ivermectin is also helpful.

Summary

- Scabies is caused by a tiny mite, the female of which burrows into the stratum corneum. It is extremely itchy and is caught by skin contact with an infected individual.

- The primary lesion is the scabies run or burrow, at the end of which sits the mite. Excoriated papules and vesicles are also seen. Affected sites include palms, soles, knees, elbow, ankles and genitalia.

- Heavy infestation occurs in immunocompromised individuals, resulting in thick, crusted areas – known as Norwegian scabies.

- Treatment is with permethrin or malathion, which should be applied over the entire skin surface below the neck after a bath and be used for all human contacts.

- Pediculosis is caused by infestation with the human louse. Head lice (*Pediculus capitis*) cause infestation of the hair and are common in schoolchildren. Eggs (or nits) are found stuck to the hair. Shampoos containing phenothrin or malathion are used in treatment.

- Pediculosis corporis is seen in the socially deprived and is transmitted by clothes and bedding. The body louse may transmit typhus.

- Pediculosis pubis (crab lice) is caused by *Phthirus pubis*, which infests pubic hair and is spread by sexual contact. Treatment is with phenothrin or malathion applications.

- Insect bites spread many disorders, including malaria, leishmaniasis and onchocerciasis. Mosquitoes, fleas, ticks, mites, bedbugs, wasps and bees cause problems by bites or stings.

Immunologically mediated skin disorders

This chapter describes several disorders with a strong immunopathogenic component.

Urticaria and angioedema

These common disorders are the result of histamine release from mast cells in the skin.

CLINICAL FEATURES

Urticaria is extremely common ('nettlerash', 'weals' and 'hives' are popular names for this disorder) and there are few individuals who do not experience it in one

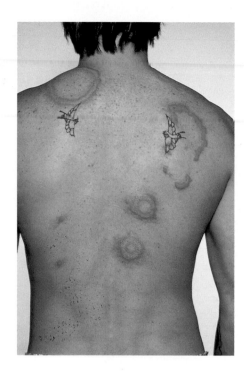

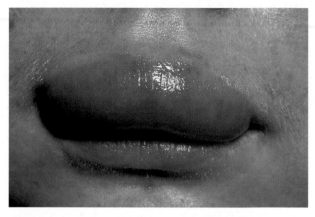

Figure 6.1 Urticarial lesions on the back of a young man.

Figure 6.2 Marked swelling of the upper lip in angioedema, which seemed to be due to fish hypersensitivity in this patient.

form or another during their lifetime. Urticarial lesions are itchy, red papules and plaques of variable size (Fig. 6.1) that arise suddenly, often within a few minutes, and last 6–24 hours. They may assume odd, polycyclic, annular and geographic forms.

An important characteristic of urticaria is its transience, but very occasionally urticarial lesions stay for days rather than hours and leave a brownish stain. This type of urticaria is due to involvement of small blood vessels and is known as urticarial vasculitis.

In many patients with urticaria and in a few people without it, firm pressure over a track with a blunt object such as a key over the skin of the back will produce blanching, then redness, then a weal. This phenomenon, which is an exaggeration of the normal 'triple response', causes itching and is known as dermographism.

In angioedema, the lesions are deeper and the swelling much more extensive than in urticaria (Fig. 6.2). Angioedema may accompany urticaria or may occur independently. The face and the tissues of the oropharynx are sometimes affected by the angioedema, which can lead to life-threatening difficulties in swallowing and breathing.

Urticaria and angioedema can last for a few days or some years. A common pattern is for the disorder to recur in a series of attacks. Chronic urticaria is a common and sometimes disabling disorder, which in most cases is of unknown origin.

Table 6.1 Some causes of urticaria

Sensitivity to exogenous antigens
Foods, e.g. fish, prawns, crabs, milk, etc.
Drugs, e.g. penicillin

Pharmacological provocation
Aspirin, opioids

Systemic disorders
Lupus erythematosus
Henoch–Schönlein purpura
Autoimmunity

'Physical' causes
Cholinergic urticaria
High pressure (dermographism)
Persistent pressure
Cold
Exposure to sunlight (solar)

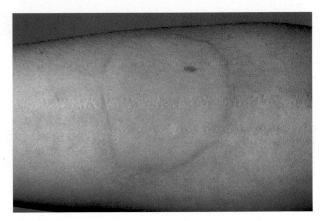

Figure 6.3 Cold urticaria elicited by a block of ice.

CAUSES

The ultimate cause of urticaria and angioedema is release of histamine from mast cell granules, but there is a large number of stimuli that can do this. Many are immunological, some are purely pharmacological and others are physical. Type I immunological reactions are involved in the production of urticarial lesions. Table 6.1 gives some of the known causes. Although the cause(s) of urticaria can be identified in some patients, in many it remains a mystery. In recent years it *has* been found that some patients have antibodies to receptors on their own mast cells.

THE 'PHYSICAL' URTICARIAS

Cold urticaria

Urticarial swelling of the hands, face and elsewhere may occur after exposure to the cold. The reaction can be elicited by an ice block (Fig. 6.3). There is a familial form.

Pressure urticaria

Urticarial lesions develop some time (up to several hours) after pressure on the skin, for example from belts or other tight clothing, or from the rungs of a ladder.

Dermographism

Many patients with urticaria mark easily when their skin is rubbed firmly, for example with a key. This is an exaggerated 'triple response' and is quite troublesome to some patients (Fig. 6.4).

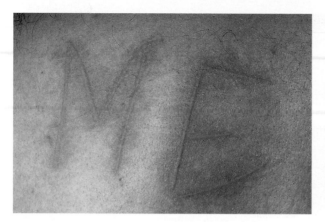

Figure 6.4 Dermographic response to firm stroking of the skin.

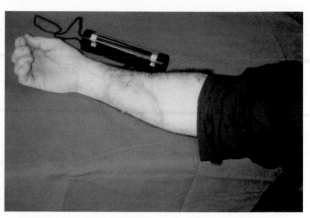

Figure 6.5 Solar urticaria. This patient was so sensitive that he developed an urticarial response to the minimal ultraviolet radiation of the A type (long-wave UVA) emitted by a battery-driven, hand-held fluorescent lamp.

Solar urticaria

Urticarial spots develop on exposed skin a few minutes after exposure to the sun. Various wavelengths may be responsible (Fig. 6.5).

CHOLINERGIC URTICARIA

Irritating, small urticarial spots develop after exercise or hot baths – stimuli that evoke sweating from the post-ganglionic cholinergically enervated sweat glands. This very common disorder can be very disabling in a few patients, as it effectively prevents them doing any kind of physical activity.

DRUG-INDUCED URTICARIA

Penicillin hypersensitivity is a common cause of urticaria. Attacks vary from the life-threatening acute anaphylactic type to crops of small urticarial papules. Opioid drugs can cause urticaria by directly stimulating histamine release. Up to one-third of patients with urticaria develop lesions after 'challenge' with aspirin, but whether this is entirely due to pharmacological stimulation of histamine release, involvement in prostanoid metabolism, or hypersensitivity is not certain.

STINGS

Nettles, jellyfish tentacles and some insect stings elicit histamine release at the site of skin contact, producing painful local reactions. Urticaria can also be a sign of an underlying systemic disorder such as lupus erythematosus and amyloidosis and a component of disorders such as dermatitis herpetiformis (see page 89) and allergic vasculitis (see page 84).

Treatment

Antihistamines of the H1 receptor blocker type are most effective at relieving symptoms in this disorder. It is better to become really familiar with just a few of these than to try to memorize the whole range available. The 'older' antihistamines such as promethazine and diphenhydramine are quite effective, but have a hypnotic effect precluding driving or using machinery. Newer antihistamines such as foxfenadine, astemizole, cetirizine and loratidine are also effective, with less hypnotic effect. A few patients obtain increased benefit by adding an H2 antagonist such as cimetidine to the H1 antagonist already being administered.

Acute severe urticaria and angioedema may require oral corticosteroids. Where the condition is life threatening, intravenous hydrocortisone should be used.

Erythema multiforme

DEFINITION

An acute and relatively short-lived inflammatory reaction of skin and mucosae, occurring in response to a variety of antigenic stimuli and resulting in scattered lesions at the dermoepidermal junction.

CLINICAL FEATURES

Individual lesions are red to purple maculopapules, some of which become annular or target-like and may blister (Figs 6.6 and 6.7). The face and upper limbs are preferentially involved, and the buccal mucosa is often involved in severely affected patients. In the worst cases, there is severe systemic upset. The front of the mouth is eroded in severely affected patients (Fig. 6.8). The conjunctivae and genital mucosae are affected in a few. The disorder starts acutely and usually lasts less than 2 weeks, although crops of new lesions often develop in the first few days.

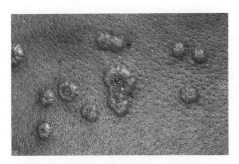

Figure 6.6 Vesiculobullous lesions of erythema multiforme. Some seem 'target-like'.

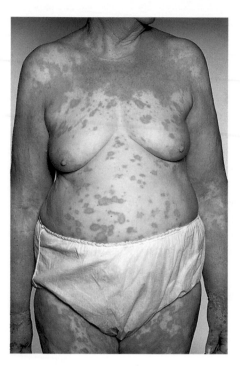

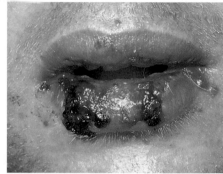

Figure 6.7 Widespread lesions of erythema multiforme.

Figure 6.8 Eroded labial mucosa in erythema multiforme. This patient's mouth was also affected.

AETIOLOGY AND PATHOLOGY

The disorder may be precipitated by infections, including herpes simplex, orf, coccidioidomycosis and histoplasmosis, drugs such as piroxicam, indomethacin and other non-steroidal anti-inflammatory compounds, sulphonamides and thiazide diuretics (Table 6.2). In a proportion of patients, it recurs for no very obvious reason. Mononuclear inflammatory cells collect at the dermoepidermal junction and fluid collects beneath the epidermis.

TREATMENT

The disorder is self-limiting and only symptomatic treatment is required. Where there is serious systemic disturbance, systemic steroids may be given.

Table 6.2 Causes of erythema multiforme

Drugs
  Non-steroidal anti-inflammatory drugs
  Psychotropic drugs
  Sulphonamides, other antimicrobial drugs

Infections
  Herpes simplex
  Orf
  Mycoplasma
  Histoplasmosis
  Coccidioidomycosis

Ultraviolet irradiation

Ulcerative colitis and Crohn's disease

Case 5

The condition started with soreness in the mouth. Sally, aged 27, thought that is was the curry she had had the previous night. Within 2 days, she had developed a widespread rash – particularly over her arms and upper trunk. Many of the lesions were annular and some showed blistering. The rash began to improve after 12 days, but the disorder had made her feel tired and ill. It was thought to be erythema multiforme – in all likelihood precipitated by an attack of labial herpes simplex some 2 weeks before the onset.

Erythema nodosum

DEFINITION

A painful inflammatory disorder in which crops of tender nodules occur in response to antigenic stimuli.

CLINICAL FEATURES

Individual lesions are red, raised and tender and vary in size from 1 to 3 cm in diameter. They occur in crops on the shins (Fig. 6.9) and, less commonly, on the forearms. There may be malaise, fever and an accompanying arthralgia of the ankles. The lesions take 2–6 weeks to resolve and leave a bruised appearance. Crops of lesions may develop over some months.

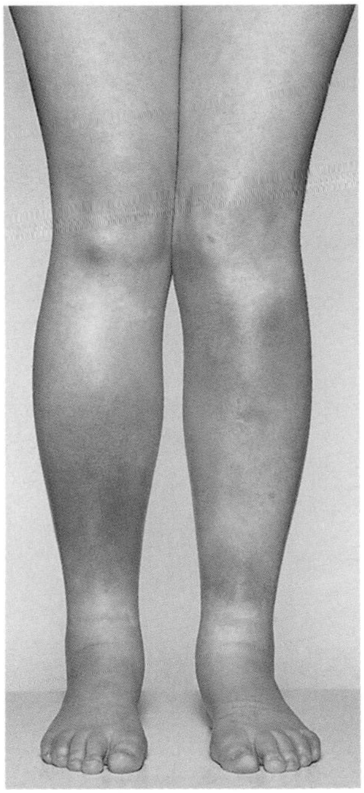

AETIOLOGY AND PATHOLOGY

There are numerous causes, including infections, drugs and systemic illnesses (Table 6.3). The most important are sarcoidosis (see page 47) and pulmonary tuberculosis. The disorder is also seen (rarely) in ulcerative colitis and leprosy. A cause is identified in some 50 per cent of patients. It is essentially a panniculitis, with inflammation and bleeding occurring in the fibrous septa between fat lobules.

TREATMENT

Treatment is mainly rest and mild analgesics and/or anti-inflammatory agents.

Annular erythemas

There are several disorders that are marked by the appearance of erythematous rings, which usually gradually enlarge and then disappear. Generally their significance is uncertain, but one, known as erythema gyratum repens, signifies the presence of an underlying visceral neoplasm (see page 281) and another, erythema chronicum migrans, indicates the presence of Lyme disease.

Autoimmune disorders

These disorders are also known as the collagen vascular disorders and the connective tissue diseases. In general terms, the immune system of an individual with

Figure 6.9 Multiple inflamed lesions of erythema nodusum.

Table 6.3 Causes of erythema nodusum

| Tuberculosis |
| Sarcoidosis |
| Brucellosis |
| Ulcerative colitis and Crohn's disease |
| Leprosy |

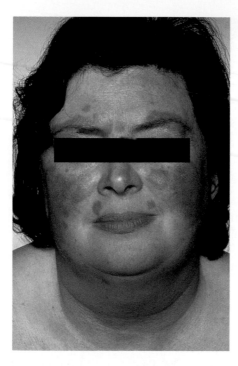

Figure 6.10 Facial erythema in a woman with severe lupus erythematosus.

autoimmune disease fails to 'recognize' the individual's own tissues and mounts an attack on them. In most of the disorders in this group, the inflammatory process seems to involve the small blood vessels in particular (vasculitis).

LUPUS ERYTHEMATOSUS

This is divided into systemic and cutaneous forms, although there is some overlap.

Systemic lupus erythematosus

Systemic lupus erythematosus (SLE) often involves the skin as well as many other organ systems, but in one type of SLE – subacute SLE – the skin is prominently affected. Antibodies to nuclear DNA occur in 80–90 per cent of patients with SLE and antibodies to other nuclear components are present in subgroups of patients. These antinuclear factors may be intimately involved in the pathogenesis of the disease.

Common components of SLE include a rheumatoid-like arthropathy, a glomerulonephritis, inflammatory disorder of the pulmonary and cardiovascular systems, a polyserositis, central nervous system involvement and skin disorder. The skin components of SLE include facial erythema across the cheeks and nose (butterfly erythema: Fig. 6.10), and discoid lupus erythematosus (DLE) occurs in the pure cutaneous form.

Mainly young women are affected. The 5-year mortality has been variously estimated to be between 15 and 50 per cent, dependent on the organ systems affected and the pace of the disease.

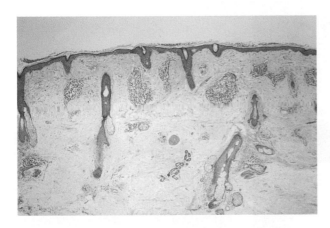

Figure 6.11 Pathology of a skin lesion in systemic lupus erythematosus. There are collections of lymphocytes perivascularly.

Pathology and laboratory findings

Affected skin shows oedema, degenerative change in the basal epidermal cells and a tight cuff of mononuclear cells around the small blood vessels (Fig. 6.11). Unexposed, uninvolved skin has deposits of immunoprotein – immunoglobulin G (IgG) or IgA – in about 60 per cent of patients at the dermoepidermal junction, detectable by direct immunofluorescent methods. Circulating antibodies to DNA or other nuclear components are found in the large majority of patients. An increase in the level of serum gamma-globulin is a frequent finding. Haematological findings include a normochromic, normocytic anaemia, a neutropenia, a lymphopenia and a thrombocytopenia.

Treatment

Patients with active, progressive disease may require systemic steroids to suppress the inflammatory process. Immunosuppressive agents such as methotrexate, azathioprine and cyclosporin may also be needed.

Chronic discoid lupus erythematosus

Lesions of chronic discoid lupus erythematosus (CDLE) can occur in the course of SLE or may be the only manifestation of the disorder. Frequently, patients with CDLE have minor haematological changes of the sort described in SLE, but no other features of SLE. In some 5 per cent of patients, CDLE transforms to SLE.

Clinical features

Irregular, red plaques appear on light-exposed skin of the face, scalp, neck, hands or arms (Fig. 6.12). The plaques develop patchy atrophy with patchy hypopigmentation and hyperpigmentation, whereas other areas are thickened and warty. On the scalp, scarring alopecia occurs in the affected areas (Fig. 6.13). The disorder may be aggravated or initiated by exposure to the sun.

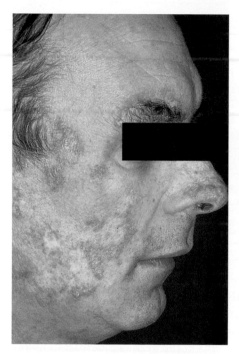

Figure 6.12 Multiple irregular, red plaques due to discoid lupus erythematosus.

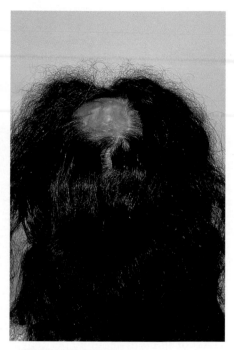

Figure 6.13 Patch of discoid lupus erythematosus causing alopecia.

Pathology

The changes are similar to those described for SLE, but the epidermal degenerative changes are more marked, with scattered cytoid body formation and patchy epidermal atrophy and thickening.

Treatment

Sun avoidance and use of sunscreens are important. Individual lesions sometimes respond to potent topical corticosteroids. Where these do not cope with the disease, hydroxychloroquine (200–400 mg per day) is often helpful. Caution must be exercised concerning the possible, although rare, toxic effects of this drug on the retina. Systemic steroids, the oral gold compound auranofin, cyclosporin and acitretin are other drugs that have been used successfully.

Systemic sclerosis

Scleroderma is an important component of systemic sclerosis. In this auto-immune disorder, the fibroblast is stimulated to produce new collagen. When other organ systems are involved, the disorder affects the vasculature as well as fibroblasts, and Raynaud's phenomenon, renal involvement with glomerular disease, gut involvement with dysphagia and gut hypomobility, a rheumatoid type of polyarthropathy and skin stiffening are all seen (Table 6.4). As with SLE, the disease is mostly seen in young women, and the pace of the disorder is extremely variable. It may start insidiously over some months or even years, with progressively worsening Raynaud's phenomenon and gradual thickening and stiffening of the skin of the hands and face. This causes a characteristic beak-like facial appearance, with narrowing of the mouth (Fig. 6.14). Telangiectatic macules appear over the face (Fig. 6.15) and deposits of calcium develop in the skin. The term CRST syndrome is used for this constellation of problems (calcinosis cutis, Raynaud's sclerosis and telangiectasia). When there is also dysphagia due to oesophageal involvement, the term CREST is more appropriate.

In more rapidly progressive systemic sclerosis, there may be more serious vascular disease affecting the fingers, resulting in tissue necrosis and even the loss of portions of the digits. Renal or pulmonary disease may eventually cause the death of the patient – the 5-year mortality rate of this disease being 30 per cent or more.

PATHOLOGY AND LABORATORY FINDINGS

Biopsy of affected skin shows excess new collagen that has an eosinophilic and almost homogeneous appearance. Antinuclear antibodies occur in up to 30 per cent of patients.

Table 6.4 Manifestations of systemic sclerosis

Raynaud's phenomenon

Skin thickening and stiffness

Ischaemic necrosis of digits

Dysphagia

Glomerulosclerosis and renal insufficiency

Hypertension

Malabsorption, constipation

Pulmonary fibrosis

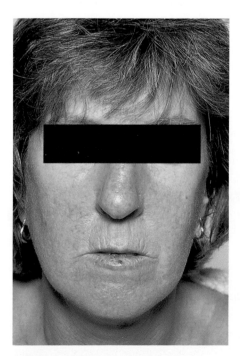

Figure 6.14 Facial appearance in systemic sclerosis. Note the 'beaked nose' with pinched cheeks and small mouth.

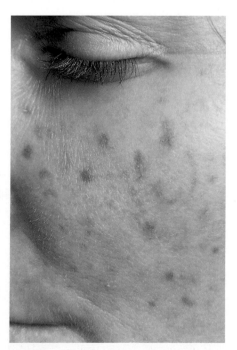

Figure 6.15 Macular telangiectasia of the facial skin in systemic sclerosis.

TREATMENT

There is no reliable way of significantly modifying the disorder. Some improvement can be obtained by skilful management of the Raynaud's phenomenon, and occasionally with penicillamine and immunosuppressive treatment with steroids and azathioprine or cyclosporin.

Morphoea

Morphoea is localized scleroderma.

CLINICAL FEATURES

One or more thickened, variably sized sclerotic plaques develop over the trunk or limbs. A mauve colour at first, they become brownish later (Fig. 6.16). It is mostly a disease of young adults, but involvement of the face and scalp in children produces an 'en coup de sabre' deformity. Morphoea generally gradually remits after a period of 2–3 years. Histologically, there is marked replacement of the subcutaneous fat with new collagen, which has a pale, homogenized appearance. There is no effective treatment.

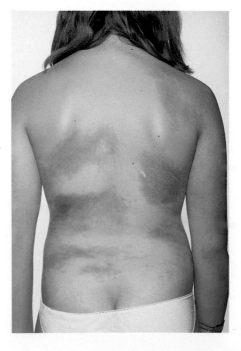

Figure 6.16 Plaques of morphoea.

VARIANTS

Generalized morphoea

This is a rare type of scleroderma that is confined to the skin but develops over wide expanses of it, causing considerable limitation of movement and even impeding breathing.

Lichen sclerosus et atrophicus

It is not certain whether or not this is a form of morphoea.

Small, irritating, whitish areas occur on the genitalia or around the anus or, less commonly, elsewhere over the skin. In men, the condition occurs on the glans penis or prepuce. It is then known as balanitis xerotica obliterans and may cause discomfort and paraphimosis. There is a characteristic pathological picture in which there is intense oedema in a subepidermal band.

Good results have been obtained with high-potency topical corticosteroids (e.g. clobetasol 17-propionate). Circumcision is recommended for the condition in men.

Dermatomyositis

Both muscle and skin are affected in this disabling disorder. Polymyositis is the identical disorder without skin involvement.

CLINICAL FEATURES

Dull red to mauve areas develop over the face, backs of the hands, elbows, knees and elsewhere. A particularly characteristic sign is the presence of a mauvish erythema on the upper lids and around the eyes, likened to the colour of the heliotrope flower (Fig. 6.17). On the backs of the hands, the erythema affects the paronychial folds and the skin over the metacarpals (Fig. 6.18).

Sometimes small areas of necrosis appear, due to an accompanying vasculitis. Calcium is deposited in long-standing skin lesions.

There is proximal myositis, which causes pain and tenderness as well as profound weakness. If progressive, pharyngeal and respiratory muscles are affected and the condition becomes life threatening. However, the disease generally remits spontaneously.

LABORATORY FINDINGS

Muscle enzymes such as phosphocreatine kinase, aldolase and lactic dehydrogenase are increased in the blood. Urine creatine is also a good indicator of disease activity. Muscle damage can also be assessed by muscle biopsy and electromyography.

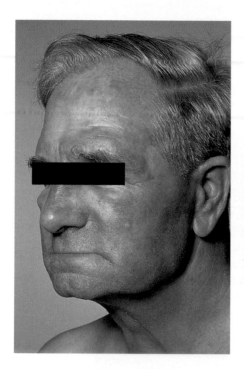

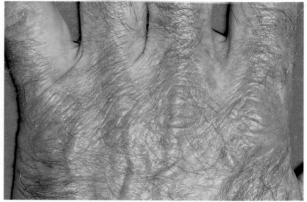

Figure 6.17 Mauve discoloration of the facial skin in dermatomyositis, with particular involvement of the periocular area.

Figure 6.18 Streaky, mauve-red appearance over the back of the metacarpals and fingers in dermatomyositis.

TREATMENT

Oral steroids are the mainstay of treatment and are given in sufficient dosage to prevent further progress of the disease. Azathioprine and other immunosuppressive drugs are sometimes prescribed.

The vasculitis group of diseases

There are several disorders in which the major focus seems to be on the vasculature, with the kidneys, respiratory system, joints and skin apparently being primarily involved. The central nervous system and the gut are also involved on occasion.

ALLERGIC VASCULITIS (HENOCH–SCHÖNLEIN PURPURA)

Although any age group can be affected, children and young adults seem especially prone to the disorder.

It starts suddenly, with fever, painful joints and a rash. The rash is both urticarial and papular, and particularly marked on extensor surfaces. It is also quite definitely purpuric in that it cannot be 'blanched' by pressure with a microscope slide (Fig. 6.19). The lesions come in recurrent crops over the first few days.

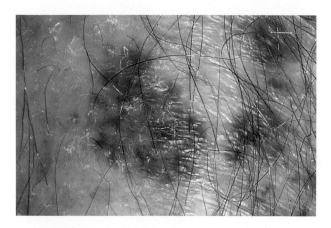

Figure 6.19 Purpura in Henoch–Schönlein purpura.

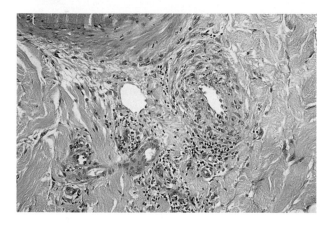

Figure 6.20 Pathology of allergic vasculitis. Polymorphonuclear cells and fragments of polymorph nuclei are seen around small damaged blood vessels (leucocytoclastic angiitis).

Joint pain with some swelling is quite commonly noted. Cramping abdominal pain and malaena occasionally develop as a result of submucosal haemorrhagic oedema. Acute glomerulonephritis causes microscopic haematuria when renal involvement is mild, but oliguria and renal failure in a very few severely affected patients. The disorder remits spontaneously in most patients, but may recur in some.

Pathology and pathogenesis

The cause is unknown, but hypersensitivity to streptococcal antigens may play a role in some patients. Immune complexes formed from streptococcal antigens and antibodies are believed to be deposited in endothelium, initiating the reaction. Histologically, collections of polymorphonuclear leucocytes and fragments of their nuclei are found around small blood vessels in the dermis (leucocytoclasis) alongside oedema and some bleeding. The endothelium is swollen and may show degenerative change (Fig. 6.20). This picture, known as leucocytoclastic angiitis, is not specific to this disease.

Treatment

Severely affected patients will need systemic steroids.

POLYARTERITIS NODOSA

Polyarteritis nodosa is a serious, rare inflammatory disorder of large and medium-sized arteries. Inflammation of the vessel wall, which dilates aneurysmally, causes rupture and ischaemic changes. Central nervous system, cardiovascular, gastrointestinal and renal problems may all arise in this potentially fatal disease. In the skin, a livedo reticularis pattern and persistent ulcers are seen.

NODULAR VASCULITIS

This is an uncommon inflammatory disorder of the cutaneous vasculature of the legs, seen predominantly in women.

Painful red and purpuric papules and nodules develop on the calves and elsewhere on the legs in recurrent crops over many years. Some may ulcerate, but generally they disappear without sequel.

OTHER TYPES OF CUTANEOUS VASCULITIS

The development of crops of purple purpuric papules with darker and occasionally crusted central areas and sometimes pustules is seen in the course of subacute bacterial endocarditis, gonococcaemia and meningococcaemia (Fig. 6.21). Drugs such as the thiazides may also cause a vasculitis. Renal involvement sometimes accompanies the skin lesions. The importance of such lesions is that they are signs of an underlying systemic disorder – demanding rapid diagnosis and treatment.

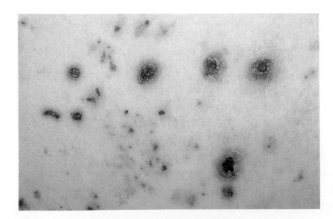

Figure 6.21 Purpuric and necrotic papules in cutaneous vasculitis.

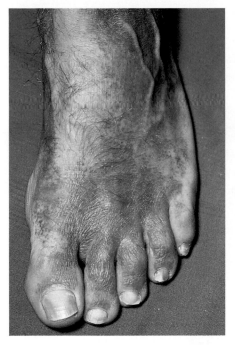

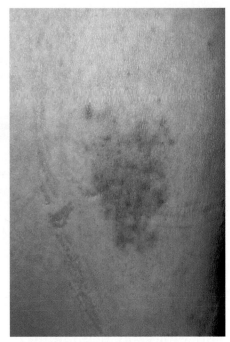

Figure 6.22 Pigmented and purpuric eruptions due to Schamberg's disease.

Figure 6.23 Patch with slight golden hue due to purpura in 'lichen aureus'.

CAPILLARITIS

There is a group of benign, persistent, mildly inflammatory skin disorders in which the focus of the abnormality appears to be in the papillary dermis and the immediately subepidermal capillary vasculature. The term persistent pigmented purpuric eruption seems appropriate, as they are persistent and because of the damage to capillaries, causing leakage of blood and pigmentation from haemosiderin staining. The lesions mostly occur on the lower legs and vary from a macular, spattered appearance (Schamberg's disease: Fig. 6.22) to an itchy, papular eruption (lichenoid purpuric eruption) or a macular golden eruption (lichen aureus: Fig. 6.23). These disorders generally cause little disability and remit spontaneously after a variable period.

Blistering diseases

Many inflammatory skin disorders can produce blistering at some stage in their natural history. In the primary blistering diseases, blistering is the major feature of the disease and a direct result of the initial pathological process. The different blistering diseases are given in Table 6.5.

Table 6.5 The 'primary' blistering disorders

Subepidermal	
Senile pemphigoid	Acute, widespread, severe
Cicatricial pemphigoid	Chronic, limited in extent, mucosae affected causing erosion and scarring
Erythema multiforme	Acute, mucosae as well, variously caused
Dermatitis herpetiformis	Itchy, persistent, associated with gluten enteropathy
Epidermolysis bullosa	Genetically and phenotypically diverse, varies from mild to lethal
Intraepidermal	
Pemphigus	
vulgaris	Suprabasal epidermal split
vegetans	
erythematosus	Subcorneal epidermal split
foliaceous	

SUBEPIDERMAL BLISTERING DISEASES

Bullous pemphigoid (senile pemphigoid)

Bullous pemphigoid (BP) is an uncommon, acute blistering disease occurring mainly in the over-60s.

Large, tense, often blood-stained blisters develop over a few days anywhere on the skin surface (Fig. 6.24) except the buccal mucosa. New crops of blisters continue to appear for many months without adequate treatment, and the disease is painful and disabling. Rarely, the disorder is a sign of an underlying malignancy.

Laboratory findings

There is a circulating antibody directed to the epidermal basement membrane zone in 85–90 per cent of patients, which can be detected using the immunofluorescence method. The titre of this antibody is to some extent a reflection of the activity of the disease. Antibodies of the IgG type and the complement component C3 are also deposited in the subepidermal zone around the lesions in the majority of patients and can also be detected using the direct immunofluorescence technique (Fig. 6.25). Biopsy reveals that there is subepidermal fluid, with polymorphs and eosinophils in the infiltrate subepidermally (Fig. 6.26).

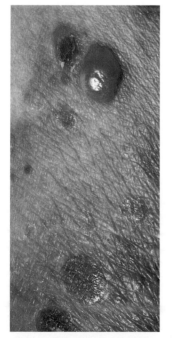

Figure 6.24 Tense blisters due to bullous pemphigoid.

Treatment

Patients with widespread blistering may need to be nursed in hospital and treated as though they had severe burns. High doses of corticosteroids (60 mg per day of prednisone, or even more) are needed to control the disease. Immunosuppressive treatment with azathioprine or methotrexate is usually started simultaneously. The blisters themselves should be treated with 'wet dressings'.

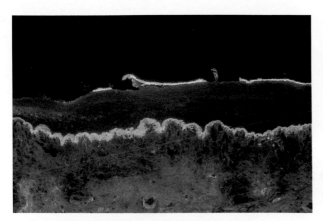

Figure 6.25 There is a fluorescent band at the dermoepidermal junction in this fluorescence photomicrograph due to deposition of immunoglobulin (IgG). A biopsy from the skin around the site of blistering was frozen and the cryostat section treated with fluorescein-tagged anti-immunoglobulin antibodies.

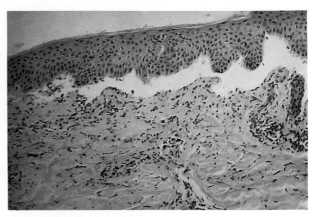

Figure 6.26 Pathology of bullous pemphigoid showing subepidermal blister.

Variants of bullous pemphigoid

There are other rare blistering diseases in which the blister forms subepidermally. These include:

- benign mucous membrane pemphigoid, in which lesions occur chronically in the mouth and in the conjunctivae as well as on the skin
- 'bullous disease of childhood', in which bullous lesions occur in infancy, particularly in the buttock and perigenital area.

In the latter disorder, and in some blistering conditions in adults, IgA is deposited instead of IgG.

Dermatitis herpetiformis

Intensely itchy vesicles, papulovesicles and urticarial papules appear in crops over the knees, elbows, scalp, buttocks and around the axillae (Fig. 6.27). Most patients with dermatitis herpetiformis (DH) have a mild gastrointestinal absorptive defect due to gluten enteropathy, as in patients with coeliac disease. Some diseases with an immunopathogenetic component are more common in patients with DH, including thyrotoxicosis, rheumatoid arthritis, myasthenia gravis and ulcerative colitis. The disorder is persistent but fluctuates in intensity.

LABORATORY FINDINGS

Small-bowel mucosal biopsy reveals partial villous atrophy in 70–80 per cent of patients with DH. Minor abnormalities of small-bowel absorptive function are

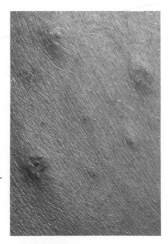

Figure 6.27
Vesiculopapules in dermatitis herpetiformis.

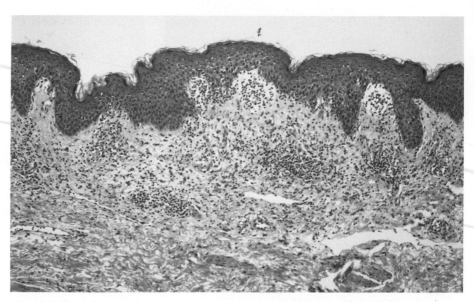

Figure 6.28 Pathology of dermatitis herpetiformis. There are collections of polymorphs in the tips of the dermal papillae where the subepidermal blistering begins.

also common. Biopsy of new lesions demonstrates that the vesicle forms subepidermally and develops from collections of inflammatory cells in the papillary tips (the papillary tip abscess: Fig. 6.28). Direct immunofluorescent examination reveals the presence of IgA in the papillary tips in the skin around the lesions in all patients.

TREATMENT

The skin lesions can be suppressed with the drug dapsone (50–200 mg per day) in most patients. Unfortunately, however, dapsone has many toxic side effects, including haemolysis, methaemoglobinaemia, sulphaemoglobinaemia and rashes such as fixed drug eruption. A gluten-free diet will improve the gastrointestinal lesion and improves the skin disorder in many patients after some months.

Epidermolysis bullosa

This is not a single disorder, but a group of similar, inherited blistering diseases. The blistering is caused by various congenital structural and metabolic defects.

EPIDERMOLYSIS BULLOSA SIMPLEX

The blistering in this rare disorder appears subepidermal, but is actually through the basal layer of the epidermis. It is usually limited to the hands and feet and the sites of trauma. It is dominantly inherited. The blisters may just be confined to the soles of the feet and not prove troublesome until adolescence. As with most geno-dermatoses, these conditions persist throughout life. There is no effective treatment other than to avoid trauma and to keep the blistered areas clean and dry.

DYSTROPHIC EPIDERMOLYSIS BULLOSA

Disorders in this rare group of conditions cause severe scarring and indeed some forms are not compatible with life. They are also subepidermal, but the split is within the upper dermis. They are mostly recessive, but there are some dominant types too. Blistering and scarring cause marked tissue loss over the hands and feet, with eventual webbing of the fingers and toes and possibly loss of these structures. There is also marked scarring of the mucosae, which affects the pharynx and oesophagus too, so that severe dysphagia is a problem. Squamous cell carcinoma develops on the most severely affected sites in some patients. This is a terrifyingly destructive and disabling group of disorders for which there is at present no adequate treatment.

Pemphigus

Pemphigus causes blistering because of a loosening of desmosomal links between epidermal cells caused by immunological attack. There are several types. They are all rare, but *pemphigus vulgaris* (PV) is the least rare. In PV, the split occurs within the epidermis just above the basal layer (suprabasal). The lesions are thin-walled, delicate blisters that usually rapidly rupture and erode (Fig. 6.29). They occur anywhere on the skin surface and very frequently occur within the mouth and throat, where they cause much discomfort and disability. The disorder is persistent, although fluctuating in intensity. Before adequate treatment became available, it was usually fatal.

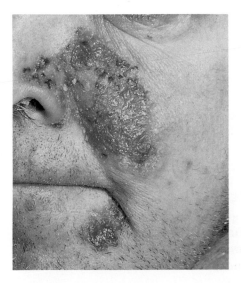

Figure 6.29 Eroded area on the face due to pemphigus vulgaris.

LABORATORY FINDINGS

In more than 90 per cent of patients, there is a detectable circulating antibody directed to the area between epidermal cells. The titre of the antibody reflects the severity of the disease. The presence of the antibody and its titre are determined by indirect immunofluorescence methods. Biopsy reveals the intraepidermal split, with rounded up epidermal cells (known as acantholysis). Direct immunofluorescence examination of the perilesional involved skin will show the presence of antibody of the IgG class and the complement component C3 between epidermal cells.

TREATMENT

The patients should be treated as though they had burns and, if severely affected, need in-patient care. Large doses of systemic steroids are required to control the blistering (doses of up to 100 mg prednisone are sometimes given). Immunosuppressive therapy with azathioprine or methotrexate should be started simultaneously. Treatment with cyclosporin and with gold, as for rheumatoid arthritis, has also been used.

VARIANTS

Pemphigus vegetans

There is a more inflammatory component to this very rare intraepidermal blistering condition in which the lesions are usually limited in extent.

Pemphigus foliaceous

This is a rare form of pemphigus in which the intraepidermal split is high within the epidermis. It can cause erosions and scaling rather than blistering and can be mistaken for sebborrhoeic dermatitis.

Pemphigus erythematodes

This rare, superficial type of pemphigus lesions have some resemblances to discoid lupus erythematosus. It occurs around the face and scalp particularly.

Drug eruptions

Most drugs have side effects as well as pharmacological effects, and skin disorders are a frequent form of drug side effect. These can mimic many of the spontaneously occurring skin disorders as well as producing quite specific changes. Drug-induced skin disorder can develop after the initial dose or after a short period of time during which sensitization has taken place. Other problems, such as pigmentations or hair anomalies, may take some months to appear. Often, a rash occurs after taking the drug for some time, without apparent reason.

It is important that drug reactions are suspected when the nature and cause of a skin disorder are in doubt, as 'drugs' in one shape or form are taken by a substantial proportion of the population. Drug eruptions do not only stem from orthodox prescribed drugs, but are also caused by cough medicines, analgesics, laxatives or other 'over-the-counter' symptomatic remedies, and enquiry must also be made about these possibilities.

The diagnosis of a drug eruption is difficult to confirm, as there are few laboratory tests available. Currently, the only useful specific laboratory tests are those dependent on there being specific IgE directed to the particular drug – penicillin is the only drug of importance that can be detected in this way (radio allergo-absorbent test, RAST).

Skin biopsy may assist in eliminating other causes of an eruption. The most useful diagnostic test is the 'challenge', in which the suspected agent is administered to determine whether the condition recurs or is aggravated. Clearly, this is not possible in the case of potentially severe or life-threatening conditions. Even when this is not the case, it should only be performed with the patient's consent and if important information may be obtained that is relevant to the care of the patient. The smallest possible dose should be given and the patient should be carefully observed subsequently.

TYPES OF DRUG ERUPTION

Severe life-threatening eruptions

Angioedema and anaphylactic shock
These are sudden in onset and IgE-mediated reactions of the immediate hypersensitivity type. They are provoked by serum-containing products and by penicillin and its derivatives when given parenterally. The patient becomes pale and collapses with severe hypotension and maybe bronchospasm. Treatment is required urgently with oxygen, intravenous hydrocortisone and adrenalin.

Erythema multiforme (Stevens–Johnson syndrome)
For a clinical description, see page 75. Sulphonamides, hydantoinates, carbamazepine, some non-steroidal anti-inflammatory agents and maybe penicillin can cause this disorder.

Toxic epidermal necrolysis
This drug reaction, which has a mortality approaching 50 per cent, occurs predominantly in middle-aged and elderly women. The drugs incriminated include sulphonamides, indomethacin, the hydantoinates and gold salts. There is erythroderma with extensive desquamation and, in places, blistering and erosion. The mucosae are also severely affected.

The patients rapidly become dehydrated and are very sick. They need to be nursed as though they had extensive burns and to have intensive support treatment with parenteral fluids, antibiotics and systemic steroids.

Exanthematic eruptions

This is probably the commonest group of drug eruptions. Red/pink macules develop over the trunk and limbs. When intense, the rash is said to be *morbilli-form* or measles-like. Ampicillin, the psychotropic drugs and the non-steroidal anti-inflammatory agents cause this type of rash.

A *lichenoid rash* (with some resemblance to lichen planus, see page 144) may be caused by gold salts, mepacrine and carbamazepine.

Vascular eruption or purpuric lesions develop over the legs and, less frequently, the arms and trunk. The thiazide diuretics and the hydantoinates are especially linked with this type of rash.

Urticarial rashes may be produced by penicillin, aspirin, tartrazine (and other dyes) and opioid drugs.

PHOTOSENSITIVITY RASHES

In this group of drug-induced conditions, the rash is confined to the light-exposed areas and is wavelength dependent, i.e. it only reacts to particular wave-lengths in the solar ultraviolet spectrum. The rash itself is red and papular or plaque-like (Fig. 6.30). Some drugs seem able to provoke a phototoxic eruption, which is seen in many patients to whom the drug is given and is dose dependent, and others cause a photoallergic rash in which a photoallergen has formed and which only affects a few individuals. Tetracyclines and sulphonamides may cause a phototoxic response. The phenothiazines may cause either a phototoxic or a photoallergic reaction.

Blistering rashes

Naproxen and frusemide may cause a 'pseudoporphyria-like' rash in the light-exposed sites. Nalidixic acid may also cause blistering. Captopril and penicil-lamine may cause a pemphigus or a pemphigoid-like eruption.

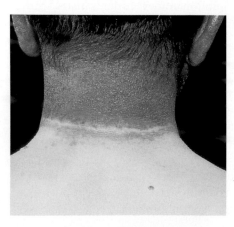

Figure 6.30 Photosensitivity rash due to the administration of a tetracycline drug.

Fixed drug eruptions

This not uncommon drug reaction causes inflammatory patches to appear within hours at the same sites on every occasion the drug is administered. The areas become inflamed, and may even blister before subsiding when the drug is stopped, leaving pigmentation (Fig. 6.31). Numerous drugs, including dapsone, the sulphonamides, tetracycline and mefenamic acid may be responsible.

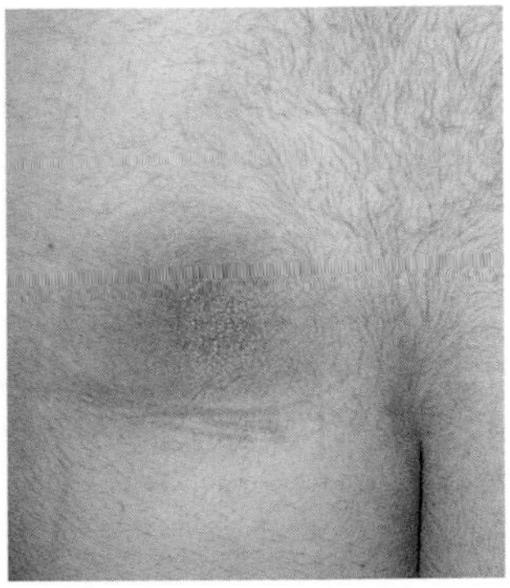

Lupus erythematosus-like rashes

These may be caused by penicillamine, hydralazine, hydantoinates and procainamide, amongst others. The drugs may precipitate or initiate lupus erythematosus.

As pointed out elsewhere, drugs can have many other effects on the skin, including changes in pigmentation and hair distribution.

Figure 6.31 Round, dusky erythematous patch on the buttock due to 'fixed drug eruption' caused by mefenamic acid.

TREATMENT

Treatment of all drug eruptions consists of identifying the causative drug and then stopping it. Care must be taken to see that the offending agent or one with cross-reacting chemical groups is not given again.

Summary

- Urticaria and angioedema result from histamine release from mast cells and are characterized by transient, itchy weals or deeper swellings. Dermographic weals are elicited by firm stroking with a blunt object.
- The cause of chronic urticaria remains undiscovered in most patients, but in a few food hypersensitivities, drug sensitivity and physical stimuli are found to be responsible. In a substantial minority, an antibody to mast cells has been found, so that the disorder can be thought of as 'autoimmune'. In cholinergic urticaria, small, itchy weals occur after exercise or hot baths.
- Antihistamines of the H1 type are the most effective in suppressing urticaria.
- Erythema multiforme is caused by infections such as herpes simplex and orf, as well as by drugs and systemic diseases. It is an acute exanthematic disorder, characterized by maculopapular lesions, some of which are annular and may blister. The mucosae are often affected.

- Erythema nodosum is characterized by the sudden appearance of large, tender, red nodules on the shins, mostly with arthralgia and systemic upset. It is a reaction to tuberculosis, sarcoidosis and, less commonly, other infections and drugs.
- Systemic lupus erythematosus is characterized by facial (butterfly) erythema, arthritis, glomerulonephritis, other visceral inflammatory disorders and circulating antinuclear factor antibodies. Histologically, degeneration of the basal layer of the epidermis and perivascular lymphocytic cuffing are typical.
- Chronic discoid lupus erythematosus occurs in the course of systemic lupus erythematosus or without other signs and is characterized by irregular red plaques in which atrophic scarring and irregular pigmentation are seen. Sun protection, hydroxychloroquine and potent steroids are used in treatment.
- In systemic sclerosis, Raynaud's phenomenon, renal glomerular disease, arthritis, gut disorder and skin stiffening of the face and hands result from the

production of excess new collagen. Raynaud's phenomenon and dysphagia are common problems.

- In morphoea, single or several mauve, indurated plaques are the sole manifestation of scleroderma. In lichen sclerosis et atrophicus, small, white patches occur over the genitalia and, less frequently, elsewhere.
- Proximal muscle tenderness and weakness accompany mauve red patches on the backs of the hands and periocularly in dermatomyositis.
- Allergic vasculitis causes fever, arthralgia and an urticarial purpuric rash. Abdominal pain, melaena and glomerulonephritis are also found. Endothelial damage and neutrophilic nuclear dust are seen histologically.
- Polyarteriitis nodosa, nodular vasculitis and vasculitis accompanying meningococcaemia and gonococcaemia are other types of vasculitis.
- Persistent, pigmented purpuric eruptions are caused by a capillaritis.

- Subepidermal blisters in senile pemphigoid are caused by circulating anti-basement membrane antibodies. Treatment is with high doses of corticosteroids and immunosuppressive agents. Cicatrical pemphigoid and bullous disease of childhood are variants.
- Dermatitis herpetiformis is an itchy vesicular disease, in which subepidermal blisters and papillary tip abscesses occur accompanied by a gluten enteropathy. Dapsone controls the skin lesions.
- Epidermolysis bullosa is a group of inherited, subepidermal blistering disorders, which can cripple and deform in the worst cases.
- Intraepidermal blistering caused by circulating antibodies to the epidermal desmosomal junctions characterizes the pemphigus group of diseases.
- Drugs can cause urticarial, erythema multiforme-like, exanthematic rashes. Photosensitivity, lupus erythematosus-like and fixed drug eruptions are other cutaneous adverse drug reactions.

Skin disorders in AIDS, immunodeficiency and venereal disease

Acquired immune deficiency syndrome (AIDS) is caused by a lymphotropic retrovirus, now known as the human immunodeficiency virus (HIV). The virus is acquired either by sexual intercourse (homosexual or heterosexual) or from the accidental introduction of material contaminated by the HIV into the systemic circulation. It was most common in homosexuals, drug addicts and the recipients of contaminated blood in the form of transfusions or concentrates, but is now spreading via heterosexual contact. The virus incapacitates the T-helper lymphocytes and thus prevents proper functioning of the cell-mediated immune response. It uses the T4 antigen as its receptor and employs the T-cell's genomic apparatus to replicate, destroying the cell as it does so. It can also infect reticuloendothelial cells (including Langerhans cells) and B-cell lymphocytes.

After gaining access, the virus usually stays latent for long periods, but may cause a systemic illness a relatively short time after infection and before or at the time of seroconversion. This illness is characterized by pyrexia, malaise and a rash, which have been described as resembling infectious mononucleosis.

For the most part, there are no symptoms for several years, even after an antibody response develops, until the virus is 'activated' by an intercurrent infection such as herpes simplex. AIDS is characterized by depressed delayed hypersensitivity, and depressing of the number of circulating T-helper cells is a constant finding. Skin disorders are prominent in AIDS and patients often present with a skin complaint.

Infections

When the disease is activated, the patient becomes subject to opportunist infections as well as to an increased incidence and severity of usually mild and commonplace infections.

FUNGUS INFECTIONS

Dermatophyte infections, including nail infection, are extensive and difficult to clear. Candidiasis is often a major problem, especially in the mouth and oropharynx. Systemic spread of *Candida* infection is unfortunately not uncommon and often a terminal event. *Pityrosporum ovale* causes extensive eruptions of pityriasis versicolor. It may also be responsible for a troublesome and persistent truncal folliculitis in some patients (Fig. 7.1) and for the common problem of severe seborrhoeic dermatitis seen in others. Various 'deep fungus' infections are common, particularly in hot and humid parts of the world.

VIRAL INFECTIONS

Viral warts may become very extensive and troublesome. Mollusca contagiosa lesions may be both larger than usual and present in very large numbers (Fig. 7.2).

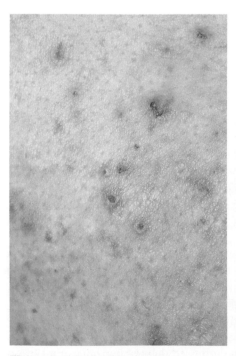

Figure 7.1 Folliculitis due to *Pityrosporum ovale* infection in a patient with HIV infection.

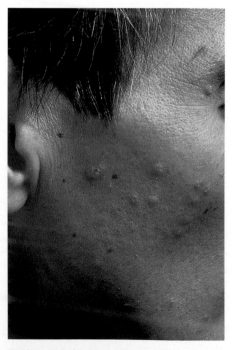

Figure 7.2 Mollusca contagiosa – multiple lesions in a patient with advanced AIDS.

Herpes simplex infection may be a particular problem, with extensive and persistent skin involvement resulting in scarring. Herpes zoster is similarly a troublesome infection in AIDS and may be the initial manifestation. It may look unlike 'ordinary' herpes zoster and may cause considerable pain and tissue destruction as well as spreading outside the dermatomes in which it began.

BACTERIAL INFECTIONS

Tuberculosis and syphilis are both major problems for individuals with AIDS. Both disorders progress rapidly and are responsible for extensive and severe disease in AIDS patients. Infections with mycobacterial species that do not generally infect humans may also be seen. Epithelioid angiomatosis is due to infection with a bacterial micro-organism similar to the bacillus causing 'cat scratch' disease. It causes Kaposi's sarcoma-like lesions (see below) and a widespread eruption of red papules.

Skin cancers

Depressed delayed hypersensitivity also results in failure of 'immune surveillance' and the development and rapid progression of many forms of skin cancer. Viral infection may also be at work in the development of the disorder known as Kaposi's sarcoma, which mainly accompanies AIDS contracted from homosexual contact. Mauve, red, purple or brown macules, nodules or plaques may ulcerate and may spread to involve the viscera. Kaposi's sarcoma is a frequent cause of death in patients with AIDS.

Case 6

Simon's dandruff gradually worsened and he developed seborrhoeic dermatitis of the skin around his ears and nose. At the age of 23, he was surprised that he was also developing numerous viral warts and mollusca contagiosa. His partner, Peter, thought that they should both have tests for HIV disease and both men were found to be positive.

Other skin manifestations

PRURITUS

The papular folliculitis rash mentioned above due to *Pityrosporum ovale* is often distressingly pruritic. The skin of patients with AIDS may become dry and ichthyotic looking, so that AIDS may be counted as one of the causes of 'acquired ichthyosis', and this is also a cause of persistent irritation.

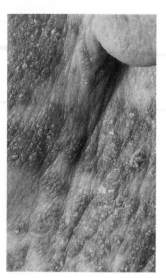

Figure 7.3 Extensive florid seborrhoeic dermatitis in a patient with HIV infection.

SCABIES

Scabies seems to spread very quickly and to cause extensive and severe involvement in patients with AIDS. It also causes severe itching.

SEBORRHOEIC DERMATITIS

Another cause of itching in AIDS is seborrhoeic dermatitis. This is common and extensive in patients with AIDS, presumably due to massive overgrowth of *Pityrosporum ovale* and whatever other micro-organisms are involved (Fig. 7.3).

Psoriasis

Pre-existing psoriasis may develop an 'explosive phase', or psoriasis may develop *de novo* as an aggressive, rapidly spreading eruption. It is not clear why psoriasis is aggravated in this manner in HIV infection.

Treatment of skin manifestations of AIDS

Treatment with zidovudine (azidothymidine, AZT) – 500–1500 mg per day in four to five divided doses – is indicated to slow the progress of the HIV infection. It causes nausea, malaise, headache, rash and many other side effects. Zidovudine is a reverse transcriptase inhibitor. Other drugs that are sometimes used include lamivudine, nevirapine, stavudine, delavudine and efavirenz.

Ganciclovir and foscarnet are indicated for cytomegalovirus complications. Aciclovir is used for herpes simplex and herpes zoster. Various antibiotics and other antimicrobials are used as indicated for the bacterial infections. Fluconazole, itraconazole and ketoconazole are particularly useful for the serious and life-threatening *Candida* infections. Recombinant interferon-alpha 2B and other interferons have been used with some success in Kaposi's sarcoma. The new retinoid tagretin is used topically to induce regression in individual lesions.

Drug-induced immunodeficiency

Patients who have organ transplants of kidneys, heart or liver are maintained on corticosteroids and azathioprine, cyclosporin or tacrolimus for the rest of their lives. Patients with autoimmune disorders such as systemic lupus erythematosus, rheumatoid arthritis or chronic renal disease, and those with psoriasis and some eczematous diseases, are also treated with immunosuppressive drugs for varying lengths of time. The cutaneous side effects from the immunosuppression are not usually as prominent as in AIDS patients, but depend on the extent and length of the immunosuppression.

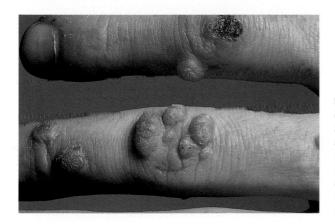

Figure 7.1 Warty lesions on the hands in a patient after 8 years on azathioprine and prednisolone following renal allograft, which are either viral warts or solar keratoses, or somewhere in between.

Patients with renal allografts have most problems, maybe because they are treated continuously for longer periods than most of the other groups. They are prone to the development of numerous warty lesions on the hands and face – after about 8 years of immunosuppression some 25 per cent were found to have warty lesions in one British study (Fig. 7.4). These are either viral warts or solar keratoses, or lesions which are somewhere in between! It may be that many of the viral warts directly transform into pre-neoplastic lesions.

It should be noted that photochemotherapy with ultraviolet radiation of the 'A' type (PUVA) treatment (see page 141) also causes depression in delayed hypersensitivity and this is probably relevant to the development of skin cancer in patients with psoriasis treated with PUVA some years previously.

Other causes of acquired immunodeficiency

Lymphoreticular diseases such as Hodgkin's disease, the leukaemias and sarcoidosis also result in depressed delayed hypersensitivity. Hypovitaminosis A, chronic malnutrition and chronic alcoholism also result in depressed immune defences.

Congenital immunodeficiencies

Infantile agammaglobulinaemia is inherited as an X-linked recessive disorder. There are no plasma cells in the marrow and the patients are susceptible to severe pyoderma and numerous warts. In severe combined immunodeficiency, there is depression of circulating lymphocytes and levels of all immunoglobulins. Patients are susceptible to all infections and usually die between the ages of 1 and 2 years. It is inherited as either a sex-linked recessive or an autosomal recessive characteristic. Ataxia telangiectasia (autosomal recessive) is characterized by cerebellar degeneration, telangiectasia on exposed skin developing progressively, lymphopenia and depressed levels of IgA.

Dermatological aspects of venereal disease

Several skin infections, although not exclusively 'venereal', are nonetheless spread by venereal contact. Such disorders include genital warts, molluscum contagiosum, scabies and pubic lice.

REITER'S SYNDROME

This disorder occurs as a sequel to non-specific urethritis in men and, less commonly, to bowel infection, and probably results from infection with a *Mycoplasma* organism. There is usually an accompanying arthritis and spondylitis and occasionally a conjunctivitis. Psoriasiform skin lesions develop on the soles and toes. These are often severe, persistent, aggressive and pustular (keratoderma blenorrhagica). Inflamed, red, scaling patches may also develop on the glans penis (circinate balanitis). There is a curious preponderance of patients with the HLA B27 haplotype.

GONORRHOEA

This venereal disease, which predominantly affects urethral epithelium, is caused by the delicate intracellular Gram-positive diplococcus – the gonococcus. The skin is only affected during gonococcaemia, when small purpuric and pustular vasculitic lesions suddenly appear in the course of a pyrexal illness (Fig. 7.5).

CHANCROID (SOFT SORE)

This venereal infection is caused by the Gram-negative bacillus *Haemophilus ducreyi*. One to 5 days post-infection, a soft sloughy ulcer appears on the penis or vulva. Other sites may be affected, and inguinal adenitis occurs in 50 per cent of patients.

Differential diagnosis includes syphilitic chancre, herpetic ulceration, granuloma inguinale and the results of trauma. The treatment of choice is erythromycin (500 mg 6-hourly for 14 days).

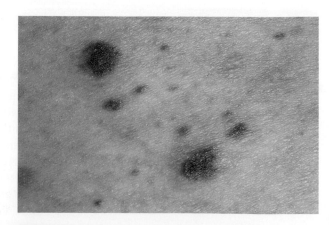

Figure 7.5 Vasculitis.

SYPHILIS

Syphilis has once again become of major importance with the emergence of AIDS. This is both because the syphilitic chancre serves as a portal of entry for the HIV virus and because the manifestations of syphilis are much more dramatic in AIDS patients.

The disease is caused by the delicate spirochaetal micro-organism *Treponema pallidum*, which is transmitted by contact between mucosal surfaces.

Clinical features

Characteristically, the incubation period is 9–90 days and the first sign is the appearance of the chancre at the site of inoculation, usually on the glans penis, prepuce or, less often, on the shaft in men and on the vulva in women. In homosexuals the chancre appears around or in the anus. The chancre is of variable size (0.5–3 cm in diameter) and has a sloughy and markedly indurated base. Untreated, it heals after 3–8 weeks.

This primary stage of the disease is followed by a brief quiescent phase of from 2 months to up to 3 years before the secondary stage occurs. In secondary syphilis there are signs of systemic upset with mild fever, headache, mild arthralgia, generalized lymphadenopathy and skin manifestations, including an early widespread macular rash, involving the palms (Fig. 7.6), and a later papular or lichenoid eruption. Thickened, warty areas (condylomalata) appear perianally and in other moist flexural sites (Fig. 7.7). Ulcers appear on the oral mucosa (snail-trail ulcers).

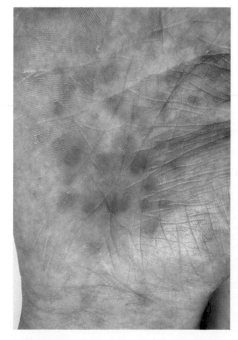

Figure 7.6 Palmar rash in secondary syphilis.

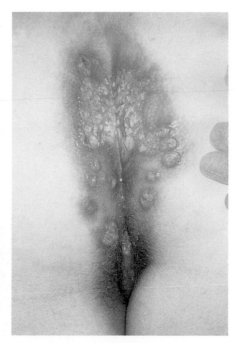

Figure 7.7 Perianal condylomata in secondary syphilis.

After resolution of the secondary stage, there is a latent period without signs or symptoms, lasting for 5–50 years. The tertiary stage takes protean forms and includes cardiovascular disease with aneurysm formation, central nervous disorder, either as tabes dorsalis or general paralysis of the insane, and ulcerative or gummatous lesions that may occur on the skin or on mucosal surfaces.

Diagnosis

Diagnosis is made by identification of the spirochaete from wet preparations of the chancre or moist secondary-stage lesions and by serological tests detecting either lipoidal substance liberated by tissues or the presence of antibodies to the micro-organism.

The older Wassermann reaction (WR) has been replaced by the Venereal Disease Reference Laboratory (VDRL) test, which is a flocculation test, which, although not specific, is quite sensitive and becomes positive early in the disease. It also responds to effective treatment by becoming negative some 6 months after therapy. The WR and the VDRL tests (and other similar tests) depend on lipoidal antigens. The *Treponema pallidum* haemagglutination assay is currently the most-used specific test depending on antibodies to the micro-organism.

TREATMENT

The treatment of syphilis is by parenteral penicillin over a 10-day period. One intramuscular injection of procaine penicillin 600 000 IU daily for 10 consecutive days is adequate. A proportion of patients develop a fever and possibly a rash after starting treatment (Jarisch–Herxheimer reaction). More serious reactions can also occur.

Summary
- AIDS is caused by a retrovirus – the Human Immunodeficiency Virus (HIV), which is transmitted by sexual contact. It is characterized by depressed delayed hypersensitivity and susceptibility to many skin infections, including candidiasis, pityriasis versicolor, molluscum contagiosum, warts, herpes simplex, herpes zoster as well as tuberculosis and syphilis. Seborrhoeic dermatitis, pruritic folliculitis and Kaposi's sarcoma are other skin disorders occurring in AIDS. Steroids and immunosuppressive drugs result in immunosuppression, and depressed delayed hypersensitivity is also seen in Hodgkin's disease, vitamin A deficiency and after UVR exposure. In some cases, immunodeficiency is inherited.
- Reiter's syndrome follows non-specific urethritis. Thick psoriasiform lesions occur on the feet and genitalia.
- Purpuric pustules are a vasculitic complication of gonorrhoea and gonococcaemia.
- Chancroid (soft sore) caused by *Haemophilus ducreyi* is characterized by soft erosions occurring on the genitalia.
- Syphilis caused by *Treponema pallidum* is spread by sexual contact. Nine to 90 days post-infection, an erosion, the primary chancre, occurs at the site of inoculation. A secondary stage with rashes and mild systemic upset develops some weeks or months later. After a latent period, a tertiary stage develops in which a destructive inflammation affects one or another organs. Treatment is with penicillin.

Eczema (dermatitis)

The term eczema includes several disorders (see Table 8.1) in which inflammation is focused on the epidermis. Typically, epidermal cells accumulate oedema fluid between them (spongiosis: Fig. 8.1), leading to vesicles in the most severe and acute cases. Inflammatory cells and vasodilatation accompany the oedema that is also present in the dermis of the affected area.

Some types of eczema stem from uncharacterized constitutional factors ('endogenous' or constitutional eczema), whereas others are the result of an external injury of some sort. The clinical picture varies according to the provocation, the acuity of the process and the site of the involvement.

Atopic dermatitis

DEFINITION

This is a very common, extremely itchy disorder of unknown cause that characteristically, but not invariably, affects the face and flexures of infants, children, adolescents and young adults.

Table 8.1 Common types of eczema

Type	Synonyms	Frequency/age group	Remarks
Atopic dermatitis	Neurodermatitis Besnier's prurigo Infantile eczema	Very common, mostly occurs in infants and the very young	Cause unknown, but appears to be immunologically mediated
Seborrhoeic dermatitis	Infectious eczematoid dermatitis	Very common in all age groups	Probably has a microbial cause, with overgrowth of normal skin flora being responsible
Discoid eczema	Nummular eczema	Uncommon, mainly in middle-aged individuals	Cause unknown
Lichen simplex chronicus	Circumscribed neurodermatitis	Quite common, mainly in young and middle-aged adults	Initial cause appears to be a localized itch causing an 'itch–scratch cycle'
Eczema craquelée	Asteatotic eczema	Uncommon, restricted to the elderly	Low humidity and vigorous washing seem responsible
Venous eczema	Stasis dermatitis Gravitational eczema	Common in the age group that has gravitational syndrome	Multiple causes, a common variety is allergic contact dermatitis to medicaments used
Allergic contact dermatitis		Common in all adult age groups except the very old	Delayed hypersensitivity response to a specific agent
Primary irritant contact dermatitis	Occupational dermatitis Housewives' eczema	Very common in all adult age groups except the very elderly	Both mechanical and chemical trauma responsible
Photosensitivity eczema		Not uncommon, mainly in adults	Both phototoxic and photoallergic types occur

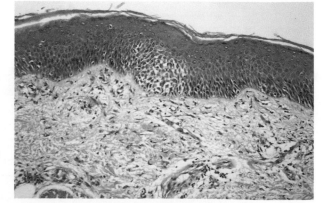

Figure 8.1 Photomicrograph to show an area of oedema of the epidermis (spongiosis) in acute eczema (H & E, ×90).

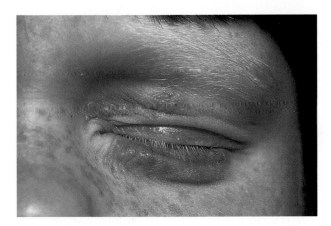

Figure 8.2 Inflamed, thickened eyelids and some loss of eyebrows and eyelashes due to perpetual eye rubbing in atopic dermatitis.

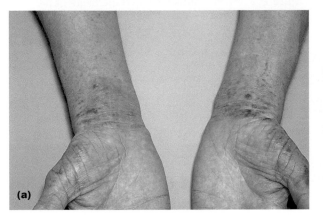

(a)

(b)

Figure 8.3 (a) Excoriations of the wrists in atopic dermatitis. (b) Excoriated, thickened eczematous area over the sacrum.

CLINICAL FEATURES

Signs and symptoms

The major issue as far as this disease is concerned is itching. The patient is constantly itchy and restless, but subject to irregular episodes of intense and quite disabling intensification of the pruritus. The itchiness is made worse by changes in temperature, by rough clothing (such as woollens) and by sundry other minor environmental alterations. This symptom greatly disturbs sleep and the whole family becomes affected. Scratching results from the severe pruritus in all except infants under the age of 2 months. Patients also rub the affected itching parts – they frequently rub their eyes with the index finger knuckles (Fig. 8.2). The incessant scratching and rubbing result in simple, linear scratch marks (excoriations: Fig. 8.3) and chronic thickening of the skin characterized by accentuation of the skin markings known as lichenification (Fig. 8.4). This is due to massive epidermal hypertrophy as well as oedema and inflammatory cell infiltrate in the upper dermis (Fig. 8.5).

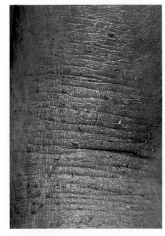

Figure 8.4 Exaggeration of skin surface marking (lichenification) due to perpetual rubbing and scratching.

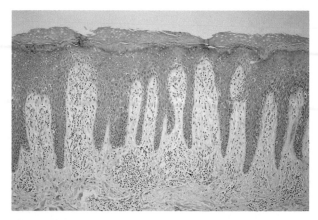

Figure 8.5 Photomicrograph showing marked epidermal thickening and inflammation in lichenification (H & E, ×45).

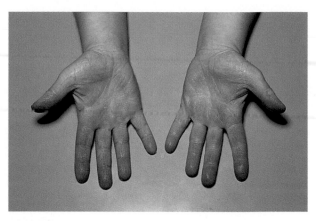

Figure 8.6 Prominent skin surface markings of the palms (hyperlinear palms) in atopic dermatitis.

Figure 8.7 Eczema of the face in an infant.

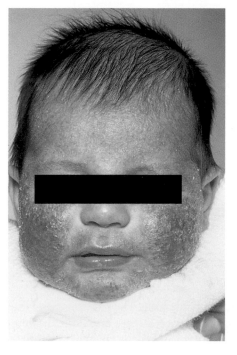

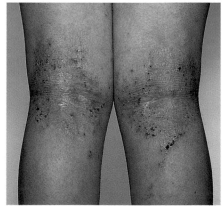

Figure 8.8 Excoriated lichenified. popliteal fossae in atopic dermatitis.

In many patients, there is a widespread fine scaling of the skin, described as 'dryness' or xeroderma, sometimes described incorrectly as ichthyosis, but really the result of the eczematous process itself. Another feature sometimes incorrectly ascribed to ichthyosis is the presence of increased prominence of the skin markings on the palms (Fig. 8.6) – the so-called hyperlinear palms. In severely affected patients, there is a background pinkness of the skin and fissuring at some sites because of the inelasticity of the abnormal stratum corneum.

Virtually any body site can be affected. The face is often involved (Fig. 8.7) as are the backs of the knees (Fig. 8.8), the antecubital fossae and the wrists.

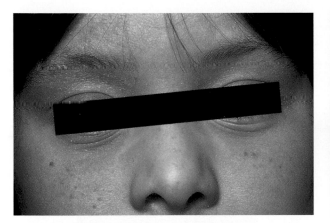

Figure 8.9 Prominent crease beneath the eyes in a child with atopic dermatitis – Denny Morgan fold.

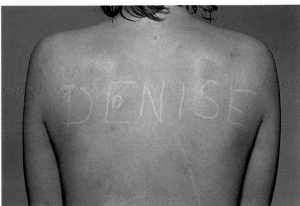

Figure 8.10 White dermographism.

The cheeks are often pale and this feature, taken together with crease lines just below the eyes (known as Denny Morgan folds) due to continual rubbing, makes the facial appearance quite characteristic (Fig. 8.9). Running a blunt instrument (such as a key) over affected skin produces a white line in about 70 per cent of patients (Fig. 8.10) – known as 'white dermatographism'. This is the reverse of the normal triple response and disappears when the condition improves. This unexplained paradoxical blanching is similar to that seen after intracutaneous injection of methacholine or carbamyl choline in atopic dermatitis patients.

CLINICAL VARIANTS

- In patients with black skin, there are often numerous follicular papules in affected areas (Fig. 8.11). In lichenified areas in black-skinned patients, there may be irregular pigmentation, with hyperpigmentation at some sites and loss of pigment at others.
- Some individuals lose their childhood eczema only to develop chronic palmar eczema in later years. This is believed also to be a manifestation of atopic disease.

ASSOCIATED DISORDERS

Patients with atopic dermatitis quite often also suffer from asthma. Some 30 per cent will also have had asthma before their skin disorder has healed. There is no particular synchronization, and worsening or remission of one has no particular implication for the other. Hay fever is also more common in atopic dermatitis patients, but the activity and severity have no link to the skin disorder.

Atopic dermatitis, asthma and hay fever seem to share pathogenetic mechanisms in which aberrant immune processes play an important part. These three 'atopic'

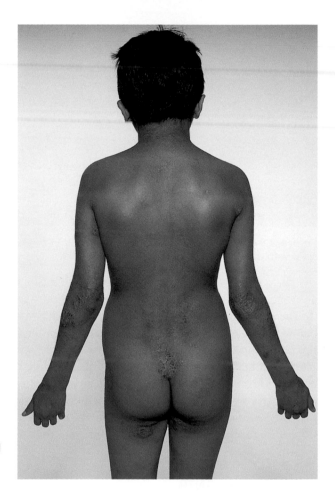

Figure 8.11 Widespread atopic dermatitis in a young Asian subject.

disorders cluster in families and the tendency to one or the other or all is inherited in an as yet uncharacterized way. Chronic urticaria (see page 71) and alopecia areata (see page 271) occur more often in atopic dermatitis patients. The skin of patients with atopic dermatitis is more vulnerable to both chemical and mechanical trauma and has an unfortunate tendency to develop irritant dermatitis.

COMPLICATIONS

Patients with atopic dermatitis are frequently troubled by skin infections. Pustules and impetiginized areas represent pyococcal infection and are the most common expression of this propensity. They are easily treated, but tend to recur. Cellulitis may also develop, giving rise to fever and systemic upset. Viral warts and mollusca contagiosa are also more frequent and more extensive than in non-eczematous subjects.

Herpes simplex sometimes causes a severe and extensive rash in atopic dermatitis patients, who may develop fever and severe systemic upset, but recover after 10–14 days.

EPIDEMIOLOGY AND NATURAL HISTORY

Atopic dermatitis occurs in families, but the mode of inheritance has been difficult to work out. It certainly does not appear to be the result of a single gene defect. Approximately 30 per cent of patients with atopic dermatitis have one affected parent and there is 90 per cent concordance in monozygotic twins.

The disorder is very common and is becoming more common. In some surveys, approximately 15 per cent of infants have been found to suffer from atopic dermatitis. The overall prevalence in the community depends, amongst other things, on the particular age structure, but in the UK it is approximately 2 per cent. Because the disorder is resistant to treatment, often disabling and long lasting, it is very common in dermatology clinics, affecting 10–15 per cent of the 'clinic population'. The disorder mostly presents at 3–5 months of age (approximately 60 per cent), with 15–20 per cent developing it before then and some 20–30 per cent subsequently. Few develop the disease in late childhood or early adult life. It affects both sexes equally and all racial and social groups. Fortunately, it tends to improve and at every decade there are fewer patients with the disease. It is said that some 75 per cent of those troubled in early childhood are free of atopic dermatitis by the age of 15 years.

LABORATORY FINDINGS AND AETIOPATHOGENESIS

- Skin biopsy reveals spongiosis, marked epidermal thickening parakeratosis and an inflammatory cell infiltrate, oedema and vasodilatation in the dermis.
- There is an elevation of serum IgE antibodies, which is correlated with the severity of the disease. These are 'reaginic', precipitating antibodies to various environmental allergens, including foods and inhaled materials, which become fixed to mast cells. When an allergen contacts its antibody fixed on mast cells, mediators, including histamine, are released, causing an urticarial response. This occurs in the positive reactions seen in scratch and prick tests. Atopic patients often have multiple 'positives' to food, house dust mite allergen and pollens, but this seems to have little relevance to the cause, prevention or treatment of their eczema.
- The susceptibility to skin infection, the association with other disorders that have an immunopathogenetic component and the elevated IgE level all suggest an abnormality of the immune system. Part of the problem may be an imbalance in the relative proportions of two subpopulations of T-helper lymphocytes – TH1 and TH2. The TH1 subset typically secretes gamma interferon and is important in turning off the secretion of immunoglobulins by B-lymphocytes. TH2 cells predominantly secrete interleukin-4 (IL4) and are thought to be dominant in atopic dermatitis.

- The importance of an enzyme (desaturase) deficiency in the blood in atopic dermatitis is uncertain. It results in a comparative deficiency of unsaturated fatty acids – particularly dihomogammalinolenic acid.

MANAGEMENT

Several points need to be kept firmly in mind.

- The disease is persistent and subject to recurrent flares, making it important to develop a good relationship with patients and their immediate relatives.
- The disorder causes much discomfort and disability because of the intense and persistent itching. The sleep disturbance that results makes the whole family unhappy.
- The affected skin needs protection from further injury. The use of bland, greasy emollients gives some symptomatic relief and provides this protection.
- Infection often seems to play some role in the precipitation or aggravation of the disease and antimicrobial treatments, both local and systemic, may rapidly terminate an exacerbation.

Topical corticosteroids

Topical corticosteroids are the most useful topical agents for the treatment of atopic dermatitis (see page 307). However, these drugs are only suppressive and need to be given over long periods. Toxic side effects, such as skin atrophy, pituitary–adrenal axis suppression and masked infection, are ever-present possibilities. Sudden withdrawal of treatment can lead to a sudden and severe 'rebound' aggravation of the eczema and it is prudent to use the least potent corticosteroid preparation that is effective. Topical corticosteroids may become less effective with continued use, but changing to another preparation of similar potency will regain control. This phenomenon of acquired tolerance is known as tachyphylaxis and is as yet unexplained.

There are many corticosteroids and less potent agents, such as hydrocortisone, clobetasone 17-butyrate, flurandrenolone and desoxymethasone, that are particularly suitable for infants with active eczema.

Creams, lotions and gels are less helpful vehicles for the corticosteroids and are less useful than greasy ointments. Application once or twice daily is quite adequate.

Recently, a topical immunosuppressive agent – tacrolimus (Protopic) – has become available. This agent is quite effective and does not have the skin-thinning or pituitary–adrenal axis suppressive activity of corticosteroids.

Emollients

Emollients have hydrating effects on the skin in eczema because of their occlusive properties. They reduce scaling and improve skin texture and appearance. They improve the extensibility of skin and reduce fissuring as well as decreasing the pruritus and inflammation via unknown mechanisms.

All emollients seem to have much the same degree of effect – providing they are sufficiently greasy and occlude the skin surface. The most important issues are how frequently they are applied and whether the patient actually uses them! They should be applied at least three times daily for the best effect and more frequently if possible – their effects only last 2 hours or so. A bath oil or an emollient skin cleanser (e.g. emulsifying ointment BP) may also help.

Tar preparations

Coal tars are used for eczema and psoriasis. The generic preparations (e.g. tar ointment or tar and salicylic acid ointment BP) are not popular because of the smell and messiness associated with their use, but modern proprietary preparations are more acceptable (e.g. Clinitar® cream). Their anti-inflammatory action is little understood and they are best employed for chronic lichenified areas of eczema. They can irritate the skin and have caused concern because of a potential for carcinogenicity.

Systemic agents

Some patients with severe disease do not respond to topical measures. For this group there are several options. These include photochemotherapy with one or another of ultraviolet radiation (see page 141), systemic steroids and cyclosporin.

Some patients improve after sun exposure, and phototherapy of some type may be of assistance for them. This may help 50–75 per cent of severely affected patients, but has to be balanced against the long-term hazards of skin cancer (see page 207 et seq.). Systemic steroids suppress the eczema, but the cost in severe long-term toxicity, including osteoporosis, skin fragility, susceptibility to infection and pituitary–adrenal axis suppression, probably outweighs the short-term benefits.

Cyclosporin is a fungal metabolite peptide with immunosuppressive effects that is found to be helpful for some patients with severe psoriasis (see page 140). It has been found to have a dramatic effect in patients with severe, generalized atopic dermatitis at a dose of 3–5 mg/kg body weight per day. As with most effective drugs, there are toxic side effects, which, in the case of cyclosporin, include nephrotoxicity and hypertension. None of these systemic drugs or photochemotherapy with UVA (PUVA) should be given without consultation with a specialist with experience in the benefits and side effects of the various treatments.

Unfortunately, cyclosporin does not work when employed topically.

Antimicrobial agents

Patients with atopic dermatitis are particularly prone to skin infection. Infection with staphylococci and possibly other bacteria cause pustules, impetiginized lesions and cellulitis and may also be responsible for flare-ups of the dermatitis. This is the reason why appropriate antibacterial measures by themselves seem to be beneficial. Bacterial swabs should be taken before starting treatment with either topical or systemic antibacterial agents. Antimicrobial bath additives such as a povidone iodine or a hexachlorophane preparation may assist. The infected area can be soaked or bathed in 1 in 8000 potassium permanganate solution or aluminium subacetate solution. Topical neomycin or mupirocin may be used, but other antibiotics should be avoided because of the problem of resistance. If there is evidence of significant infection in several sites that may be aggravating the atopic state, systemic antibiotics should be given, taking into account local and current policy with regard to penicillin resistance.

Seborrhoeic dermatitis

DEFINITION

This is a common eczematous disorder that characteristically occurs in hairy areas, on the flexures and on the central parts of the trunk, and is now believed to be at least in part due to overgrowth of the normal skin flora in the regions affected.

CLINICAL FEATURES

Signs and symptoms

Reddened, itchy patches appear at the affected sites, which may become either scaly or exudative and crusted. Scaling is a common feature when the condition develops insidiously. Often, mild scaling occurs without erythema, as it does, for example, on the scalp as 'dandruff'. When severe, the eyebrows may also be affected. Other facial areas may become involved such as the nasolabial folds, the paranasal sites, the external ears and the retroauricular folds (Figs 8.12 and 8.13).

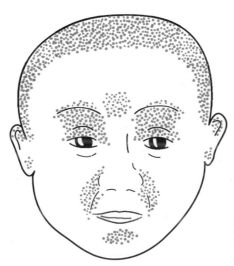

Figure 8.12 Diagram to show frequently affected sites in seborrhoeic dermatitis.

Figure 8.13 Scaling area in the ear due to seborrhoeic dermatitis.

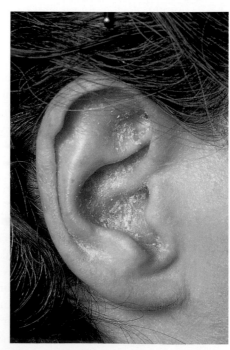

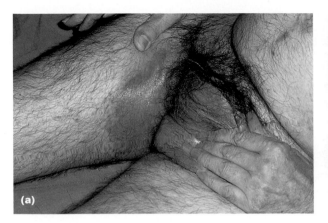

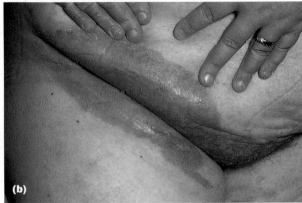

Figure 8.14 (a) Exudative lesions of seborrhoeic dermatitis in the groin area. (b) Seborrhoeic dermatitis of intertriginous areas in the groin of an obese woman.

Scaling and erythema of the eyelid margins (marginal blepharitis) may also occur. Another type of lesions seen in seborrhoeic dermatitis is a form of folliculitis. This seborrhoeic folliculitis is marked by numerous small papules and papulopustules originating in the hair follicles. The usually commensal yeast-like micro-organism *Pityrosporum ovale* seems to have taken on an aggressive role, causing the inflammatory lesions seen.

OTHER SITES INVOLVED

The condition may also erupt suddenly and cause exudative lesions in the flexures (Fig. 8.14). This is especially likely to occur in the summer months in overweight individuals. In the elderly, seborrhoeic dermatitis sometimes spreads rapidly, becoming generalized. This 'erythrodermic' picture is quite disabling, but fortunately quite uncommon.

The disorder causes considerable itchiness, as do all the eczematous disorders. It also gives rise to soreness and much discomfort when it is exudative and affects the major flexures.

Round or annular scaling patches over the central chest (Fig. 8.15) and upper back are particularly common in middle-aged and elderly men, as are erythematous areas in the groins, especially in the overweight. When acute and severe, the condition becomes exudative and other flexural sites such as the axillae and the umbilicus also become involved (sometimes known as infectious eczematoid dermatitis).

DIFFERENTIAL DIAGNOSIS

In the groin area, it is important to distinguish flexural psoriasis (see page 129) and ringworm infection (tinea cruris; Table 8.2). Ringworm rashes are usually

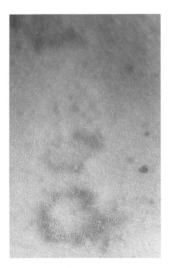

Figure 8.15 Annular lesion on the chest in seborrhoeic dermatitis.

Table 8.2 Differential diagnosis of rashes in the groin

	Clinical features	Tests
Ringworm	Often not symmetrical, very itchy, rapidly spreading	Microscopy and culture of scales
Seborrhoeic dermatitis/ intertrigo	Tends to be symmetrical and to involve apices of groins, other areas may be affected	None available
Clothing dermatitis	May resemble seborrhoeic dermatitis, likely to affect other areas	Patch testing

asymmetrical and do not reach up right into the groin apices. There is usually a raised advancing edge to ringworm and a tendency to clear centrally. Mycological testing is so simple and useful and the results of misdiagnosis so embarrassing that all should become proficient at skin scraping and recognition of fungal mycelium (see page 38).

NATURAL HISTORY AND EPIDEMIOLOGY

The condition is common at all ages and in both sexes. Severe and widespread seborrhoeic dermatitis is a particular problem for elderly men, but the milder forms are no more common in the elderly than in younger age groups. 'Cradle cap' occurring in the newborn is probably not seborrhoeic dermatitis, but a minor and transient abnormality of scalp desquamation. There is no racial predilection for the disorder and it appears to affect all social groups and occupations. The disorder has become notorious as a sign of acquired immune deficiency syndrome (AIDS) and presumably this is a result of the underlying immunosuppression (see page 100). Left untreated, the condition waxes and wanes over many years.

TREATMENT

The major aims in the treatment of seborrhoeic dermatitis are the removal of the precipitating microbial cause and the suppression of the eczematous response. For this purpose, topical preparations containing both 1 per cent hydrocortisone and an imidazole such as miconazole or clotrimazole may be all that is required for patients with limited disease. A preparation containing lithium succinate has also been useful. Sulphur and salicylic acid preparations are antimicrobial and keratolytic and, although inelegant, appear quite effective when all else fails!

Exudative intertriginous areas in the major body folds rapidly respond to bed rest to avoid further friction between opposing skin surfaces and bland lotions or weak, non-irritating antibacterial solutions for bathing and wet dressings.

Broad-spectrum systemic antibiotics should also be employed: ampicillin or a tetracycline is suitable.

Discoid eczema (nummular eczema)

DEFINITION

Discoid eczema is a quite common eczematous disorder of unknown cause, distinguished by the appearance of reddened, scaling, rounded areas on the arms and legs.

CLINICAL FEATURES

Signs and symptoms

Slightly raised, pink-red, scaly discs, varying in diameter from 1 cm to 4 cm, appear on the arms and legs and, less frequently, on the trunk (Fig. 8.16). The disorder is usually quite itchy and the skin on the arms and legs is often dry as well.

NATURAL HISTORY AND EPIDEMIOLOGY

Discoid eczema is one of the less common eczematous conditions, but is by no means rare. It is most common in the middle aged and elderly. The condition usually lasts for a few months only.

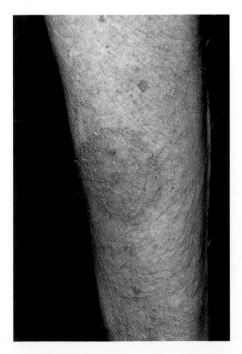

Figure 8.16 Discoid eczema.

Table 8.3 Differential diagnosis of round, red, scaling patches

Disease	Features
Psoriasis	Well-defined, thickened, scaly plaques, usually multiple
Discoid eczema	Only a moderately well-defined edge; slightly scaly, pink patches, limited in number
Ringworm	May be annular with central clearing; microscopy and culture of scales will reveal fungal mycelium
Bowen's disease	Often slightly irregular in shape; edge is well defined; biopsy is decisive

DIFFERENTIAL DIAGNOSIS

The condition has to be distinguished from psoriasis, in which the margins are more distinct; from ringworm, which usually spreads peripherally and has a raised margin; and from Bowen's disease, which is mostly restricted to the light-exposed areas and is usually one or two solitary red, scaling patches (Table 8.3).

TREATMENT

Weak and moderately strong corticosteroid preparations (e.g. 1 per cent hydrocortisone, clobetasone or desoximethasone are all suitable) applied once or twice daily usually suppress the disorder. Emollients and emollient cleansers are also helpful as adjuncts.

Eczema craquelée (asteatotic eczema)

DEFINITION

Eczema craquelée is an uncommon eczematous disorder that occurs on the extensor aspects of the limbs of elderly subjects and is characterized by a 'crazy paving' appearance.

CLINICAL FEATURES

Signs and symptoms

The most common affected sites are the shins, the fronts and sides of the thighs, extensor aspects of the upper arms and forearms, and the back. Involved skin is pink, roughened and superficially fissured, giving a crazed appearance (Fig. 8.17). The areas affected are more sore than itchy. The condition has a very

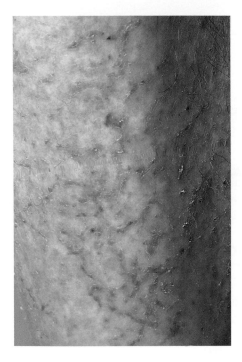

Figure 8.17 Eczema craquelée – note the 'crazed appearance'.

characteristic appearance and it is uncommon for it to be mistaken for any other disorder.

NATURAL HISTORY AND EPIDEMIOLOGY

The disorder is restricted to the elderly and is mainly seen in the newly hospitalized or institutionalized individual where there is low ambient relative humidity and after unaccustomed vigorous bathing.

It seems to be an unusual response of already vulnerable skin to minor mechanical and chemical trauma.

TREATMENT

The condition responds to emollients and, if necessary, 1 per cent hydrocortisone ointment – when the atmosphere is humidified and vigorous washing stops.

Lichen simplex chronicus (circumscribed neurodermatitis)

DEFINITION

This is an intensely pruritic rash, sharply localized to one or a few sites, which is characterized by thickening and exaggeration of the skin surface markings.

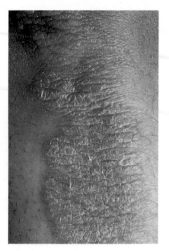

Figure 8.18 Lichen simplex chronicus – note the exaggerated skin surface markings.

CLINICAL FEATURES

Signs and symptoms

The medial aspect of the ankle, the back of the scalp, the extensor aspects of the forearms, the wrists and the genitalia are predisposed to this disorder. The condition is extremely itchy and patients complain bitterly about the intense local irritation. The lesions are characteristically raised, irregular, red plaques with well-defined margins, which have exaggerated skin markings (lichenification) over the scaling surface (Fig. 8.18). If the itching is persistent and intense and the resultant scratching vigorous, the affected sites may become very thickened, raised and excoriated The resultant lesion is known as a prurigo nodule (Fig. 8.19). When many such nodules occur over the surface, the condition is known as prurigo nodularis.

NATURAL HISTORY AND EPIDEMIOLOGY

The disorder is quite common in middle-aged subjects of either sex and all races. It may be more common in the Indian subcontinent. It is a very stubborn and persistent disorder, which may stay unchanged for many years. Prurigo nodularis is similarly stubborn and persistent.

DIFFERENTIAL DIAGNOSIS

Hypertrophic lichen planus (see page 145) may be difficult to distinguish, although this disorder tends to be more mauve and be less regularly lichenified than lichen simplex chronicus. Biopsy may be needed to distinguish these disorders with certainty. Lichen simplex chronicus may also resemble a patch of psoriasis.

PATHOLOGY AND PATHOGENESIS

Histologically, there may be striking epidermal hypertrophy, which, in extreme cases, may resemble epitheliomatous change (pseudoepitheliomatous hyperplasia).

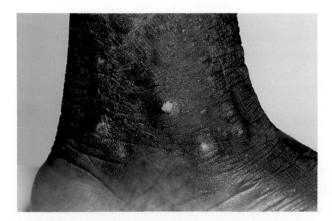

Figure 8.19 Prurigo papules on the ankle.

The persistent scratching causes an increased rate of epidermal cell production and accounts for the hypertrophy. The cause of the pruritus is unknown.

TREATMENT

The condition tends to persist regardless of the treatment prescribed. High potency topical corticosteroids, intralesional corticosteroids or preparations of coal tar are sometimes helpful.

Case 7

The persistent itching of the thickened, scaling patches around the ankles and at the back of the neck was extremely distressing for 68-year-old Michael. A biopsy showed only thickening of the epidermis and some inflammation, which was diagnosed as lichen simplex chronicus. Michael had had the condition for at least 6 years and nothing seemed to help. One Tuesday morning he woke up with much less itching and by the end of the week it was clear that the condition had gone into remission – for no known reason!

Contact dermatitis

Contact dermatitis may be caused by a direct toxic action of a substance on the skin – the so-called primary irritant dermatitis – or by a substance inducing a delayed hypersensitivity reaction – allergic contact dermatitis. Both are common and cause considerable loss of work and disability.

PRIMARY IRRITANT DERMATITIS

Definition

Primary irritant dermatitis is an eczematous rash that results from direct contact with toxic 'irritating' materials.

Clinical features

Scaly, red and fissured areas appear on the irritated skin (Figs 8.20 and 8.21). The hands are most frequently affected. The palmar skin and the palmar surfaces of the fingers are often affected, but the areas between the fingers and elsewhere on the hands may also be involved. The condition may become exudative and very inflamed if the substances contacted are very toxic. This form of contact dermatitis causes considerable soreness and irritation. The fissures make movement very difficult and effectively disable the victims.

Differential diagnosis

The condition must be distinguished from allergic contact dermatitis by a carefully taken history and patch testing (see below). Psoriasis of the palms may resemble

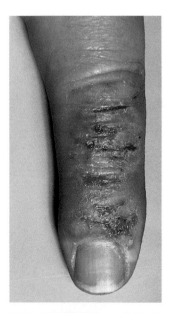

Figure 8.20 Primary irritant contact dermatitis affecting the back of the finger.

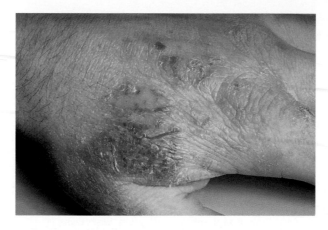

Figure 8.21 Primary irritant contact dermatitis affecting the back of the hand.

contact dermatitis, but is usually accompanied by signs of psoriasis elsewhere. Ringworm usually affects one palm only and is marked by diffuse erythema and silvery scaling. If there is any doubt, scales should be examined for fungal mycelium under the microscope.

Natural history and epidemiology

An 'irritant' substance will injure anyone's skin if there is sufficient contact. However, some individuals are more prone to develop primary irritant contact dermatitis – especially atopic subjects and those with fair skins who sunburn easily.

The disorder is seen particularly often in manual workers (occupational dermatitis) and housewives (housewives' eczema). Builders, mechanics, hairdressers, cooks and laundry workers are some of the groups that are frequently affected. The condition causes considerable economic loss from loss of work. Contact with alkalis, organic solvents, detergent substances, cement and particulate waste is often responsible.

Prevention and management

The identification of potential hazards, use of non-toxic substances, prevention of skin contact, use of protective gloves, use of emollients and worker education are all important in prevention. When present, the cause must be identified and further contact prevented. When the condition is severe, rest from manual work is required. Emollients are an important part of treatment to make affected skin more supple and to minimize fissuring. Weak and moderately potent corticosteroids should accelerate healing.

ALLERGIC CONTACT DERMATITIS

Definition

Allergic contact dermatitis is an eczematous rash that develops after contact with an agent to which delayed (cellular) hypersensitivity has developed.

Clinical features

The rash develops at the sites of skin contact with the 'allergen', but occasionally spreads outside these limits for unknown reasons. The vigour and speed of the reaction vary enormously depending on the particular individual. When very acute, the reaction develops within a few hours of contacting the responsible substance – such a speedy response is seen, for example, in the condition of 'poison ivy', which is common in the USA. Itching is noticed at first and then the area involved becomes red, swollen and vesicular. Later, the area becomes scaled and fissured.

An enormous number of substances are capable of causing allergic contact dermatitis. Nickel dermatitis is one of the commonest examples – some 5 per cent of women in the UK are said to be nickel sensitive. Affected individuals cannot wear stainless-steel jewellery because of the nickel in the steel (Fig. 8.22) and develop a rash beneath steel studs, clips and buckles. Patients who are nickel sensitive may also react to 'dichromate' and other chromate salts.

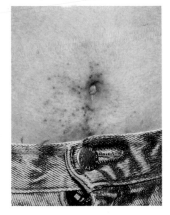

Figure 8.22 Allergic contact dermatitis to nickel in the metal studs in a pair of jeans.

Other examples include allergy to chemicals in rubber, for example mercaptobenzthiazole (MBT) and thiouram, and to formalin. These allergies may cause dermatitis when wearing particular clothes, as, indeed, may sensitivities to dyes. Allergies to lanolin (in sheep-wool fat and in many ointments and creams) and to perfumes can cause dermatitis after the wearing of cosmetics. Lanolin, ethylene diamine, vioform, neomycin and local anaesthetics may cause a dermatitis after using a cream or an ointment. Dyes (such as the black hair dye paraphenylene diamine) can also be the cause of allergic contact dermatitis (Fig. 8.23). Some materials are notorious for causing sensitivity and are not often used topically because of this, for example penicillin and sulphonamides.

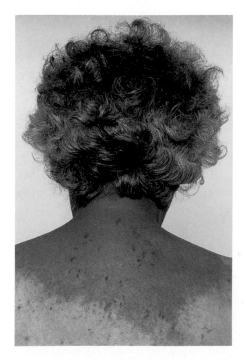

Figure 8.23 Allergic contact dermatitis due to paraphenylene diamine hair dye.

Natural history and epidemiology

Allergic contact dermatitis is quite common, but not as common as primary irritant dermatitis. It is rare in children and uncommon in the elderly. It is seen in all racial groups, although less so in black-skinned individuals.

Diagnosis of allergic contact hypersensitivity

Accurate history taking and careful examination identifying all involved areas are very important. The definitive technique for diagnosing allergic contact hypersensitivity is patch testing. In this test, possible allergens are placed in occlusive contact with the skin for 48-hour periods and the area is inspected 48 hours after removal of the patch. A positive test is revealed by the development of an eczematous patch with erythema, swelling and vesicles at the site of application. In practice, low concentrations of allergen are applied to avoid false-positive primary irritant reactions.

In most cases, a battery of the commonest allergens in appropriate concentrations is applied. Such a battery is shown in Table 8.4.

Table 8.4 Common antigens used in patch testing and concentrations in which they are used

Antigen	%
Nickel sulphate	5
Balsam of Peru	25
Colophony	1
Chlorocresol	1
PPD base	1
MBT	2
Formalin	1
Potassium dichromate	0.5
Wool alcohols	30
Epoxy resin (Araldite)	1
Chloroxylenol	1
Neomycin	20
Cobalt chloride	1
Dowicil 200	1
Parabens	15
Thiuram-mix	1
Mercapto-mix	2
Perfume-mix	8
Kanthon CG	0.67
Primin	0.01
Ethylene diamine	1
Benzocaine	5

PPD = paraphenylene diamine; MBT = mercaptobenzthiazole.

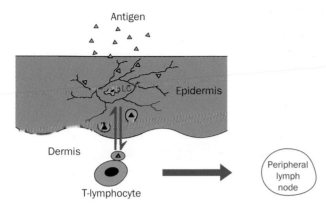

Figure 8.24 Diagram to show the processes in allergic contact dermatitis. Antigen is processed by Langerhans cells in the epidermis and then presented to T-lymphocytes.
▲ = antigen;
▲ = antigen processed by Langerhans cell;
LC = Langerhans cell.

Pathology and pathogenesis

The sensitizing chemical (antigen) crosses the stratum corneum barrier and is picked up by the Langerhans cells in the epidermis (Fig. 8.24). The antigen is then 'processed' by the Langerhans cell and passed on to T-lymphocytes in the peripheral lymph nodes. Here, some of the T-lymphocytes develop a specific 'memory' for the particular antigen and the population of these expands. This process of sensitization takes some 10–14 days in humans. After this period, when the particular antigen contacts the skin, the primed T-lymphocytes with the 'memory' for this chemical species rush to the contacted site and liberate cytokines and mediators that injure the epidermis and cause the eczematous reaction.

Treatment

It is vital to identify the sensitizing material and prevent further contact. The eczema will subside rapidly in most cases after removal from the antigen. The use of weak or moderately potent topical corticosteroids and emollients will speed the resolution of the eczematous patches.

Venous eczema (gravitational eczema; stasis dermatitis)

DEFINITION

Venous eczema occurs on the lower legs and is the result of chronic venous hypertension.

CLINICAL FEATURES

Itchy, pink, scaling areas develop on a background of the changes of chronic venous hypertension (Fig. 8.25). The affected areas are often around venous ulcers, but the margins of the eczematous process are poorly defined. Occasionally, the process spreads to the contralateral leg and even to the thighs and arms.

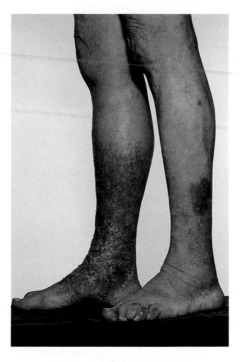

Figure 8.25 Gravitational eczema.

In most cases, venous eczema is actually an allergic contact hypersensitivity to one of the substances used to treat the venous ulcer. Such substances include lanolin, neomycin, vioform, ethylene diamine and rubber additives. It has been suggested that some patients develop a sensitivity to the breakdown products of their own tissues (autosensitization).

TREATMENT

Contact hypersensitivity must be identified and the patient advised to stop using the agent responsible. The simplest of topical applications should be used – white soft paraffin is suitable as an emollient and 1 per cent hydrocortisone ointment is suitable as an anti-inflammatory agent.

Summary

- Eczema (synonymous with dermatitis) is characterized by epidermal oedema (spongiosis) and may be caused by external factors or result from poorly understood 'endogenous' or constitutional factors. The former types of eczema include allergic contact dermatitis and primary irritant contact dermatitis, whereas amongst the latter are atopic dermatitis, seborrhoeic dermatitis, discoid eczema and lichen simplex chronicus.

- Atopic dermatitis is a very common, chronic, remittent, extremely itchy dermatosis starting in infancy. There is a marked tendency to occur in families, probably via the inheritance of susceptibility genes. The disease is strongly associated with asthma and hay fever. There is depression of cell-mediated immunity, enhancement of immediate hypersensitivity and elevated serum IgE. An imbalance between H1 and H2 populations of T-lymphocytes with dominance of TH2 cells has been proposed as the underlying problem.

- Clinical features of atopic dermatitis include a predilection for flexural distribution of the eczema, excoriations and lichenification, generalized xeroderma, white dermographism, hyperlinear palms and Denny Morgan folds beneath the eyes. The skin often becomes infected with *Staphylococcus aureus*, which may play a role in relapses. There is a susceptibility to virus infections, including multiple viral warts, mollusca contagiosa and extensive herpes simplex.
- Topical corticosteroids are the most effective topical agents, but cause skin thinning and pituitary–adrenal axis suppression as well as rebound when their use ends. Emollients also have major benefits and most patients can be managed with a combination of emollients and corticosteroids. Very severely affected patients may benefit from some kind of phototherapy or oral immunosuppressive drugs such as cyclosporin or azathioprine, where the risk of severe side effects is outweighed by the benefits. Antimicrobial agents may also be helpful.
- Seborrhoeic dermatitis occurs on hairy sites and flexures or on the central trunk. Common signs are severe dandruff and scaling, pink areas in the facial flexures. It affects major flexures, particularly in the elderly. Milder forms are very common. It appears to be due to overgrowth of the normal follicular flora and is often seen in the immunosuppressed (e.g. AIDS). Treatment with weak corticosteroids combined with antimicrobial agents such as the imidazoles is often helpful.
- Discoid eczema mainly occurs in the middle aged and elderly and is characterized by round, coin-sized, red scaling patches. It has to be distinguished from psoriasis and Bowen's disease. Treatment is with emollients and corticosteroids.
- Eczema craquelée (asteototic eczema) occurs particularly on the legs of elderly subjects with very dry skin and is marked by a red rash with a 'crazy paving' pattern. It responds to frequent emollients.
- Lichen simplex chronicus is an intensely pruritic disorder, occurring in particular locations such as the back of the neck and the medial aspects of the ankles. Affected sites are well-defined, raised, red, excoriated and lichenified plaques. The condition is stubbornly persistent, but potent topical corticosteroids may assist. Histologically, there is marked epidermal thickening.
- Primary irritant contact dermatitis is due to toxic damage to the skin from alkalis and surfactants and is mostly seen on the hands of housewives and those who work with their hands. Allergic contact dermatitis is due to the development of delayed hypersensitivity to a particular chemical substance such as nickel, neomycin or a rubber additive in a few exposed individuals.
- Venous eczema occurs on the lower legs of elderly individuals with venous hypertension. In some, it seems to be due to allergic contact dermatitis to agents used to treat venous ulcers.

Psoriasis and lichen planus

Psoriasis

Psoriasis is important because of its frequency, its recurrent nature and its tendency to disable a proportion of its victims.

DEFINITION

Psoriasis is a common, genetically determined, inflammatory skin disorder of unknown cause, which, in its most usual form, is characterized by well-demarcated, raised, red scaling patches that preferentially localize to the extensor surfaces.

CLINICAL FEATURES

The lesions

Typical lesions are red, raised and scaly and have well-demarcated margins (Fig. 9.1). Plaques vary enormously in size and shape. They often start out discoid, but end up polycyclic (Fig. 9.2) as several lesions coalesce.

Sites affected

Psoriasis affects the extensor aspects of the trunk and limbs preferentially. The knees, elbows and scalp are especially frequently affected (Fig. 9.3), although the mucosae seem to be spared.

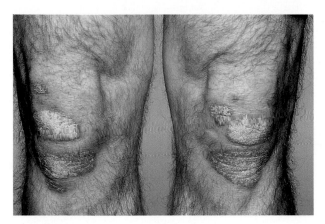

Figure 9.1 Typical red, scaling plaques of psoriasis on the knees.

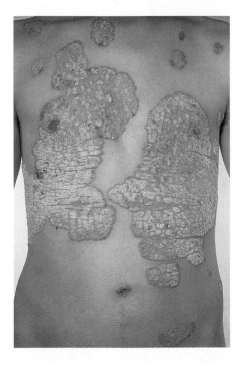

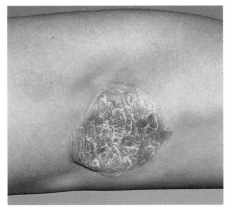

Figure 9.3 Psoriatic patch on the elbow – a site of predilection.

Figure 9.2 Polycyclic plaque of psoriasis.

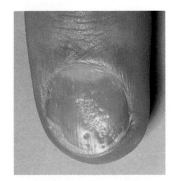

Figure 9.4 A minor degree of involvement of the nail plate with pitting and onycholysis.

The nails are often affected and may show the so-called thimble pitting, separation of the nail plate from the nail bed (onycholysis), subungual debris, brownish-black discolourations and deformities of the nail plate (Fig. 9.4).

Flexural lesions, which occur in some patients, are most often seen in the major body folds in the elderly, especially in those who are overweight. The groins and genitalia, axillae, inframammary folds in women and the skin of abdominal folds and the umbilicus in either sex are affected. The moistness of the flexural areas decreases the scaling and produces a moist and glazed appearance (Fig. 9.5).

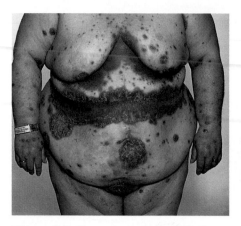

Figure 9.5 Flexural psoriasis affecting the body folds in an obese patient.

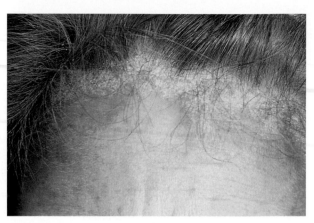

Figure 9.6 Psoriasis of the scalp margin.

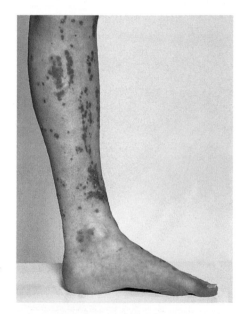

Figure 9.7 Psoriasis appearing at sites of injury (from scratching) – the isomorphic response.

The face is not usually severely affected in psoriasis, although the scalp margin, paranasal folds and retroauricular folds are quite often involved (Fig. 9.6).

Psoriasis sometimes appears at the site of a minor injury such as a scratch or a graze (Fig. 9.7). This reaction, known as the isomorphic response or the Koebner phenomenon, mostly occurs when the psoriasis is in active spreading phase. The development of a skin disorder at the site of injury is characteristic of psoriasis, but is also seen in lichen planus (see page 144) and discoid lupus erythematosus (see page 79). Its cause is unknown.

NATURAL HISTORY AND EPIDEMIOLOGY

Surveys in the UK, the USA and Scandinavia have all reported that psoriasis is found in between 1 and 3 per cent of the population. It has been claimed that the disorder is less common in African and Asian groups, but detailed figures are not available. It seems less of a problem in the Japanese and other Asian populations, but may be becoming more frequent with the trend to Westernization.

The disease is more common in men than in women. There are two main peaks of incidence, the first of which is in the second half of the second decade of life. Recently, it has been recognized that psoriasis may also occur for the first time in the seventh decade. In general, the younger the age of onset, the worse the outlook as far as frequency, severity and persistence of the disease are concerned.

Psoriasis is a life-long disorder subject to unpredictable remissions and relapses. Single episodes are uncommon and in the most frequent variety an episode in the teenage years is followed by a series of attacks, each lasting weeks or months, in the succeeding years.

GENETICS

Psoriasis is often familial, but does not appear to be inherited in any regular dominant, sex-linked or recessive way. With one parent affected, there is an approximately 30 per cent chance of a child being affected. With both parents suffering from psoriasis, the chance that a child will develop the condition rises to 60 per cent. In a recent survey in Sweden, it was found that 6.4 per cent of relatives of families in which there was a patient with psoriasis were affected, compared to 1.94 per cent of controls. Non-identical twins have an approximately 20 per cent chance of both being affected, and the concordance rate for identical twins seems to be in the order of 70 per cent. Recent research indicated that, although no one gene is responsible for the disease, the direct inheritance of 'susceptibility genes' is necessary for its development.

Psoriasis is associated with HLA groups HLA-B13, HLA-B17 and HLA-B37 as well as with the class II antigen DR7. It is even more strongly associated with CW6 – increasing the risk of the disease some 13 times in Caucasians.

DIFFERENTIAL DIAGNOSIS

Any red, scaling disorder can be mistaken for psoriasis, and vice versa (Table 9.1). On the scalp, the most frequently seen disorder to be mistaken for psoriasis is seborrhoeic dermatitis (see page 114), although this usually affects the scalp diffusely rather than in distinct plaques. Lichen simplex chronicus (see page 119) of the scalp typically presents with a red, scaling patch on the occiput, which can look very psoriasis-like. The intense itching and lichenified surface should serve to distinguish the two disorders.

Multiple patches of ringworm may appear very like psoriasis (Fig. 9.8), but the lesions are often more ring-like than psoriasis and can be distinguished by microscopical examination of potassium hydroxide (KOH)-treated skin scrapings (see page 38). Mycosis fungoides – a T-cell lymphoma of skin – often evolves through a phase in which there are many red psoriasiform lesions on the trunk, but these differ from psoriasis by being more irregular in shape and persistent.

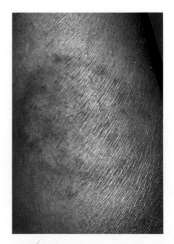

Figure 9.8 Psoriasiform plaque in the leg due to ringworm.

Table 9.1 Differential diagnosis of red, scaling rashes

	Discriminants
Psoriasis	Nail changes, family history, multiple patches on extensor surfaces
Discoid eczema	Round, scaly patches on arms and legs
Lichen simplex chronicus	Itchy, lichenified, persistent patches
Bowen's disease	Plaques tend to be smaller and more limited in number; biopsy decides
Superficial basal cell carcinoma	Thin, slightly raised edge; biopsy decides
Mycosis fungoides	Multiple psoriasiform patches, but irregularly thickened; biopsy helps
Ringworm	Often annular, spreads peripherally; microscopy and culture of scale important

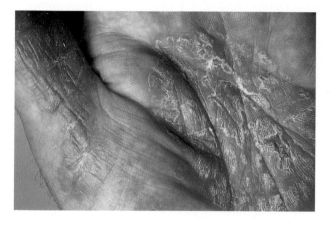

Figure 9.9 Red, scaling patch on the palm due to psoriasis. Such a presentation can be very difficult to distinguish from eczema.

On the legs, raised, round, red, scaling psoriasiform patches often turn out to be Bowen's disease in the elderly, or discoid eczema. Lichen simplex chronicus around the ankles may also be difficult to distinguish.

Psoriasis of the palms (Fig. 9.9) is difficult to distinguish from eczema affecting these sites. Even after biopsy, the clinician may remain uncertain.

Superficial basal cell carcinoma lesions are sometimes several centimetres in diameter and quite psoriasiform in appearance, but have a fine, raised, 'hair-like' margin.

CLINICAL VARIANTS

Guttate psoriasis

This disorder is mainly seen in children aged 7–14 years. Often, it develops some 2–4 weeks after an episode of tonsillitis or pharyngitis, mostly due to beta-haemolytic

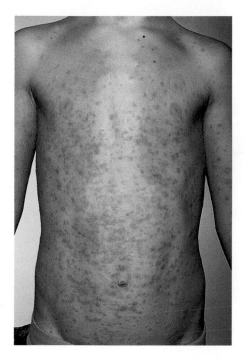

Figure 9.10 Multiple small patches of guttate psoriasis seen after a streptococcal tonsillitis.

streptococci. It behaves like an exanthem, as the characteristically 'drop'-sized lesions develop suddenly (Fig. 9.10) and at the same time. The lesions do not usually last longer than 8–10 weeks.

Napkin psoriasis

Infantile napkin dermatitis (see page 229) sometimes takes on a very psoriasis-like appearance and typical psoriatic lesions develop on the scalp and trunk. The true relationship with psoriasis is unknown.

Erythrodermic psoriasis

Psoriasis sometimes progresses to generalized skin involvement. Typical plaque-like lesions disappear, the skin is universally red and scaly and the condition is known as erythrodermic psoriasis. Patients who are seriously ill suffer from:

- heat loss, and are in danger of hypothermia because of the increased blood supply to the skin
- water loss, leading to dehydration because of the disturbed barrier function of the abnormal stratum corneum
- a hyperdynamic circulation, because effectively there is a vascular shunt in the skin; when the patient's myocardium is already compromised because of other factors, there is a danger of high output failure
- loss of protein, electrolytes and metabolites via the shed scales and exudates; patients may develop deficiency states.

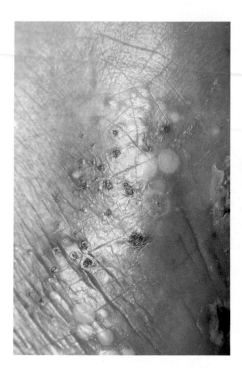

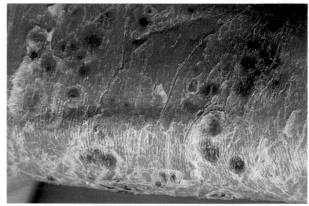

Figure 9.11 Typical pustular psoriasis affecting the sole of the foot.

Figure 9.12 Pustular psoriasis of the sole of the foot with several older, brown, scaling lesions that were pustules.

Pustular psoriasis

Most dermatologists consider this to be a manifestation of psoriasis, although there are some who believe it is a separate disorder. It seems probable that pustular psoriasis is indeed a type of psoriasis, with exaggeration of one particular component of the disease (see Pathology below). There are two main types.

Palmoplantar pustulosis

Patients with palmoplantar pustulosis develop yellowish white, sterile pustules on the central parts of the palms and soles (Figs 9.11 and 9.12). Older lesions take on a brownish appearance and are later shed in a scale at the surface. The affected area can become generally inflamed, scaly and fissured and, although relatively small areas of skin are affected, the condition can be very disabling.

The disorder tends to be resistant to treatment (see below) and is subject to relapses and remission over many years.

Generalized pustular psoriasis

This is also known eponymously as Von Zumbusch disease, and is one of the most serious disorders dealt with by dermatologists. In its classical form, attacks occur suddenly and are characterized by severe systemic upset, a swinging pyrexia, arthralgia and a high polymorphonuclear leucocytosis accompanying the skin disorder.

The skin first becomes erythrodermic and then develops sheets of sterile pustules over the trunk and limbs (Fig. 9.13).

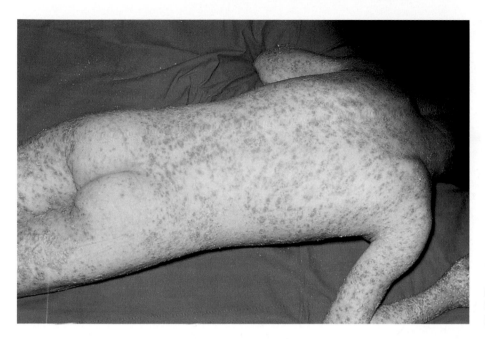

Figure 9.13 A 10-year-old boy with severe generalized pustular psoriasis.

Sometimes, the pustules become confluent so that 'lakes of pus' develop just beneath the skin surface. In other areas, there is a curious type of superficial peeling without pustules forming.

These patients are very unwell and require hospitalization. They can usually be brought into remission by modern treatments (see below), but are subject to recurrent attacks. The disorder sometimes affects infants and small children.

Other forms of pustular psoriasis

Occasionally, pustules may develop after strong topical or systemic corticosteroids have been used and then abruptly withdrawn. Other rare variants of pustular psoriasis include:

- acrodermatitis continua, in which there is a recalcitrant pustular erosive disorder on the fingers and toes around the nails and occasionally elsewhere
- pustular bacterid, in which sterile pustules suddenly appear on the palms, soles and distal parts of the limbs after an infection.

Arthropathic psoriasis

There is a higher prevalence of a rheumatoid-like arthritis with symmetrical involvement of the small joints of the hands and feet, wrists and ankles in patients with psoriasis (5–6 per cent) compared to a matched control population (1–2 per cent). This 'rheumatoid arthritis-like' disorder differs in one important respect from ordinary rheumatoid arthritis – there is no circulating rheumatoid factor.

In addition, there is a distinctive and destructive form of joint disease that seems specific to psoriasis. In this 'psoriatic arthropathy', the distal interphalangeal joints, the posterior zygohypophysial, the temporomandibular and the sacroiliac

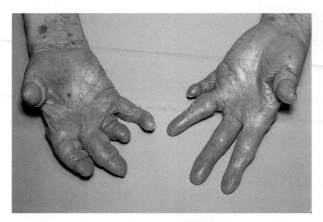

Figure 9.14 The results of psoriatic arthropathy (arthritis mutilans).

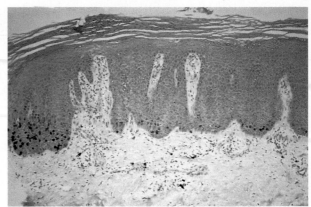

Figure 9.15 Regular epidermal thickening in psoriasis with parakeratosis. There are cells at the base of the epidermis that are darkly labelled by the process of autoradiography after incubation in radiolabelled thymidine, indicating that they are in the DNA synthesis phase of cell division.

joints are particularly affected. The disorder is more destructive than rheumatoid disease. Bony erosion and destruction take place, leading to 'collapse' of affected digits (Fig. 9.14), justifying the term often used for this dreadful disease – arthritis mutilans.

Treatment may temporarily improve these joint complications of psoriasis, but they tend to run a progressive course subject to remissions and relapses.

PATHOLOGY AND PATHOGENESIS

The histopathological appearance of psoriasis is distinctive but not specific. The main features may be subdivided into (1) the epidermal thickening, (2) the inflammatory component, and (3) the vascular component, but of course all are closely interlinked.

The epidermal thickening

The epidermis shows marked exaggeration of the rete pattern and elongation of the epidermal downgrowths with bulbous, club-like enlargement of their ends (Fig. 9.15). The average thickness is increased from about three to four cells in the normal skin to approximately 12–15 cells in the psoriatic lesion. Many mitotic figures can be seen and the rate of epidermal cell production seems to be greatly enhanced. The turnover time of psoriatic epidermis and stratum corneum is consequently very much shortened. Normally, it takes some 28 days for new cells to ascend from the basal layer and travel through the epidermis and the stratum corneum and reach the surface. In psoriasis, it takes some 4 days! Epidermal nuclei are retained in the inefficient horny layer that results (parakeratosis).

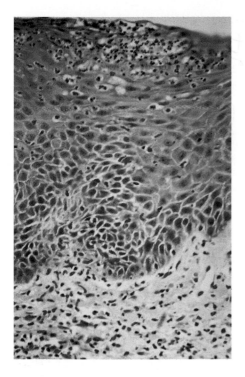

Figure 9.16 Photomicrograph showing many inflammatory cells in the thickened epidermis in psoriasis.

The inflammatory component

Interspersed between the 'parakeratotic' horn cells are collections of desiccated polymorphonuclear leucocytes known as Munro microabscesses. The epidermis is oedematous and is itself infiltrated by inflammatory cells. The dermis immediately below the epidermis also contains many inflammatory cells, mostly lymphocytes. In pustular psoriasis, the epidermal component is much less in evidence and there are collections of inflammatory cells within the epidermis (Fig. 9.16).

The vascular component

The papillary capillaries are greatly dilated and tortuous to a degree not seen in other inflammatory skin disorders. Ultrastructurally it can be seen that there are larger gaps than usual between the endothelial cells. These abnormal capillaries are the last of the features to go during resolution.

AETIOLOGY

The cause of psoriasis is unknown, despite the enormous research effort that has been made in the past three decades. Various hypotheses have been popular at different times. One very obvious abnormality in psoriasis is the hyperplastic epidermis with increased mitotic activity, and one line of intense investigation was directed at the control of epidermal cell production in this disease. Attention has moved away from this possibility in recent years and focused more on the inflammation and possible immunopathogenesis. The disorder often responds to immunosuppressive agents such as cyclosporin and methotrexate and currently psoriasis is thought of as a 'lymphocyte driven' disease.

Various potentially heritable biochemical abnormalities have been suggested and/or described that could explain both the increased epidermal proliferation and the inflammatory component. At different times, alterations in the skin content or activity of cyclic nucleotides, polyamines, eicosanoids, cytokines and growth factors have been described, but in most cases these changes are secondary to the underlying and fundamental less well-characterized events.

Infection has been considered as a cause and in recent years the involvement of retroviruses has been suggested. It is worth noting that in acquired immune deficiency syndrome (AIDS) patients, a very acute and aggressive form of psoriasis may develop.

Case 8

Jessie's mother and aunt had psoriasis and at the age of 19 Jessie thought that she was getting it too, as she had scaling patches on her knees and elbows and in her scalp. She also noticed some separation of the nail plates from the nail beds and pitting of three of her fingernails. Her GP diagnosed psoriasis and started her on a tar preparation, which she didn't like because it burnt and soiled her clothes. However, she did quite well with a later treatment – calcipotriol (Dovonex). The rash disappeared after 6 weeks, but unfortunately recurred the following year.

TREATMENT

- Patients with just a few plaques affecting the knees, elbows or elsewhere require little treatment. In other patients, simple treatment with an emollient such as white soft paraffin, by itself or with 2 per cent salicylic acid, is sufficient when used once or twice daily.
- With more lesions and symptoms, more active topical treatment is needed. Tar-containing preparations are less popular than previously, but may suit some patients who can put up with the stinging, the unpleasant smell and the staining. Tar has anti-inflammatory and cytostatic activity and certainly has mild anti-psoriatic effect. Proprietary tar preparations have some advantages over the British National Formulary formulations. Tar shampoos for scalp involvement are still popular.
- Analogues of vitamin D3 are effective topical treatments; calcipotriol used once or twice daily improves some 60 per cent patients after 6 weeks' treatment. Used alongside medium-potency corticosteroids, the efficacy is increased and the skin imitation decreased. A preparation of calcipotriol formulated together with betamethasone-17-valerate is now available as 'Dovobet', and does appear quite effective. Tacalcitol is another vitamin D3 analogue, which, although effective when employed topically, is not as potent as calcipotriol. Apart from skin irritation, there is the concern that sufficient of these D3 analogues will be absorbed to cause hypercalcaemia. Fortunately, this has not proved to be a problem thus far.

- Anthralin (dithranol) is a potent reducing agent that has marked therapeutic activity in psoriasis. It is generally used in ascending concentrations, starting at 0.1 or 0.05 per cent. To make dithranol treatment suitable for out-patients, the tendency has been to use either dithranol in white soft paraffin or one of the proprietary preparations such as Dithrocream®, which is available in different strengths. Dithranol often irritates and burns the skin and care must be taken to match the concentration used to the individual patient's tolerance. It also causes a distinctive brown-purple staining of clothes, towels and skin (Fig. 9.17). Apart from the irritation and staining, dithranol has no serious side effects.
- There is only a very limited role for topical corticosteroids in the treatment of psoriasis. They are useful for patients with flexural lesions for which other irritant preparations are not suitable. For the same reason, weak topical corticosteroids are also suitable for lesions on the genitalia and the face. Potent topical corticosteroids should *not* be used, because frequent use is likely to lead to side effects (see page 307) and because eventual withdrawal may lead to severe rebound and even the appearance of pustular lesions. Potent topical steroids (such as fluocinolone acetonide or betamethasone dipropionate) may be suitable for use on the scalp and their use is sometimes justifiable on the palms and soles if other treatment is not helping.
- Another quite new treatment is a topical retinoid analogue called tazarotene (0.05 or 0.1 per cent). This is really very effective – giving some 65 per cent improvement in 6 weeks. When used alongside medium-potency topical corticosteroids, its efficiency is increased and the irritation experienced by some 15 per cent of users is decreased.

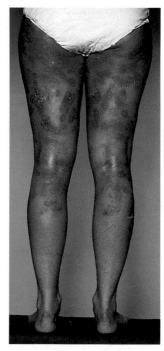

Figure 9.17 Brownish-purple staining on the skin due to dithranol.

Both the vitamin D3 analogues and tazarotene may improve psoriasis by modulating gene activity and redirecting differentiation and by reducing the epidermal proliferation. When more than 15 per cent of the body surface area is involved, topical treatment becomes very difficult. The same is true of erythrodermic psoriasis and generalized pustular psoriasis. All these types require systemic treatments.

Methotrexate

The antimetabolite methotrexate is a competitive antagonist of tetrahydrofolate reductase, blocking the formation of thymidine and thus DNA. It is thought that this antiproliferative activity may be important in reducing epidermal and lymphocyte proliferation. Whichever way it works, it is a highly effective treatment for patients with severe psoriasis. Unfortunately, it is also quite toxic, producing hepatotoxicity in most patients who stay on the drug for long periods. The drug also suppresses haematopoiesis and may cause gastrointestinal upset.

It is given once weekly in doses of 5–25 mg orally or intramuscularly. To minimize the possibility of serious side effects, patients must be monitored frequently (preferably monthly) by blood counts and blood biochemistry. It is recommended that a liver biopsy is performed both before treatment begins and after a cumulated dose of 1.5 g methotrexate.

Methotrexate is also a teratogen, and fertile women should use contraceptive measures. It is mainly suitable for those who would otherwise be disabled by the disease, and for some elderly patients with severe psoriasis.

The retinoids

Retinoids are analogues of retinol (vitamin A) and have been found to exert important actions on cell division and maturation. The orally administered acitretin is of particular value in psoriasis. The drug benefits patients with all types of severe psoriasis after 3–4 weeks, but is of most help when used in combination with ultraviolet treatment. Its major drawback is that it is teratogenic and can only be given to fertile women if they use contraception and are prepared to continue using the contraceptive measures for 3 years after stopping treatment. Other significant toxicities include hyperlipidaemia and a possibility of hyperostosis and extraosseous calcification. In addition, it does have some hepatotoxicity in a few patients (Table 9.2). These 'significant' toxicities are not common, but minor mucosal side effects occur in all patients, including drying of the lips and the buccal, nasal and conjunctival mucosae. Minor generalized pruritus and slight hair loss also occur. Oral retinoids should only be prescribed by dermatologists, i.e. those who are familiar with their effects.

Cyclosporin

Cyclosporin is an immunosuppressive agent used in organ transplantation. It appears to work by inhibiting the synthesis of cytokines by T-lymphocytes. It is

Table 9.2 Toxic side effects of etretinate and acitretin

Toxic side effect	Comment
Major	
Teratogenicity	Contraception necessary for fertile women; should be continued for 3 years after stopping
Hyperlipidaemic effect	Causes a rise of serum lipids in about 30% of patients; low-fat diet required
Hepatotoxicity	Possible but uncommon
Bone toxicity	Disseminated interstitial skeletal hyperostosis and other changes in chronic use
Minor	
Drying and cracking of lips	In most patients
Drying of eyes and nose	In about 25% of patients
Increased rate of hair loss	In about 25% of patients
Pruritus, peeling palms and soles	In about 10% of patients

also dramatically effective in psoriasis when given in doses of 3–5 mg/kg per day. Its toxic side effects include severe renal damage and hypertension. Its place in the treatment of disabling and severe psoriasis is assured, but great care and constant monitoring are required.

Treatment with ultraviolet radiation

Ultraviolet radiation (UVR) has long been known to have therapeutic effects in a number of skin disorders, including psoriasis. A form of UVR treatment known as PUVA is mainly used. PUVA is an acronym for photochemotherapy with ultraviolet radiation of the A (long-wave) type. The UVA is supplied by special fluorescent lamps that emit at wavelengths of 300–400 nm, housed in cabinets or special frames over beds.

A photosensitizing psoralen drug is given orally 2 hours before exposure. The main psoralen used is 8-methoxy psoralen, but 5-methoxy psoralen and trimethoxy psoralen are sometimes used. The dose of 8-methoxy psoralen is 0.6 mg/kg. Alternatively, the patient bathes in water containing a psoralen and is then exposed to UVR a few minutes later.

Ordinary 'sun lamps' emitting UVB (290–320 nm) can also be used to treat psoriasis. The dangers of burning may be greater and the dangers of skin cancer are similar to PUVA.

Both PUVA and UVB can be combined with topical dithranol, calcipotriol and tazarotene or oral acitricin. These combinations reduce the danger of side effects from UVR and reduce the likelihood of toxicity from the accompanying agent.

The dose of UVA is calculated (in Joules) from the output of the lamps and the time of exposure. The dose required for clearance is approximately 50–100 J/cm^2 and care is taken to keep the dose as low as possible and certainly below a total cumulated dose of 1500 J/cm^2 to reduce the possibility of long-term side effects.

There are several long-term side effects (Table 9.3).

- Increased incidence of squamous cell carcinoma of the skin (see page 207) – up to 10 or 12 times that in a control group of psoriatics after 10 years. Carcinoma of the external genitalia in men is a particular problem. There is an increased incidence of basal cell carcinoma and melanoma as well.
- Increased solar elastotic degenerative change, with the appearance of ageing and alteration of skin elasticity.
- Cataracts can develop and all patients who receive PUVA must wear effective UVA protective goggles or sunglasses during exposure and for 24 hours afterwards.

In the short term, nausea is often experienced and, if too long an exposure is given, burning can occur. Patients who are 'sensitive to the sun' or who coincidently have a disorder that can be aggravated by UVA exposure, such as lupus erythematosus or porphyria cutanea tarda, should not be treated by PUVA.

So-called 'narrow-band UVR' is UVR at a wavelength of 311 nm. It has recently been introduced as an effective and less hazardous form of UVR treatment (although there is uncertainty on this issue).

Table 9.3 Side effects of PUVA treatment

Side effects	Comment
Major (long term)	
Skin cancer	Considerable increase in incidence of squamous cell carcinoma and, to a lesser extent, other types of skin cancer
Cataract	UVA-screening spectacles must be used during and 24 hours after exposure
'Photoageing'	Damage to the dermis results in the appearance of ageing and altered elastic properties
Minor (short term)	
Nausea	Probably due to the psoralen if taken orally
Burning	In some sensitive people, or if the dose of UVR is too great
Pruritus and xeroderma	Emollients are helpful

Other treatments

Numerous other treatments have been investigated in the past few years. These range from propylthiouracil to fumaric acid derivatives and new immunosuppressive agents such as tacrolimus.

Pityriasis rubra pilaris

DEFINITION

Pityriasis rubra pilaris is an uncommon skin disorder of unknown cause, which often has a superficial resemblance to psoriasis as it is characterized by redness and scaling, but has a distinctive histological appearance and a distinctive component of follicular involvement.

CLINICAL FEATURES

The commonest type of pityriasis rubra pilaris occurs in the late middle-aged or elderly and is often of sudden onset. Usually, the disease begins on the face and scalp, with pinkness and scaling, and spreads within a few days or a week or two to involve the rest of the body. There is a characteristic orange hue to the redness, and on the thickened palms there is a characteristic yellowish discoloration (Fig. 9.18). Scattered amongst the red, scaling eruptions are islands of spared

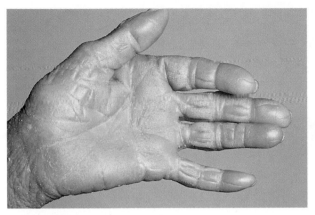

Figure 9.18 Palmar thickening due to hyperkeratosis in pityriasis rubra pilaris.

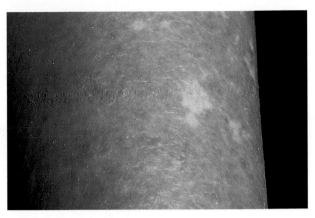

Figure 9.19 An island of white spared skin in pityriasis rubra pilaris.

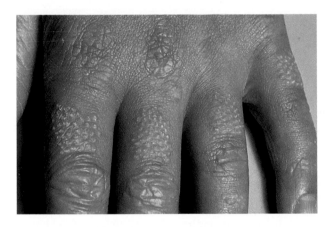

Figure 9.20 Follicular distribution of eruption in pityriasis rubra pilaris.

white skin (Fig. 9.19), and on the hands, thighs and sometimes elsewhere there is a typical follicular accentuation due to the presence of hyperkeratotic spines (Fig. 9.20).

There is also an infantile type which, although similar in many ways to the adult form, tends to be much more stubborn and resistant to treatment.

The histological appearance is distinctive in that, although there is considerable epidermal thickening, the accentuation of the dermal papillae and the undulations of the dermoepidermal junction are much less marked than in psoriasis.

TREATMENT

Many patients respond well to oral retinoids by mouth (see page 140) given in the same manner as for psoriasis. Treatment by methotrexate has also been advocated.

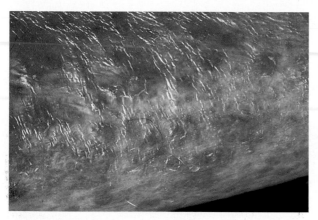

Figure 9.21 Red-mauve papules of lichen planus. Some of these have a faint white network pattern on the surface (Wickham's striae).

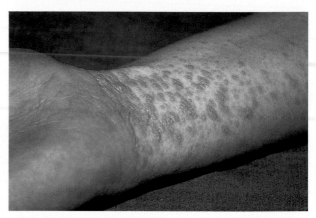

Figure 9.22 Many papules of lichen planus affecting the wrist.

Lichen planus

DEFINITION

Lichen planus is an inflammatory disorder of skin of unknown origin but with a prominent immunopathogenetic component. It is characterized by an eruption of variable extent of typical mauve or pink, flat-topped, itchy papules.

CLINICAL FEATURES

The typical lesion of lichen planus is a mauve or pink, flat-topped, polygonal papule, which often has a whitish lacework pattern on its surface (Wickham's striae) (Fig. 9.21). The papules are often aggregated in some sites, for example the front of the wrist (Fig. 9.22), but may also occur scattered sparsely over the skin of the limbs and trunk. Usually, only a few lesions develop, but in some cases the eruption may be dense and generalized.

The mucosae are often affected and lesions occur in the mouth in some 30 per cent of patients. A white lacework pattern on the buccal mucosa is the most frequently observed type of lesion (Fig. 9.23), but the tongue and elsewhere in the mouth may also be involved, with white lacework, whitish macule or punctuate lesions. The male genitalia are also sometimes affected (Fig. 9.24). The nails develop longitudinal ridges in 5–10 per cent of patients (Fig. 9.25). Less commonly, a destructive process develops in which the nail plate is lost and the nail-forming tissue (the nail matrix) is damaged.

The scalp is sometimes affected and then localized patches of hair loss and scalp scarring occur.

As lesions heal, they flatten and often leave a pigmented patch, which persists for some weeks.

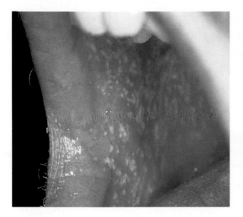

Figure 9.23 White lacework pattern on the buccal mucosa due to lichen planus.

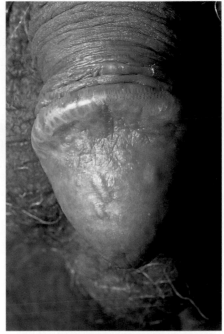

Figure 9.24 Lichen planus papules affecting the glans penis.

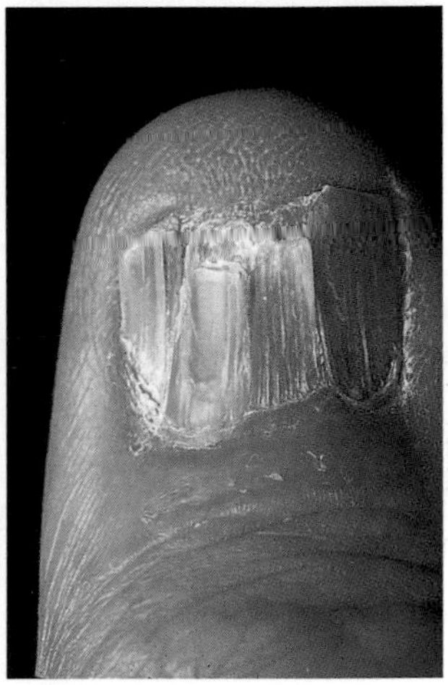

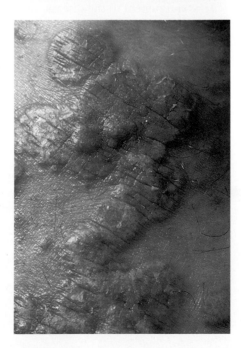

Figure 9.25 Longitudinal ridging of the nails in lichen planus.

Figure 9.26 Thickened patch of hypertrophic lichen planus.

The commonest variant is *hypertrophic lichen planus*, in which thickened, mauvish papules or nodules of irregular shape with a warty or scaling surface develop (Fig. 9.26). Solitary hypertrophic lesions may appear in the course of ordinary lichen planus or develop as solitary lesions.

Annular lichen planus describes the situation in which lichen planus lesions have fused to give a ring-type configuration. This odd variant sometimes occurs on the male genitalia and lower abdomen, but rarely elsewhere.

Lichen nitidus is a rare variant of lichen planus in which numerous tiny, pink, flat-topped papules develop.

Bullous lichen planus is a very rare variant in which blistering occurs on some lesions.

Lichen plano-pilaris predominantly involves the hair follicles. Affected sites lose their terminal hair and develop horny spines, which project from the affected hair follicles.

AETIOPATHOGENESIS

Lichen planus appears to be in the general category of autoimmune diseases and patients affected by it have a higher frequency of other autoimmune disorders than a comparable unaffected population. Myasthenia gravis and vitiligo seem particularly associated.

The disease is not uncommon in Europe, possibly accounting for some 2–4 per cent of new patients in skin clinics, but is quite uncommon in the USA. It appears to be a more frequent problem in parts of Asia. There does not seem to be a major genetic component to the disease.

Most patients are free of lesions after a year. Hypertrophic lesions tend to last for many years.

There are characteristic histopathological changes (Fig. 9.27).

- A band of lymphocytes and histiocytes immediately subepidermally. Amongst the inflammatory cell infiltrate are clumps of melanin pigment as a result of damage to the epidermis.

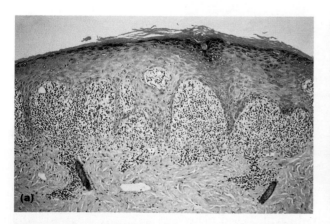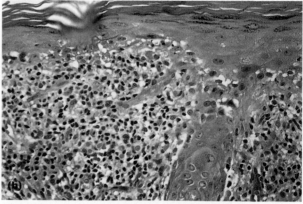

Figure 9.27 (a) Pathology of lichen planus showing typical changes, with a band of lymphocytes and histiocytes in the subepidermal region (lichenoid band) and epidermal thickening with hypergranulosis, but a 'sawtooth' pattern of erosion in the basal epidermal region. (b) Detail of the pathology of lichen planus showing the basal epidermal region with erosion, cytoid bodies and a dense lymphocytic infiltrate.

- Damage to the basal epidermal cells causing a 'sawtooth' profile, vacuolar degenerative change and scattered eosinophilic cytoid bodies representing dead epidermal cells.
- Variable epidermal thickening with increase in thickness of the granular cell layer.

Immunofluorescence studies show a dense, ragged band of fibrin at the dermo-epidermal junction and clumps of IgM deposit.

The basic process is thought of as an immunological attack on the basal layer; the presence of inflammatory cells and the other epidermal alterations are believed to be secondary events.

TREATMENT

The disease mostly remits spontaneously, so that most patients require very little treatment. Weak topical corticosteroids may be helpful in relieving the pruritus. When patients are severely affected with a generalized eruption, systemic corticosteroids are sometimes helpful, as is the oral retinoid acitretin.

Summary

Psoriasis
- Psoriasis is a genetically determined, persistent and/or recurring inflammatory dermatosis, which occurs in 1–2 per cent of the population. It usually starts between the ages of 15 and 25, but in some patients it develops in the 60s.
- It is characterized by raised, red, rounded, scaling patches of variable size that tend to occur on the elbows, knees, scalp and other extensor surfaces.
- Nail involvement occurs in many patients and is characterized by 'thimble pitting', subungual debris and areas of discoloration.
- Variants include guttate psoriasis with myriads of tiny psoriatic patches, flexural psoriasis, generalized pustular psoriasis and a localized form of pustular psoriasis occurring on the palms and soles, and erythrodermic psoriasis.
- Psoriasis needs to be distinguished from other red scaling conditions, including eczematous disorders such as seborrhoeic dermatitis, lichen simplex chronicus and discoid eczema, ringworm infections and neoplastic disorders such as Bowen's disease and superficial basal cell carcinoma.

- A seronegative rheumatoid arthritis-like condition occurs in 5–6 per cent of patients with psoriasis. In addition, in a few psoriatics, a distinctive arthropathy affects the terminal interphalangeal joints (arthritis mutilans) as well as other small and medium-sized joints.
- Histologically, the epidermis is greatly thickened and hyperplastic, with accentuation of the rete pattern. There is increased mitotic activity and decreased epidermal replacement time. The epidermis is surmounted by an incompletely differentiated stratum corneum in which the nuclei are retained. Also within the stratum corneum are collections of nuclei from polymorph leucocytes (Munro microabscesses). Polymorphs also infiltrate the thickened epidermis and there is a variable degree of lymphocytic infiltrate beneath the epidermis. The papillary capillaries are dilated and tortuous.
- The cause of psoriasis is unknown, but it is currently thought of as a lymphocyte-driven disorder in genetically susceptible individuals.
- Topical treatments include tar preparations (1–6 per cent), anthralin (0.1–5 per cent) vitamin D analogues (calcipotriol and tacalcitol)

and a novel stable acetylenic retinoid known as lazarotene.

- Some patients with extensive psoriasis benefit from treatment with one or another form of UVR. Sensitization with psoralens and radiation with long-wave UVR (known as PUVA) is an effective method, but may cause skin cancers when used over the long term.

- Severely affected patients may require oral treatments such as methotrexate, cyclosporin and acitretin, all of which may cause serious adverse side effects.

Lichen planus

- Lichen planus is a self-limiting, not uncommon inflammatory disorder of skin and mucosae of unknown origin, but with a prominent immunopathogenetic component.

- Mauve, flat-topped, itchy, angulated papules develop, on which a white lacework tracery (known as Wickham's striae) may be seen. The number of papules varies from just a few to myriads.

- A white network appears on the buccal mucosa in about 30 per cent of patients and lesions may also appear on the genitalia.

- Micropapular and hypertrophic variants are seen. The condition may also affect the scalp, causing areas of alopecia as well as involving the nails.

- Histologically, there is damage to the basal layer of the epidermis, with the formation of cytoid bodies as well as a prominent infiltrate of lymphocytes and histiocytes subepidermally. The disorder is thought to be autoimmune in nature.

- Treatment with topical corticosteroids may help to relieve the itch, but the condition is self-limiting.

Acne, rosacea and similar disorders

The disorders described in this chapter are common, inflammatory, characterized clinically by papules and occur on the face pre-eminently. These features do not imply a common aetiopathogenesis.

Acne

Acne is one of the commonest skin disorders – if not the commonest. It has been estimated that 70 per cent of the population have some clinically evident acne at some stage during adolescence!

DEFINITION

Acne (acne vulgaris) is a disorder in which hair follicles develop obstructing horny plugs (comedones), as a result of which inflammation later develops around the obstructed follicles, causing tissue destruction and scar formation.

CLINICAL FEATURES

The lesions

The earliest feature of the disorder is an increased rate of sebum secretion, making the skin look greasy (seborrhoea). Blackheads or comedones usually accompany the greasiness. They often occur over the sides of the nose and the forehead, but can occur anywhere (Fig. 10.1). Comedones are follicular plugs composed

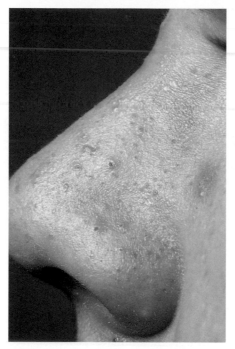

Figure 10.1 Multiple comedones and seborrhoea in acne.

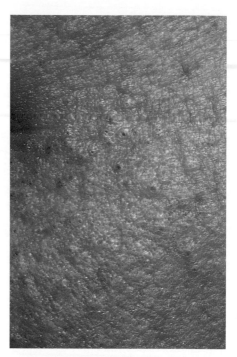

Figure 10.2 Multiple comedones in acne. Note the blackened tips from melanin.

of follicular debris and compacted sebum. They have pigmented tips from the melanin pigment deposited by the follicular epithelium at this level (Fig. 10.2). Accompanying the visible comedones are numerous invisible comedones, many of which do not have pigmented tips.

Inflamed, reddened papules develop from blocked follicles. These are often quite tender to the touch and may be set quite deep within the skin (Fig. 10.3). Sometimes they develop pus at their tips (pustules), but these may also arise independently. In a few patients, some of the papules become quite large and persist for long periods – they are then referred to as nodules.

In severely affected patients, the nodules liquefy centrally so that fluctuant cysts are formed. In reality, the lesions are pseudocysts, as they have no epithelial lining. This type of severe acne is known as cystic or nodulocystic acne and can be very disabling and disfiguring.

When the large nodules and cysts eventually subside, they leave in their wake firm, fibrotic, nodular scars, which sometimes become hypertrophic or even keloidal (Fig. 10.4a). The scars are often quite irregular and tend to form 'bridges' (Fig. 10.4b). Even the smaller inflamed papules can cause scars and these tend to be pock-like or are triangular indentations ('ice-pick scars': Fig. 10.5).

There is a very rare and severe type of cystic acne known as acne fulminans in which the acne lesions quite suddenly become very inflamed. At the same time the affected individual is unwell and develops fever and arthralgia. Laboratory

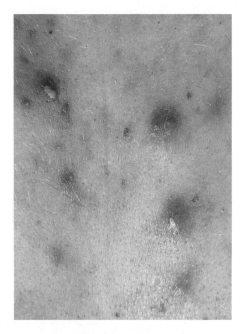

Figure 10.3 Acne papules.

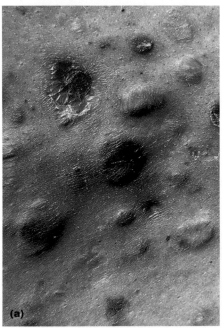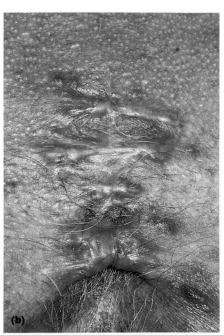

Figure 10.4 (a) Nodular scars in acne. These lesions developed following the resolution of inflamed acne papules. (b) Hypertrophic scarring in a bridging pattern.

investigation reveals a polymorphonuclear leucocytosis and odd osteolytic lesions in the bony skeleton. The cause of this disorder is not clear, although it has been suggested that it is due to the presence of a vasculitis that is somehow precipitated as a result of the underlying acne.

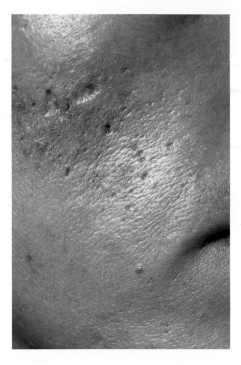

Figure 10.5 Pock scarring of acne.

SITES AFFECTED

Any hair-bearing skin can develop acne, but certain areas are much more prone than others (Fig. 10.6). These acne-prone areas tend to have hair follicles with small terminal hairs and larger sebaceous glands (sebaceous follicles). The face and particularly the skin of the cheeks, lower jaw, chin, nose and forehead are usually affected. The scalp is not involved, but the back of the neck, front of the chest, the back and shoulders are all 'favoured areas' for the development of lesions.

In patients with severe acne, it is quite common for other areas to be affected, including the outer aspects of the upper arms, the buttocks and thighs.

CLINICAL COURSE

For most of those affected, the disorder is annoying and may be troublesome, but is not of enormous significance because it is limited in extent and only lasts a few months or at the most a year. For the unfortunate few, the condition is a disaster, as it is disfiguring, disabling and persistent, with wave after wave of new lesions. Although the natural tendency is for resolution, it is difficult to know in any individual patient when the condition will improve. The majority have lost their acne by the age of 25 years, but some tend to have the occasional lesion for very much longer. In some women there is a pronounced premenstrual flare of their acne some 7–10 days before the menses begin.

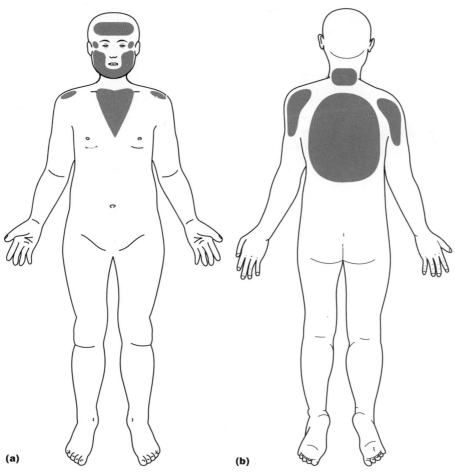

Figure 10.6 Diagram to show common sites of involvement due to acne on (a) the front of the trunk and face, and (b) the back of the trunk.

Acne improves in the summertime and sun exposure seems to improve the condition of many patients. However, the heat does not produce improvement and, indeed, can make it much worse. Soldiers with acne in hot, humid climates often become disabled by it suddenly worsening, with large areas of skin covered by inflamed and exuding acne lesions, and have to be evacuated home or to a cooler climate.

EPIDEMIOLOGY

Some 70 per cent of the population develop some clinically evident acne at some point during adolescence and early adult life, but perhaps only 10–20 per cent request medical attention for the problem. This proportion varies in different parts of the world, depending on the racial mixture, the affluence and the sophistication of medical services.

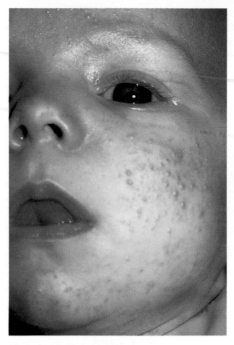

Figure 10.7 Infantile acne.

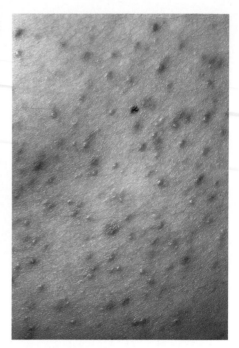

Figure 10.8 Steroid acne. The lesions tend to be more uniform in appearance than in 'ordinary' acne.

The variations in incidence in different ethnic groups have not been well characterized, although it does appear that Eskimos and Japanese suffer less from acne than do Western Caucasians.

Onset is usually at puberty or a little later, although many patients do not appear troubled until the age of 16 or 17 years. Men appear to be affected earlier and more severely than women. Older age groups are not immune and it certainly is not rare to develop acne in the sixth, seventh or even eighth decade.

Acne lesions sometimes appear on the cheeks and chin of infants a few weeks or months of age and even a little later than that (Fig. 10.7). This infantile acne is usually trivial and short lived, but can occasionally be troublesome.

SPECIAL TYPES OF ACNE

Acne from drugs and chemical agents

Androgens provide the normal 'drive' to the sebaceous glands. It is the increased secretion of these hormones that is responsible for the increased sebum secretion at puberty. When given therapeutically for any reason, they can also cause an eruption of acne spots.

Glucocorticoids, such as prednisolone, when given to suppress the signs of rheumatoid arthritis or some other chronic inflammation, can also induce troublesome acne (Fig. 10.8). Why this should be so has never been adequately

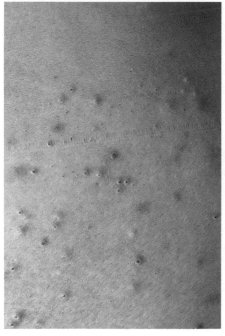

Figure 10.9 Comedones and inflamed follicular papules from tar application.

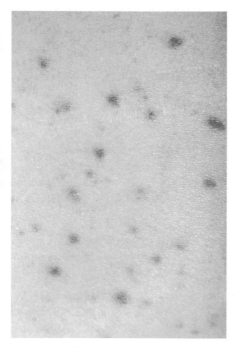

Figure 10.10 Acne due to cosmetics.

explained. Glucocorticoids do not seem to increase the rate of sebum secretion, and the acne that results is curiously monomorphic in that sheets of acne lesions appear (unlike ordinary acne) all at the same stage of development. Interestingly, corticosteroid creams can, uncommonly, also cause acne spots at the site of application.

Oil acne

Workers who come into contact with lubricating and cutting oils develop an acne-like eruption at the sites of contact, consisting of small papules, pustules and comedones. This is often observed on the fronts of the thighs and forearms, where oil-soaked overalls come in contact with the skin. A similar 'acneiform folliculitis' sometimes arises at sites of application of tar-containing ointments during the treatment of skin diseases (Fig. 10.9).

Some cosmetics seem to aggravate or even cause acne. This is because they sometimes contain comedo-inducing (comedogenic) agents, such as cocoa butter and derivatives and some mineral oils, that can induce acne. This cosmetic acne is less of a problem now that cosmetic manufacturers are aware of it (Fig. 10.10).

Chloracne

Chloracne is an extremely severe form of industrial acne due to exposure to complex chlorinated naphthalenic compounds and dioxin. Epidemics have occurred after industrial accidents such as occurred in Serveso in Italy, in which the population around the factory was affected. The compounds responsible are extremely potent, and lesions continue to develop for months after exposure. Typically, numerous large, cystic-type lesions occur in this form of industrial acne.

Excoriated acne

This disorder is most often seen in young women. Small acne spots around the chin, forehead and on the jaw line are picked, squeezed and otherwise altered by manual interference. The resulting papules are crusted and often more inflamed than routine acne spots. Often, the patients have little true acne and the main cosmetic problem is the results of the labour of their fingers!

PATHOLOGY, AETIOLOGY AND PATHOGENESIS

Histologically, the essential features are those of a folliculitis with considerable inflammation. The exact histological picture depends on the stage reached at the time of biopsy. Usually, it is possible to make out the remnants of a ruptured follicle. In the earliest stages, a follicular plug of horn (comedone) can be identified. Later, fragments of horn appear to have provoked a violent mixed inflammatory reaction with many polymorphs and, in places, a granulomatous reaction with many giant cells and histiocytes (Fig. 10.11). In older lesions, fibrous tissue is deposited, indicating scar formation.

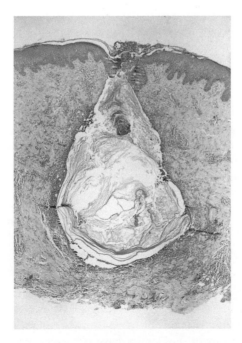

Figure 10.11 Pathology of inflamed acne papules showing a ruptured follicle and a dense inflammatory cell infiltrate composed predominantly of polymorphs.

What do we believe is the sequence of events? In the first place, patients with acne have a higher rate of sebum secretion rate (SER) compared to matched control subjects and, furthermore, there is some correlation between the extent of the increase in the SER and the severity of the acne.

Acne first appears at puberty, at which time there is a sudden increase in the level of circulating androgens. Eunuchs do not get acne, and the administration of testosterone provokes the appearance of acne lesions. Sebaceous glands are predominantly 'androgen driven' and few other influences are as important. Follicular obstruction also plays an important role. Comedones are early lesions and microscopically it is commonplace to find horny plugs in the follicular canals. Changes have been described in the follicular epithelium suggesting that there is abnormal keratinization at the mouth of the hair follicle.

Pathogenic bacteria are not found in acne lesions and are not involved in the pathogenesis. It is possible, nonetheless, that the normal flora has a role to play. The flora consists of Gram-positive cocci – the micrococci (also known as *Staphylococcus epidermidis*) – and Gram-positive bacteria – *Propionibacterium acnes*. In addition, there are also yeast-like micro-organisms known as *Pityrosporum ovale*. The *Propionibacteria* are microaerophilic and lipophilic, so that they are ideally suited to living in the depths of the hair follicle in an oily milieu, and it is not surprising that they increase in numbers during puberty when their food supply, in the form of sebum, increases. The normal follicular flora may be responsible for hydrolysing the lipid esters of sebum, liberating potentially irritating fatty acids. The constituents of sebum and of skin surface lipid (after bacterial hydrolysis) are given in Table 10.1.

How can these observations be linked? An acceptable hypothesis is set out in Figure 10.12, in which it is suggested that the important inflammatory lesions of acne are the result of follicular rupture.

Table 10.1 Main constituents of sebum and skin surface lipid

Sebum
Triglycerides
Cholesterol ester
Squalene
Wax esters
Skin surface lipid
Sebum lipids
Fatty acids
Monoglycerides
Diglycerides

TREATMENT

Typically, unasked for advice from the family is given in which the sufferer is blamed in one way or another for having the disorder and accused of doing too much of one thing or not enough of the other. Consequently, many forms of familial or folk treatments seem to be more in the nature of punishments than anything else. Dietetic and social restrictions are typical, as is more frequent washing, which is another tactic adopted by well-meaning but misguided family and friends.

Fortunately, most acne patients improve spontaneously after a few months. Those who do not, find their way to the pharmacist and purchase preparations containing benzoyl peroxide or other antimicrobial compounds, or sulphur or salicylic acid. Many with milder degrees of acne will be helped by these medications. It is only those with resistant, recalcitrant and more severe types of acne who reach the physician. Perhaps only 10 per cent of those with clinical acne in the UK see their practitioner.

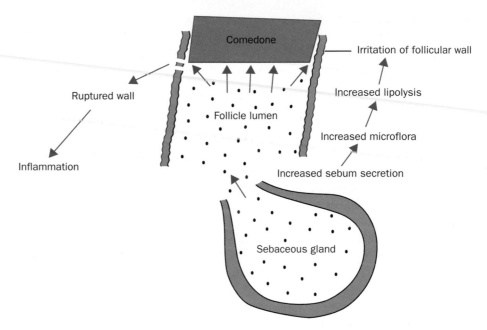

Figure 10.12 Diagram to show suggested events in the pathogenesis of acne.

Basic principles

Treatment may be aimed at:

- reducing the bacterial population of the hair follicles to cut down the hydrolysis of lipids (antimicrobial agents)
- encouraging the shedding of the follicular horny plugs to free the obstruction (comedolytic agents)
- reducing the rate of sebum production, either directly by acting on the sebaceous glands or indirectly by inhibiting the effects of androgens on the sebaceous glands (anti-androgens)
- reducing the damaging effects of acne inflammation on the skin with anti-inflammatory agents (Table 10.2).

General measures

Patients with acne are often depressed and may need sympathetic counselling and support. There is no evidence that particular foodstuffs have any deleterious effect or that washing vigorously will help remove lesions. These and other myths should be dispelled and replaced with a straightforward explanation of the nature of the disorder, its natural history and treatment.

Topical treatment

Currently, the most popular form of topical preparation is a gel, cream or alcohol-based lotion.

Table 10.2 Treatments for acne

Topical		Oral	
Antimicrobial	**Comedolytic**	**Antimicrobial**	**Sebum suppressive**
Benzoyl peroxide	Tretinoin	Tetracycline	Isotretinoin
Tetracycline	Isotretinoin	Minocycline	Cyproterone and ethinylestranol
Erythromycin	Adapalene	Doxycycline	
Clindamycin		Erythromycin	Spironolactone
Azelaic acid			

Topical retinoids

These are comedolytic. Tretinoin-containing preparations are not bactericidal, but are nonetheless effective. The *cis*-isomer of tretinoin – isotretinoin – is also used successfully for the treatment of acne. Adapalene is a recently introduced, effective topical retinoid that is also useful.

The side effects from the use of retinoid preparations include some pinkness and slight scaling of the skin surface, especially in fair, sensitive-skinned individuals. For the most part, this 'dryness' of the treated area is tolerable and decreases after continual usage. It is less marked with adapalene.

Sulphur (as elemental sulphur 2–10 per cent) has been used traditionally as a treatment for acne. It seems to be helpful for some patients, but has dropped out of fashion. Its efficacy probably depends on both its antimicrobial action and its comedolytic activity.

Other agents employed to remove blackheads include abrasive preparations. These contain particles of substances such as aluminium oxide or polyethylene beads, which literally abrade the skin surface and 'liberate' the comedones.

Topical antibiotics

Erythromycin (1–2 per cent) and clindamycin (2 per cent) preparations are quite effective for mild and moderate types of acne. Tetracycline preparations (2 per cent) are slightly less effective. Fortunately, these antibiotics have a low tendency to sensitize and are not often responsible for allergic contact dermatitis, although they may cause a minor degree of direct primary irritation.

Other antimicrobial compounds

Bacterial resistance to erythromycin frequently develops and may prove a problem in the future.

Systemic treatment

Antibiotics
Tetracyclines

Systemic tetracyclines have been the sheet anchor of treatment for moderate and severe acne for many years. Patients with many papular lesions involving several sites are suitable for systemic tetracyclines. It is usual to start treatment with a dose of 250 mg t.i.d. or 6-hourly, and then, when there is a response, to reduce the dose to that required to keep the patient free of new lesions. The improvement usually begins 4–8 weeks after starting treatment and continues over the next 2–3 months. Some 70 per cent of patients can be expected to improve on this regimen. Treatment may have to be maintained for several months or, exceptionally, even longer. With tetracycline and oxytetracycline, the drug should be given 30 minutes before a meal to prevent interference with absorption. The newer minocycline and doxycycline are given in smaller doses (50 mg or 100 mg) once or twice per day and their absorption does not seem to be affected by food.

Side effects with the tetracyclines are few and not usually serious. Gastrointestinal discomfort and diarrhoea occasionally occur. Photosensitivity was mainly a problem with older, now no longer used, analogues. Fixed drug eruption and, rarely, other acute drug rashes develop. Minocycline can cause a dark-brown pigmentation of the skin or acne scars or acral areas on the exposed part of the skin after long-continued use in a small number of patients.

Tetracyclines must not be given to pregnant women, as they are teratogenic, and must not be given to infants, as they cause a bone and tooth dystrophy in which these structures become deformed and discoloured.

Erythromycin

The efficacy of erythromycin in acne is similar to that of the tetracyclines. The starting dosage is 250 mg 6-hourly for the first few weeks, with reduction after a response has begun. Subsequently, management is as for the tetracyclines. Side effects are usually minor and restricted to nausea.

Other antibiotics and antimicrobials

Clindamycin, the quinolines and the sulphonamides are other drugs that have been used systemically for acne. None is more effective than the tetracyclines, but they may be suitable for patients who are either intolerant or who no longer respond to the tetracyclines or erythromycin. Side effects are more common and sometimes of a serious nature (e.g. blood dyscrasias).

Isotretinoin (13-*cis*-retinoic acid)

The large majority of patients with acne will respond to topical or some combination of topical and systemic drugs. However, some severely affected patients may not, and for them there is another drug that can offer relief. This agent is the retinoid isotretinoin (the same *cis*-isomer of tretinoin used topically). It reduces sebum secretion by shrinking the sebaceous glands and may also alter keratinization of the mouth of the hair follicle and have an anti-inflammatory action.

It is given in a dose of 0.5–1.0 mg/kg body weight per day, usually for a 4-month period. The response after a few weeks is to inhibit new lesions in more than 80 per cent of patients. Patients with many large cystic lesions affecting the trunk as well as the head and neck region take longer to respond and may need more than one 4-month course.

Unfortunately, toxic side effects are frequent. They range from the trivial, of which the most common is drying and cracking of the lips, to the very serious, which include teratogenicity, hepatotoxicity, bone toxicity and a blood lipid-elevating effect. The teratogenic effects are very worrisome, as the acne age group is almost identical to the reproductive age group. The effects on the fetus include facial, cardiac, renal and neural defects and are most likely to arise if the drug is taken during the first trimester. Some 30–50 per cent of pregnancies during which the drug was taken have been affected. Because of this, it is strongly recommended that if it is planned to prescribe isotretinoin for women who can conceive, effective contraceptive measures must also be planned and used during and for 2 months after stopping the drug.

Hepatotoxicity is rare, although a small rise in liver enzymes is common. A rise in triglycerides and cholesterol, such that the ratio of very low-density lipoproteins to high-density lipoproteins is increased, regularly occurs, and overall there is a 30 per cent rise in lipid levels. This is not likely to be a problem for most patients with acne, but may be for older patients. The same is true for the bone toxicity. A variety of bone anomalies have been described, including disseminated interstitial skeletal hyperostosis and osteoporosis, but these are not likely to be a problem for acne subjects. The drug has also been accused of causing severe depression, leading to suicide in some cases. The evidence for this is not strong, as severe acne patients are often depressed before starting treatment. *Because of the toxicities of this important drug it can only be prescribed from hospitals in the UK.*

Case 9

Julia was 15 when she started to develop embarrassing acne. She had noticed that her skin had been very greasy skin for the last few months. New spots appeared every day and she spent hours in front of the mirror trying to squeeze out blackheads and get rid of pustules. It made her quite depressed and matters were made worse by her parents telling her that she didn't wash her face enough and that going to discos didn't help her skin. Fortunately, her GP was more sympathetic and prescribed a benzoyl peroxide preparation and oral doxycycline, which made a big improvement after about 6 weeks.

Anti-androgens

Anti-androgens inhibit androgenic activity and reduce sebum secretion. Currently, only one anti-androgen preparation is available – Dianette. This is a mixture of an anti-androgen, cyproterone acetate (2 mg), and an oestrogen, ethinyl oestradiol (35 μg). It is a central anti-androgen, blocking the pituitary drive to androgen secretion. It also suppresses ovulation and acts as an oral contraceptive. It is not suitable for men because of its feminizing properties. It improves acne after some 6–8 weeks of use, but is not as effective as isotretinoin. It is associated with a number of minor side effects, essentially those associated with taking oral contraceptives.

Spironolactone, the potassium-sparing diuretic, has also been found to have anti-androgenic effects and has occasionally been used as a treatment for acne.

Rosacea

DEFINITION

Rosacea is a chronic inflammatory disorder of the skin of the facial convexities, characterized by persistent erythema and telangiectasia punctuated by acute episodes of swelling, papules and pustules.

CLINICAL FEATURES

Sites affected

The cheeks, forehead, nose and chin are the most frequently affected areas, making a typical cruciate pattern of skin involvement (Fig. 10.13). The flexures and periocular areas are conspicuously spared. Uncommonly, the neck and the bald area of the scalp in men are also affected. Sometimes only one or two areas are affected, and this makes diagnosis quite difficult.

The lesions

The most characteristic physical sign is that of persistent erythema, often accompanied by marked telangiectasia (Fig. 10.14). The disorder may not progress

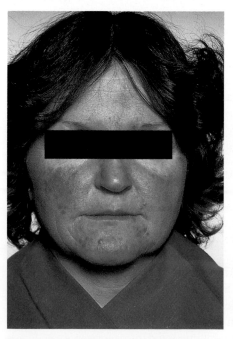

Figure 10.13 Typical rosacea with involvement of the cheeks, forehead and chin.

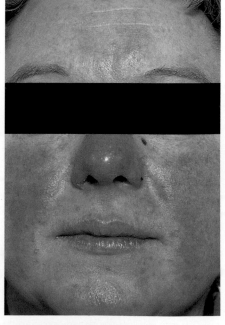

Figure 10.14 Erythema and telangiectasia in rosacea.

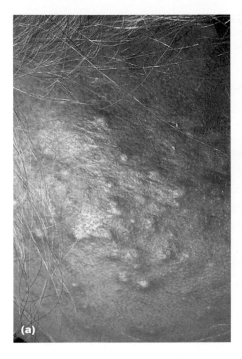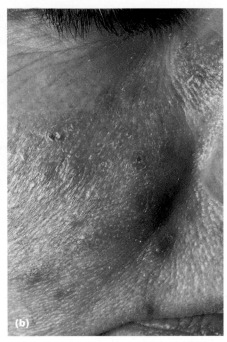

Figure 10.15 (a) and (b) Papules of facial skin in rosacea.

beyond this 'erythemato-telangiectatic' state but, even if it does not, the bright red face causes considerable social discomfort and often marked depression. Such patients also complain of frequent flushing at the most trivial stimuli.

Superimposed on this persistent background of erythema are episodes of swelling and papules, which develop for no very obvious reason (Fig. 10.15). The papules are a dull red, dome shaped and non-tender, in contrast to acne, in which they tend to be irregular and tender. Pustules also occur, but are less frequent than in acne; blackheads, cysts and scars do not.

DIFFERENTIAL DIAGNOSIS

Any red rash of the face may be confused with rosacea (Table 10.3).

Papular rashes of the face seem to cause most problems. Acne occurs in a younger age group and is usually distinguished by the greasy skin, comedones and scars as well as lesions on sites other than the face. However, in some patients, the presence of persistent erythema can make differentiation quite difficult. Perioral dermatitis (see page 168) should not be difficult to differentiate, as this disease is mainly distributed around the mouth and there is no background of erythema. Systemic lupus erythematosus may superficially resemble rosacea, become of the symmertrical butterfly erythema but there are no symptoms of systemic disease in rosacea. Dermatitis of the face (including seborrhoeic dermatitis) is marked by scaling, which is not characteristic of rosacea.

Polycythaemia rubra vera gives the face a plethoric appearance. The carcinoid syndrome is characterized by reddened areas on the face in the same

Table 10.3 Differential diagnosis of rosacea

Disorder	Positive discriminants
Skin disorders	
Acne	Scars, seborrhoea, cysts, back and chest involvement
Seborrhoeic dermatitis	Scaling involvement of flexures
Perioral dermatitis	Micropapules, perioral and paranasal involvement
Systemic disorders	
Systemic lupus erythematosus	Rash on light-exposed areas, arthropathy, positive antinuclear factor, haematological findings
Dermatomyositis	Mauve-lilac rash around the eyes, with swelling, rash on backs of fingers, muscle tenderness, pain and weakness, positive laboratory findings
Carcinoid syndrome	Marked telangiectasia, flushing attacks, hepatomegaly
Polycythaemia rubra vera	General facial redness and suffusion, possibly hepatosplenomegaly

distribution as in rosacea, but the condition is accompanied by severe systemic symptoms.

Dermatomyositis is characterized by mauvish erythema around the eyes, but the pain, tenderness and weakness of limb girdle muscles should quickly distinguish this disease.

COMPLICATIONS

Rhinophyma

This occurs mainly in elderly men, although it occasionally occurs in women too. The nose becomes irregularly enlarged and 'craggy', with accentuation of the pilosebaceous orifices (Fig. 10.16). At the same time, the nose develops a mauve or dull-red discoloration with prominent telangiectatic vessels coursing over it (Fig. 10.17). Popular names for this include 'whisky-drinkers nose' and 'grog blossom', but it is not due to alcoholism.

Lymphoedema

Persistent lymphoedema is another unpleasant, though uncommon, complication of rosacea seen predominantly in men. The swollen areas are usually a shade of red and may persist when the other manifestations of rosacea have remitted.

Ocular complications

Some 30–50 per cent of patients with acute papular rosacea have a blepharoconjunctivitis. This is usually mild, but some patients complain bitterly of soreness and

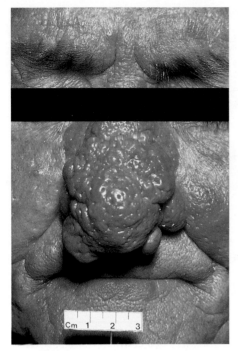

Figure 10.16 Severe, irregular, craggy enlargement of the nose due to rhinophyma.

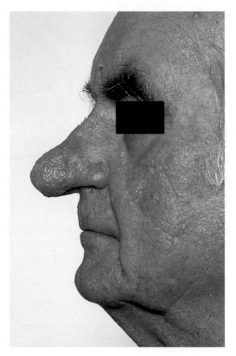

Figure 10.17 Rhinophyma with prominent telangiectasia.

grittiness of the eyes. Some of this may be the result of keratoconjunctivitis sicca, which appears to be quite common in rosacea. Styes and chalazion are also more common in rosacea. Keratitis is a rare, painful complication occurring in men, in which a vascular pannus moves across the cornea, producing severe visual defects.

NATURAL HISTORY

Rosacea tends to be a persistent disease and the tendency for patients to develop episodes of acute rosacea remains for many years after appropriate treatment has calmed down an attack.

EPIDEMIOLOGY

Rosacea is quite a common disorder, but its exact prevalence is not known and varies in different communities. The disorder is essentially one of fair-skinned Caucasians. It seems particularly common in Celtic peoples and in individuals from northwest Europe. It is only occasionally seen in darker-skinned and Asian skin types and is rare in black-skinned individuals. It has been claimed that it is more common in women, but this may be merely a reflection of the disorder being of more concern to women.

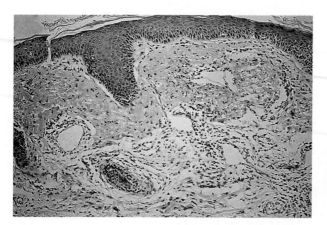

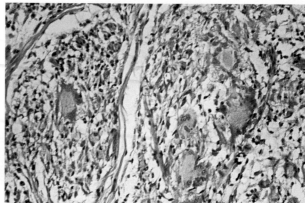

Figure 10.18 Pathology of rosacea showing marked telangiectasia, dermal oedema and marked solar degenerative change.

Figure 10.19 Pathology of rosacea showing inflammatory cell infiltrate with many lymphocytes and giant cells around blood vessels.

PATHOLOGY

There is no single pathognomonic feature, but there is a characteristic constellation of features in histological sections that makes skin biopsy a useful test when the clinical diagnosis is uncertain. A feature common to all rosacea skin samples is the presence of disorganization, solar damage, oedema and telangiectasia in the upper dermis (Fig. 10.18). When there are inflammatory papules, the blood vessels are encircled by lymphocytes and histiocytes, amongst which giant cell systems are sometimes found (Fig. 10.19). In rhinophyma, apart from abnormalities in the fibrous dermis and inflammation, there is also marked sebaceous gland hyperplasia.

AETIOLOGY AND PATHOGENESIS

The cause of rosacea remains uncertain. Historically, dietary excess, alcoholism, gastrointestinal inflammatory disease, malabsorption and psychiatric disturbance have all been though to be responsible, but controlled studies fail to implicate these agencies. The role of the mite *Demodex folliculorum*, a normal commensal of the hair follicle, is also unclear. Although it is found in increased numbers in rosacea, this increase may result from the underlying disorder in which there is follicular distortion and dilatation.

Environmental trauma appears to play an important role in the development of rosacea. The disorganization of upper dermal collagen, the excess of solar elastotic degenerative change and the predominance in fair-skinned types all point to the importance of damage to the upper dermis. Inadequate dermal support to the vasculature, which then dilates, allows pooling of the blood in this site. This pooling may then itself compromise endothelial function and ultimately result in episodes of inflammation (Fig. 10.20).

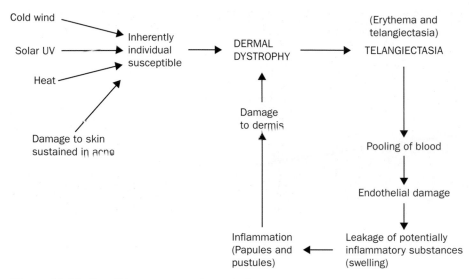

Figure 10.20 Possible sequence of events in rosacea.

Depressed delayed hypersensitivity and deposits of immunoprotein in facial skin have also been reported, suggesting that the immune system is involved in the pathogenesis.

TREATMENT

Systemic treatment

The acute episodes can be calmed with systemic tetracycline, erythromycin or metronidazole, using the full antibacterial dosage until the condition improves and then a dose sufficient to maintain improvement. Initial improvement usually occurs within the first 3–4 weeks of treatment. It would be typical for a patient to start tetracycline 250 mg 6-hourly for 3 weeks and then receive the drug three times daily for a further 3 or 4 weeks. At that time, reduction to twice-daily dosage would be made and maintained until stopping (perhaps at 10 or 12 weeks) did not result in the appearance of further papules. Minocycline or doxycycline 50 mg once or twice per day is more convenient. Erythromycin is also effective and the same dose regimen applies as for tetracycline. Metronidazole is not often given because of its side-effect profile. It has a disulfiram-like effect, causing alcohol intolerance. Other side effects include nausea and blood dyscrasias.

Isotretinoin may help some patients, particularly those who have rhinophyma, as it has been shown that it reduces the size of the enlarged nose as well as reducing the numbers of papules present.

Topical treatments

Topical corticosteroids are definitely contraindicated. Although they may suppress the inflammatory papules, they tend to make the face redder and more telangiectatic,

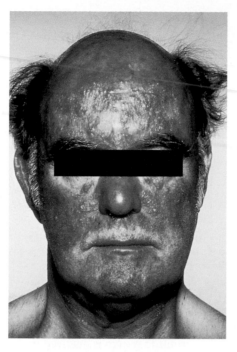

Figure 10.21 Intense erythema and telangiectasia in rosacea due to mistreatment with potent topical corticosteroids.

presumably because they cause even more upper dermal wasting and exposure of the subpapillary venous plexus (Fig. 10.21).

Facial skin may be sore and uncomfortable in rosacea and the use of emollients can give some symptomatic relief as well as discouraging the use of topical corticosteroids! Sunscreens are of help in preventing further solar damage. Preparations of 0.75–1.5 per cent metronidazole in either a cream or gel base seem capable of reducing the inflammatory papules as efficiently and as quickly as systemic tetracycline. Topical azelaic acid (20 per cent) has also been shown to be effective.

How systemic antibiotics, or metronidazole, systemic or topical, achieve their effects in rosacea is not clear. Treatment with the pulsed dye laser can greatly improve the erythema in rosacea.

Perioral dermatitis

DEFINITION

Perioral dermatitis is a not uncommon, inflammatory disorder of the skin around the mouth, characterized by the occurrence of micropapules and pustules.

CLINICAL FEATURES

Many minute, pink papules and pustules develop around the mouth, sparing the area immediately next to the vermillion of the lips (Fig. 10.22). Lesions sometimes

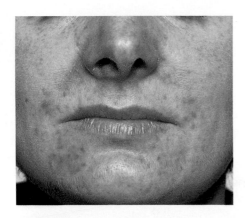

Figure 10.22 Perioral dermatitis. There are many tiny papules around the mouth.

involve the nasolabial grooves and, in severely affected patients, also affect the skin at the sides of the nose. There is no background of erythema, distinguishing the condition from rosacea.

The condition develops insidiously and seems to persist until treated. Recurrence is uncommon.

Perioral dermatitis is most common in young women aged 15–25 years, being quite rare in men and in older women. Its exact incidence is unknown, but it is of interest to know that it was first recognized in the late 1960s, seemed quite common in affluent Western communities in the 1970s and then appeared to become less frequently observed in the 1980s, reappearing once again in the 1990s. Many have suspected that the use of topical corticosteroids is to blame. Patients usually respond to a course of systemic tetracycline as for rosacea for a period of 4–8 weeks. No topical treatments are indicated.

Summary

- Acne occurs in most individuals during adolescence. It is characterized by increased sebum secretion and the formation of comedones.
- Comedones are dilated hair follicles containing horny plugs, the tips of which are black due to melanin (blackheads). These blocked follicles often leak and may rupture, causing inflammatory papules and pustules, and when several are involved, give rise to acne cysts (pseudocysts in reality) form. The inflammation causes tissue destruction and hypertrophic, keloidal, pock-like or ice-pick scars.
- The face (cheeks, chin, forehead, lower jaw and nose), back of the neck, back, shoulders and chest are the commonest sites involved.
- The disorder is not troublesome for most, but discomforting and embarrassing for many, and a complete disaster in a few. It may only last a few months, but can persist for years. Older subjects are not immune and mild acne occasionally occurs in infants. Oils and greases can aggravate or even cause acne.
- The rate of sebum secretion is increased by the surge in testosterone levels at puberty. *Propionibacterium acnes* – a major component of the normal follicular flora – is microaerophilic and lipophilic. These bacteria greatly increase in numbers in the dilated and plugged follicle. The inflammation of acne may well be caused by the leakage of follicular content and bacterial degradation products, including irritating fatty acids, into the dermis.
- Only a small proportion of acne sufferers (perhaps 10 per cent) are seen by their general practitioners.

The basic principles of treatment are to reduce the bacterial population, encourage shedding of follicular plugs (comedolysis), reduce the rate of sebum production and reduce the degree of inflammation.

- Topical retinoids (tretinoin, isotretinoin and adapalene) are comedolytic agents. They are quite effective but irritating. Topical antibiotics (erythromycin, clindamycin and tetracycline) are quite useful, as are preparations of benzoyl peroxide, which are both antimicrobial and comedolytic.

- When the acne is severe, systemic treatments are needed. Systemic tetracyclines (oxytetracycline, doxycycline or minocycline) and erythromycin are most often used. They may need to be given over some months. Systemic isotretinoin is the most effective agent for severe acne, but is capable of causing many adverse side effects, including fetal deformities if given to pregnant women. An anti-androgen preparation containing cyproterone acetate and ethinyl oestradiol is also used in female patients and may be helpful.

- Rosacea may be defined as a chronic inflammatory disorder of the convexities of facial skin, characterized by persistent erythema and telangiectasia, punctuated by acute episodes of swelling, papules and pustules. It is quite common, affecting mainly fair-complexioned adults aged 30–60.

- The cheeks, chin, nose and forehead are mainly affected, but the neck and the bald scalp of men my occasionally be involved. The papules are unlike those of acne, being non-tender and dome shaped. Blackheads, cysts and scars are not seen. Rhinophyma (irregular nasal swelling), keratitis and persistent lymphoedema of facial skin are complications seen mainly in men.

- Rosacea needs to be distinguished from acne, seborrhoeic dermatitis and other disorders with reddened facial skin, such as lupus erythematosus and dermatomyositis.

- The cause is unknown, but the occurrence in fair-skinned individuals on light-exposed sites and the presence of a marked degree of solar damage histologically suggest that photodamage plays a major role.

- The condition tends to persist, but acute episodes usually respond to oral tetracycline or erythromycin or topical metronidazole. Topical corticosteroids tend to aggravate the disorder.

- Perioral dermatitis is a disorder in which micropapules and papulopustules occur periorally and paranasally in young women. It responds to oral tetracycline but not to topical preparations.

Wound healing and ulcers

Principles of wound healing

Wound healing is a complex and fundamental activity of all damaged body structures. The same principles underlie the healing of cuts, abrasions, ulcers and areas damaged by chemical attack, invasion by micro-organisms or immune reactions.

Healing of the skin damaged by a physical insult may be divided into:

- an immediate haemostatic phase,
- an early phase of re-epithelialization,
- a later phase of dermal repair and remodelling (Fig. 11.1).

It is hoped that better understanding of the complex interactions and their controls will result in new techniques and substances for the treatment of non-healing wounds. Persistent non-healing ulcers of the skin are very common and cause much unhappiness, disablement and economic loss.

FACTORS IMPORTANT IN THE HEALING OF WOUNDS

- Adequate supplies of nutrients and oxygen are required for efficient healing; when the blood supply is compromised, healing is delayed. Vitamin C and zinc deficiencies are amongst the deficiency states also associated with delayed wound healing.

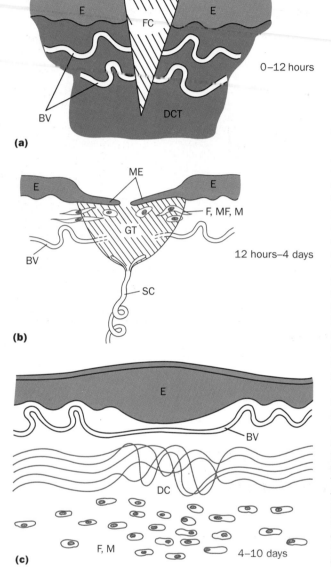

(a) 0–12 hours

(b) 12 hours–4 days

(c) 4–10 days

Figure 11.1 The sequence of events after incisional wounding of the skin. (a) *0 to 12 hours*. Initially, the small blood vessels constrict and then platelets plug the endothelial gaps. The extravasated blood clots form a temporary plug for the wound. White cells accumulate at the interface between the damaged and the normal tissue. (b) *12 hours to 4 days*. After some 18–24 hours, epidermal cells actively move on to the surface of the defect. Epidermal cells at the sides of the wound divide some hours later to make good the loss. Epidermis also sprouts from the cut ends of the sweat coils and hair follicles. After 2–4 days, new capillaries start to sprout and vascularize the granulation tissue in the wound cavity. Damaged connective tissue is destroyed and removed by macrophages, and new collagen is secreted by fibroblasts. Myofibroblasts are fibroblastic cells that develop the power to contract and are responsible for wound contraction. (c) *4 to 10 days*. Between 4 and 10 days after wounding, the wound cavity has become covered with new epidermis, whose stratum corneum does not possess normal barrier efficiency until the end of this period. The granulation tissue has been replaced by a new dermis whose collagenous fibres are not yet orientated. In the later stages, remodelling takes place so that orientation of the dermal collagenous bundles to the original lines of stress occurs. Scar formation occurs when there has been significant damage to the dermis. The epidermis ultimately develops a normal profile and the vasculature is also restored to normal contractility. E = epidermis; DCT = dermal connective tissue; BV = blood vessel; FC = fibrin clot; ME = migrating epidermis; F = fibroblasts; MF = myofibroblasts; M = macrophages; DC = dermal collagen; GT = granulation tissue; SC = sweat coil.

- Persistent infection with tuberculosis, *Mycobacterium ulcerans* or syphilis causes ulcerative conditions directly due to an infection. Any ulcerated area becomes contaminated by microbes in the environment and often this 'secondary infection' causes further tissue destruction.
- In some uncommon congenital disorders, there is delayed wound healing because the orderly sequence is disrupted. These disorders include factor XIII deficiency, in which there are abnormalities of cross-linking of fibronectin and

Table 11.1 Common causes of persistent ulcers

Condition	Aetiopathogenesis	Site(s)	Features
Venous ulcer	Venous incompetence, venous hypertension, tissue oedema and inflammation	Medial malleolus commonly and ankle nearby	Sloughy; signs of venous hypertension
Ischaemic ulcer	Atherosclerosis in most instances	Mostly feet and lower legs	Painful; occurring in atrophic skin
Ulcer due to vasculitis	Polyarteritis nodosa and Henoch–Schönlein purpura are examples of vasculitic disorders causing ulcers	Commonly on the legs, but anywhere can be affected	Lesions often start as purpuric patches or nodules
Neuropathic ulcer	Inadvertent repetitive injury because of sensory loss – common in diabetes and leprosy	Soles of feet particularly	Deeply perforating ulcers are characteristic
Decubitus ulcer	Pressure on skin of dependent parts in unconscious or paralysed patients	Sacrum ischial region, heels, scapular region, back of head, elbows	Deep sloughy ulcers

collagen, protein C deficiency and Marfan's syndrome, in which there are abnormalities of dermal connective tissue repair.

The common causes of persistent leg ulcers are given in Table 11.1.

Venous hypertension, the gravitational syndrome and venous ulceration

VENOUS HYPERTENSION

Epidemiology

It has been estimated that between 0.5 and 1.0 per cent of the population of the UK suffers from venous ulcers at any one time. The disorder is most often seen after the age of 60 and women are more often affected – particularly the multiparous. It is mostly a problem of the poor and underprivileged. Interestingly, it does not occur with equal prevalence in all racial groups, for example it is rare in Arabic peoples.

Pathology and pathogenesis

When venous return is impeded, hypertension develops in the venous circulation behind the blockage. This results in the development of dilatation of the small

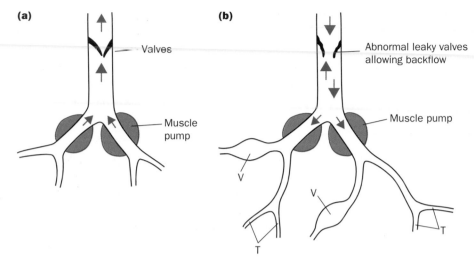

Figure 11.2 (a) Normal venous return from the legs. (b) Venous hypertension due to leaky valves.
V = varicosities
T = telangiectatic vessels

venules and, because of the changed pressure relationships at the tissue level, exudation into the tissues and oedema.

This situation arises in the leg veins when the venous valves are faulty. Blood leaks back through these faulty valves after being pushed towards the heart by the 'muscle pump' of the lower leg (Fig. 11.2). The valves become faulty because venous thrombosis destroys them, but are sometimes congenitally faulty. Venous hypertension caused by the back pressure is transmitted back to the smaller superficial veins via perforating veins, causing varicosities and telangiectasia (Figs 11.3 and 11.4).

The increased pressure at the venous end of the capillaries leads to transudation and the deposition of fibrin perivascularly (Fig. 11.4). The tissue oedema and

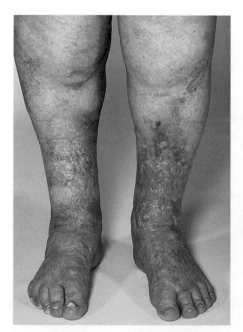

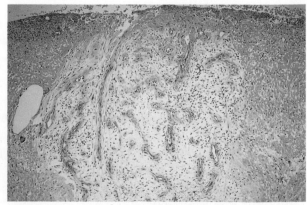

Figure 11.3 The results of venous hypertension – 'the gravitational syndrome'. Note the pigmentation, telangiectasia and visible varicosities.

Figure 11.4 Pathology of venous hypertension showing thickening and increase in number of small blood vessels in the dermis.

the fibrin cause hypoxaemia, inflammation and eventually fibrosis. Extravasation of red blood cells results in the deposition of haemosiderin pigment in dermal macrophages, imparting a brownish pigmentation to the skin.

The small blood vessels thicken and proliferate in response to the hypoxaemia, giving rise to a characteristic histological picture that can, because of the vascular proliferation, in extreme cases resemble Kaposi's sarcoma (see page 223).

Clinical features

The earliest signs are of pitting ankle oedema and distended superficial long veins in the lower leg. A network of smaller veins appears around the foot. Later, brownish discoloration develops and the swelling becomes firmer and eventually woody to the touch because of the fibrosis (Fig. 11.5). Ulceration may occur at any stage, usually after a minor injury that does not heal but steadily enlarges.

Venous ulcers are usually seen around the medial malleolus, but sometimes occur elsewhere and are usually single (Figs 11.6 and 11.7). Large ulcers may encircle the leg. The base of venous ulcers is often lined by a yellowish grey slough and the edges are for the most part flush with the skin surface and irregular in outline (Fig. 11.7).

Course and prognosis

Many ulcers heal, but may take many months to do so. Unfortunately, when healed, they tend to recur. Some never completely heal, but run a remittent course.

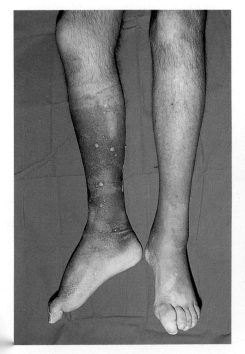

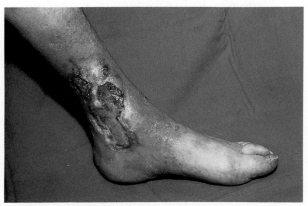

Figure 11.5 Venous hypertension. Note the pigmentation and appearance of the skin, suggesting that it is bound down to underlying tissues.

Figure 11.6 Typical venous ulcer.

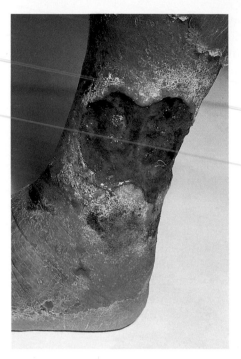

Figure 11.7 Venous ulcer with exudative base and sloughy appearance of surrounding skin.

Complications

- *Infection.* They may become severely infected with either Gram-positive cocci or Gram-negative micro-organisms.
- *Bleeding.* Uncommonly, large veins may rupture and cause severe bleeding.
- *Eczema.* An eczematous rash is common in patients with venous ulcers. In two-thirds to three-quarters of patients, this is the result of allergic contact hyper-sensitivity to one of the medicaments used in treatment (e.g. neomycin, Vioform) or one of the constituents of the vehicle (e.g. lanolin or ethylene diamine; see page 123). In a few patients, autosensitization is thought to occur in which sensitivity to the breakdown products from the ulcerated area develops. Venous eczema develops on the opposite leg, the lateral aspects of the thighs and the upper arms and at other scattered sites.
- *Malignant change.* Rarely, squamous cell carcinoma or basal cell carcinoma develops in long-standing lesions.
- *Anaemia.* Patients with persistent ulcers often develop a normochromic anaemia and are generally debilitated. The loss of protein, salts and metabolites in the exudates from the open area and absorption of products of tissue degradation and bacterial activity are probably responsible.

Treatment

The most useful approach is to try to improve venous drainage by:

- Elevation of the legs above the head level at regular periods during the day (two 1-hour periods).

- Compression bandaging, using either specially made elasticated stockings or elasticated bandage. The pressure should be graduated so that it is greatest at the ankle and least at the top of the bandage or stocking. Care must be taken to ensure that there is no restriction of arterial blood supply.
- Gentle regular exercise to ensure that the 'calf muscle pump' assists in the return of blood towards the heart.
- Weight reduction.

Dressings

Non-adherent, non-toxic, non-sensitizing dressings should be used. Antibacterial properties are also helpful. In addition, dressings should ideally be partially absorptive and semi-occlusive to provide high humidity at the wound interface. This promotes re-epithelialization. 'Hydrocolloid' dressing materials, gels and some paste bandages are suitable. Tulle dressings are also acceptable.

Topical treatments

The ulcer base may be irrigated with normal saline, dilute potassium permanganate solution or very weak chlorhexidine or hypochlorite solutions. Many 'traditional' agents are damaging to the healing tissues and must not be left in contact with the wound surface.

Surgery

Split skin fragment grafts may speed ulcer healing in the short term, but may not improve the long-term outlook. Grafts with skin cultivated *in vitro* have also been used with some success. Surgical management of the incompetent veins may assist in some cases.

Case 10

Andrew was fed up. At the age of 79 he had been all through the 1939–45 war without serious injury, but now he had a large, non-healing ulcer on his right ankle (just above the medial malleolus). It hurt quite a bit, but he found that the oozing and unpleasant smell it caused were even more troublesome. Andrew had the ulcer for 3 months and wanted to get rid of it. His ankles were swollen and there was some brown discoloration around both of them. The dermatologist told him that the ulcer was due to the veins not draining the blood back from his legs efficiently. Andrew was told to lose weight, to use elasticated stockings and to elevate his legs for at least 2 hours per day. Arrangements were made for the district nurse to dress his ulcer three times a week with a non-adherent dressing, and he was happy when it started to heal a few months later.

Ischaemic ulceration

Ulceration due to ischaemia is a common clinical problem, though less often seen than that due to venous hypertension.

PATHOGENESIS

Atherosclerosis accounts for the majority of cases. This affects major vessels and mostly occurs gradually, so that the ulceration occurs in chronically ischaemic skin. Embolism may cause acute ulceration and gangrene.

Diabetes predisposes to atherosclerosis and impairs wound healing, making the problem particularly common. Disease of the medium-sized or small blood vessels also causes ulceration in allergic vasculitis.

It should be noted that 'ischaemic' and 'venous' ulcers are often due to both processes, although one predominates, as venous hypertension and atherosclerotic arterial disease are common and often coexist.

CLINICAL FEATURES

Ischaemic ulcers are painful and irregular, occurring anywhere around the feet or lower legs. The skin around the ulcerated area is pale, cool, smooth and hairless. Light pressure with a finger on the skin makes it a deathly white and the pink colour takes longer to return than normal.

TREATMENT

Medical treatment is only helpful in the earliest and mildest cases. Keeping the affected part warm and protecting it from injury are important. Peripheral vasodilating drugs are only marginally useful (e.g. pentaerythritol tetranitrate, glyceryl trinitrate, isosorbide dinitrate, nifedipine). Drugs promoting vascular flow, such as hydroxyethyl rutosides and oxpentifylline, are rarely helpful.

Sympathectomy removes sympathetic vasoconstrictor tone and causes some vasodilatation, but rarely results in much clinical benefit. Of greater help is endarterectomy, either by open surgical technique or percutaneously, or arterial grafting.

Decubitus ulceration

These lesions are the result of localized ischaemia due to long-continued pressure on skin at contact points with bedclothes and occurs in the unconscious or paralysed patient.

CLINICAL FEATURES

Classically, ulcers occur over the sacrum or ischial regions (Fig. 11.8), the heels, the back of the head, the scapulae and the elbows. The ulcers are often deeply penetrating and sloughy.

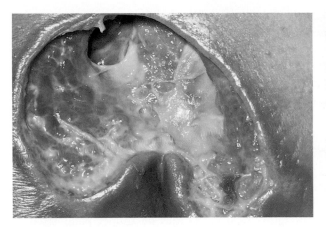

Figure 11.8 Ischial ulceration in a paralysed patient.

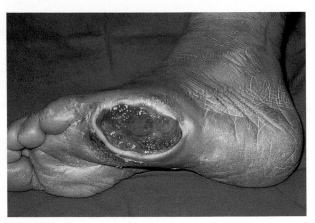

Figure 11.9 Neuropathic ulcer.

PROPHYLAXIS AND TREATMENT

Meticulously careful nursing, with regular turning and the use of sheep's fleece bedding or 'ripple' mattresses that constantly change pressure points, helps prevent decubitus ulcers. Maintenance of nutrition and general health as much as possible will also aid in the prevention of 'pressure sores'.

The individual ulcerated lesions need cleaning with non-toxic antibacterial solutions and dressing with non-adherent, non-toxic dressings (as for venous ulcers).

Neuropathic ulcers

Neuropathic ulcers result from repeated, inadvertent injury to hypoanaesthetic or anaesthetic areas of skin subsequent to nerve injury. They are most often seen in diabetes in the UK and Europe, but leprosy is a common cause in some parts of the world.

CLINICAL FEATURES

These lesions may be very deeply penetrating. They occur mostly on the soles of the feet, but may also be seen elsewhere on the foot (Fig. 11.9).

TREATMENT

Local treatment is unlikely to make any impact on these lesions. The only effective treatment is to protect the damaged area with padding and appliances and, if possible, to restore sensation to the anaesthetic area.

Less common causes of ulceration

PYODERMA GANGRENOSUM

This is a rare, serious ulcerative disorder that is often due to serious underlying systemic disease.

Clinical features

Usually, an acutely inflamed, purplish nodule rapidly becomes an ulcer, which then spreads with frightening speed (Fig. 11.10). The ulcer characteristically has bluish-mauve, undermined margins. Such ulcers may be 'dinner plate' sized or even larger. Eventually, they become static in size and may then spontaneously heal. Some patients have multiple lesions and may succumb to the disorder. Lesions may recur or new ones may develop after a quiescent phase.

Aetiopathogenesis

The disorder may occur in the course of ulcerative colitis, Crohn's disease, rheumatoid arthritis or myeloma, although in about half the cases no predisposing cause is found. It has been suggested that the tissue destruction is caused by a vasculitis, although it is difficult to find evidence of this.

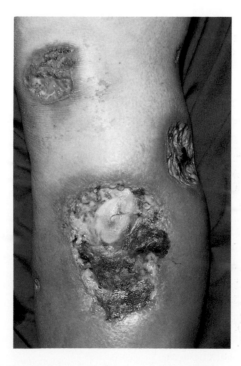

Figure 11.10 Multiple ulcers of the leg in pyoderma gangrenosum, which developed over a 3-day period.

Treatment

Drugs, including cyclosporin, minocycline and dapsone, have been reported as promoting the healing of pyoderma gangrenosum lesions.

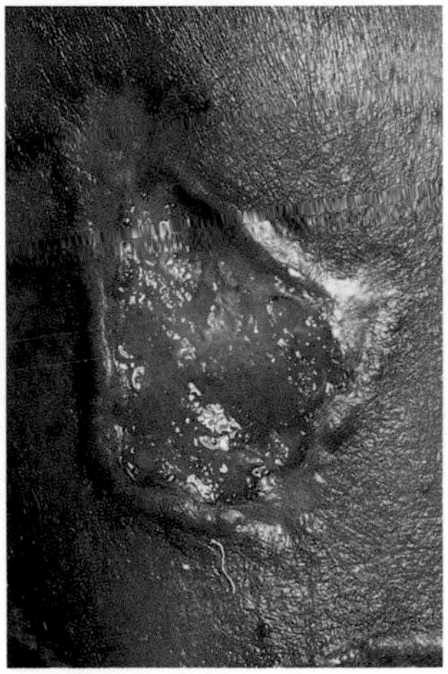

VASCULITIC ULCERS

Ulcers may develop in the course of a disorder in which small blood vessels become inflamed and thrombosed (vasculitic). Rheumatoid vasculitis is one such condition in which ulceration may occur. Ulcers often occur on the legs (Fig. 11.11), but may develop anywhere. They may start from a patch of purpura. Treatment is directed towards the underlying illness.

HAEMATOLOGICAL CAUSES

Leg ulcers are more common in patients with sickle cell disease and idiopathic thrombocytopenic purpura.

INFECTIVE CAUSES

Tuberculosis, tertiary syphilis and deep fungus infections can all result in persistent ulcers.

ARTERIOVENOUS MALFORMATION

Shunting of the blood at deeper levels may deprive the overlying skin and cause ulcers (Fig. 11.12).

Figure 11.11 Vasculitic ulcer.

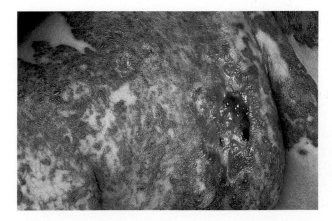

Figure 11.12 Ulcerated area in a vascular birthmark.

MALIGNANT DISEASE

This is an uncommon, but important to recognize, cause of persistent ulceration. The lesions are usually squamous cell carcinoma or basal cell carcinoma. They have raised edges and are slowly but relentlessly progressive.

Diagnosis and assessment of ulcers

Before treatment is planned, it is important to reach a definitive diagnosis and assess the social background of the patient. The history and the appearance of the lesion and surrounding skin are the most important sources of diagnostic information.

A biopsy from the margin may provide useful information and will do no harm. Bacterial swabs are not often helpful unless the ulcer is obviously clinically infected, as an open wound will always harbour a large number of microbes. Haematological tests will identify underlying anaemia, a leucocytosis due to infection and rare haematological disorders.

Venography, arteriography, measurement of blood pressure at the ankle and ultrasound Doppler blood flow studies are amongst the tests that may assist in assessment. Laser Doppler devices can even image capillary blood flow in the skin, providing potentially important information.

Summary

- Non-healing may be due to inadequate nutrition, infection or a congenital disorder (e.g. factor XIII deficiency). Leg ulcers are a very common cause of disability. The commonest cause of leg ulcers is venous hypertension due to faulty venous valves, which is most often seen in the elderly. The inadequate venous return causes venous hypertension, resulting in oedema, extravasation of blood into the tissues, thickening of the small vessels, perivascular deposition of fibrin and inflammation leading to fibrosis.
- Oedema, telangiectasia and brown discoloration usually precede ulceration. Such ulcers are sloughy and of varying size. They occur around the medial malleolus and tend to persist, but elevation, compression bandaging and weight reduction are important in their treatment. Dressings should be non-adherent, absorptive and non-toxic.
- Ischaemic ulceration is due to inadequate blood supply to the skin and usually the result of atherosclerosis. Often, there is an element of ischaemia in venous ulceration. Affected skin tends to be pale, smooth and hairless and the ulcer itself is painful and may occur anywhere over the foot. Treatment must be directed towards increasing the blood supply.
- Decubitus ulceration is due to localized ischaemia resulting from pressure on the skin at certain points, such as over the sacrum and on the heels, in unconscious or paralysed patients. It can be prevented by careful nursing.
- Neuropathic ulcers are due to repeated trauma to anaesthetic skin in patients with diabetes or leprosy. They are often deeply penetrating and often occur on the soles of the feet.
- Pyoderma gangrenosum may occur anywhere over the skin in patients with ulcerative colitis, rheumatoid arthritis or no identifiable underlying problem. The ulcers occur on inflamed skin and may enlarge rapidly.
- Vasculitis, sickle cell disease and malignant disease are other causes of ulceration.

Benign tumours, moles, birthmarks and cysts

Introduction

The many cell and tissue types in skin is responsible for the enormous number of benign tumours that may arise from it. Despite the large number of such lesions, they have a limited number of clinical appearances and, because of this, accurate clinical diagnosis is difficult. The treatment of all the lesions included is discussed together at the end of the chapter.

Tumours of epidermal origin

SEBORRHOEIC WARTS

Also known as basal cell papillomas, seborrhoeic warts are extremely common, benign tumours of ageing skin. Most patients over the age of 40 years have seborrhoeic warts – some have literally hundreds. They seem to be most common in Caucasians, but similar lesions are seen in black-skinned and Asian peoples.

Clinical appearance

Their commonest clinical appearance is that of a brownish, warty nodule or plaque on the upper trunk (Fig. 12.1) or head and neck regions. Their pigmentation varies from light fawn to black. They may occur as solitary lesions, but are usually multiple and quite often present in vast numbers (Fig. 12.2). They often have a greasy and 'stuck on' look. In black-skinned people, they may appear as multiple, blackish, dome-shaped warty papules over the face, a condition known as dermatosis papulosa nigra. The differential diagnosis of warty lesions is given in Table 12.1. When deeply pigmented, they are sometimes mistaken for malignant melanoma.

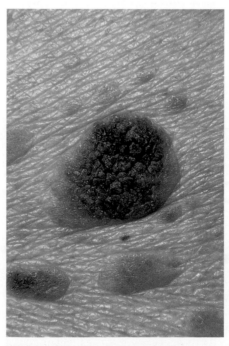

Figure 12.1 Typical brown/black, 'stuck-on' warty lesions known as seborrhoeic warts.

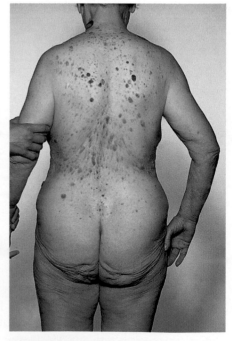

Figure 12.2 Large numbers of seborrhoeic warts.

Table 12.1 Differential diagnosis of warty tumours

Lesion	Comment
Seborrhoeic wart	Mostly in elderly individuals and multiple; may have a greasy, 'stuck-on' appearance
Viral wart	Not usually pigmented; mostly in younger individuals on hands, feet, face and genitalia
Solar keratosis	Flat, pink and scaly usually, but can have a horny or warty surface; mostly on the backs of hands and face
Epidermal naevus	Usually since birth; anywhere on body; often a linear arrangement

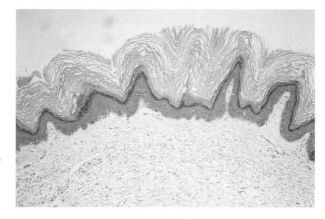

Figure 12.3 Pathology of a flat seborrhoeic wart showing 'church spire' arrangement.

They usually cause no symptoms, but patients complain that they catch in clothing and are unsightly. They may also irritate and, less frequently, become inflamed and cause soreness and pain.

Histologically, there is epidermal thickening, the predominant cell being rather like the normal basal epidermal cell. Surmounting the thickened epidermis there is a warty hyperkeratosis whose arrangement has been likened to a series of church spires (Fig. 12.3). Within the lesion are foci of keratinization and horn cysts.

EPIDERMAL NAEVUS

Epidermal naevus is the name given to a wide variety of uncommon, localized malformations of the epidermis. Congenital in origin, they are classified as hamartomata and are usually present at birth.

Clinical appearance

Many epidermal naevi are arranged linearly and are warty. Sometimes they track along a limb and adjoining trunk and are extensive and disfiguring. This type is known as naevus unius lateris (Fig. 12.4). Histologically, there is regular epidermal thickening and hyperkeratosis, often in a church-spire pattern.

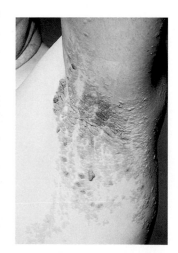

Figure 12.4 Naevus unius lateris – linear warty lesion.

185

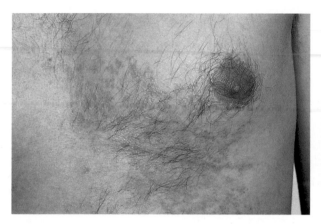

Figure 12.5 Becker's naevus on the chest wall. The affected area is pigmented, thickened and hairy.

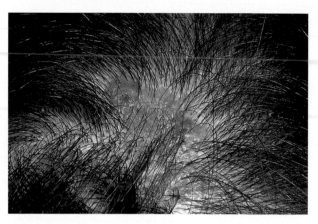

Figure 12.6 Typical orange plaque of naevus sebaceous on the scalp.

VARIANTS

Becker's naevus is an odd type of hamartomatous lesion that develops in adolescence or early adult life. It usually occurs around the shoulders or upper arms, but is not unknown elsewhere. A comparatively large area of skin is affected by a brownish and sometimes hairy plaque (Fig. 12.5). It consists of hypertrophy of all the epidermal structures, including the hair follicles and melanocytes.

Naevus sebaceous lesions are yellowish orange plaques on the scalp, which contain hypertrophied and deformed structures of epidermal origin in various amounts. They are either present at birth or shortly afterwards, and may enlarge, thicken and develop other lesions in them, such as basal cell carcinoma in adult life (Fig. 12.6).

Benign tumours of sweat gland origin

The more common benign tumours of sweat gland origin are listed in Table 12.2. The most common are described below.

SYRINGOMA

Syringoma lesions are multiple, small, white or skin-coloured papules that occur below the eyes (Fig. 12.7) in young adults. Uncommonly, they are also evident on the arms and lower trunk. Histologically, there are tiny, comma-shaped epithelial structures, some of which appear cuticle lined, forming microcysts (Fig. 12.8).

CYLINDROMA

This is a benign tumour arising from apocrine sweat glands that, like syringoma, is often multiple. Smooth, pink and skin-coloured nodules and papules occur over

Table 12.2 Benign tumours of sweat gland origin

Syringoma	Multiple white papules beneath eyes; composed of tiny cysts and comma-shaped epithelial clumps
Cylindroma	Solitary or multiple nodules on face or scalp; clumps of basaloid cells with eosinophilic colloid material
Syringocystadenoma papilliferum	Mostly develop in naevus sebaceous on scalp or on mons pubis
Nodular hidradenoma	Skin coloured or, rarely, pigmented solitary nodule of epithelial cells and ducts
Eccrine poroma	Solitary nodule on palms or soles or, rarely, elsewhere; basaloid clumps in upper dermis
Eccrine spiradenoma	Tender and painful solitary nodule

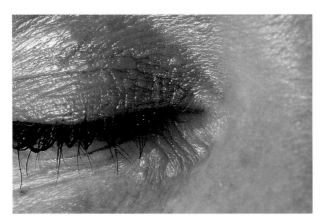

Figure 12.7 Syringoma lesions beneath the eye.

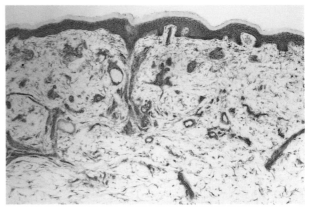

Figure 12.8 Pathology of syringoma showing many comma-shaped epithelial structures and tiny cysts.

the scalp and face in young adults. Oval and rounded masses of basaloid epidermal cells surrounded by an eosinophilic band of homogeneous connective tissue characterize the histological appearance.

NODULAR HIDRADENOMA

This is a rare benign tumour of sweat gland epithelium. It is usually solitary and may be pigmented. Histologically, it consists of clumps of small epithelial cells amongst which are duct-like structures.

ECCRINE POROMA

Eccrine poroma describes an eccrine sweat duct-derived tumour that arises predominantly on the palms and soles in adults. Histologically, the lesion appears contiguous with the surface epidermis and consists of basaloid cells in which there are cuticularly lined duct-like structures.

Benign tumours of hair follicle origin

PILOMATRIXOMA

Pilomatrixoma (calcifying epithelioma of Malherbe) develops around the head, neck and upper trunk in young adults as a solitary, smooth, skin-coloured or bluish nodule. Clumps of basal cells progressively become calcified and eventually ossified, leaving behind their cell walls only (ghost cells).

TRICHOEPITHELIOMA

Trichoepithelioma is more often multiple than solitary and usually occurs over the scalp and face. Histologically, it consists for the most part of clumps of epithelial cells and horn-filled cysts.

SEBACEOUS GLAND HYPERPLASIA

Sebaceous gland hyperplasia is a common feature of elderly skin and has been suspected to be due to chronic solar damage rather than ageing. One or, more often, several yellowish, skin-coloured papules develop over the skin of the face, some of which have central puncta (Fig. 12.9). They are often mistaken for basal cell carcinomata or dermal cellular naevi. Histologically, they consist of hypertrophied lobules of normal sebaceous gland tissue.

CLEAR CELL ACANTHOMA (DEGOS ACANTHOMA)

Clinically, this is usually a moist, pink papule or nodule on the upper arms, thighs or trunk that has been present, unchanging, for several years. The name derives from the epidermal thickening composed of large cells that, when stained with periodic acid-Schiff reagent, are found to be stuffed with glycogen (Fig. 12.10) and infiltrated with polymorphonuclear leucocytes.

Melanocytic naevi (moles)

These are developmental anomalies consisting of immature melanocytes in abnormal numbers and sites within the skin. They are very common and, on average, white-skinned Caucasians have 16 over the skin surface. Melanocytic naevi come in a wide variety of shapes and sizes and the main types are summarized in Table 12.3.

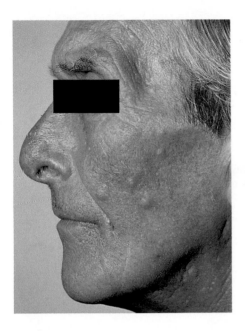

Figure 12.9 Sebaceous gland hyperplasia. Note the multiple yellowish papules on the face.

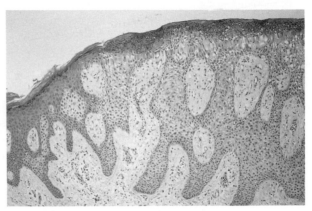

Figure 12.10 Pathology of clear cell acanthoma showing hypertrophied epidermis with areas of large, pale epithelial cells.

Table 12.3 Main varieties of melanocytic naevi

Type	Clinical features	Comment
Congenital/simple	Present since birth, tend to be larger than acquired naevi	Increased tendency for malignant transformation
Girdle	Cover large areas around pelvic or pectoral zone (bathing trunk or cape naevus)	Compare to acquired naevi
Acquired	Develop mainly in late childhood and early adolescence	
Junctional	Macular, brown/black	Anywhere on skin or mucosae
Dermal cellular	Papular or nodular, may be hairy; usually light brown or skin coloured	Very common on face and scalp
Compound		Combination of dermal, cellular and junctional
Naevus spilus	Large, speckled, light-brown naevus	Uncommon
Dysplastic naevus syndrome	Many moles with irregular margins and pigmentation; may be sporadic but also familial	Increased tendency to malignant melanoma
Juvenile melanoma	Orange-pink nodule or plaque in childhood	Histological picture may simulate melanoma
Blue naevus	Blue due to depth of pigment in dermis	
Cellular blue naevus	Bluish nodule on scalp, hands or feet	
Mongolian spot	Large, flat, greyish blue macule	Present at birth over sacrum; may fade
Naevus of Ota or Ito	Flat, blue-grey areas on face and neck	Predominantly in Asians

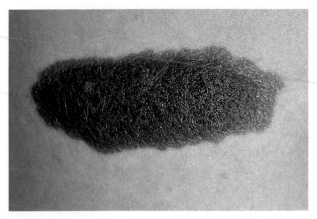

Figure 12.11 Large congenital melanocytic naevus.

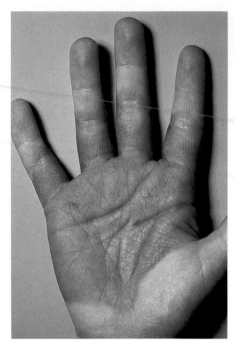

Figure 12.12 Congenital naevus affecting most of one hand.

CONGENITAL NAEVI

These lesions, which are present at birth, are usually solitary and dark brown, and are more than $1\,cm^2$ in size. They are plaque-like or nodular (Fig. 12.11). They share with the limb girdle naevus the increased tendency to malignant transformation. It has been suggested that 10 per cent of the larger congenital naevi develop malignant melanoma.

The most deforming congenital melanocytic naevi are those that cover large tracts of skin on the pelvic region and adjoining back (bathing trunk naevi) or over the shoulder region and upper limb (cape naevi: Fig. 12.12). Histologically, these lesions consist of numerous 'packets' (theques) of naevus cells (Fig. 12.13), which may be small and basophilic (lymphocytoid), large and less intensely staining (epithelioid) or spindle shaped. They may also coalesce to form naevus giant cells or, after they have been present for many years, may show degenerative changes, including fatty degeneration and calcification. Naevus cells tend to be faceted together in a rather characteristic way.

ACQUIRED NAEVI

Acquired naevi appear after birth, usually during adolescence or young adult life. Potential difficulty arises when an adult notices a brown lesion for the first time. Has it been there for many years before being noticed? Or is it a new benign mole,

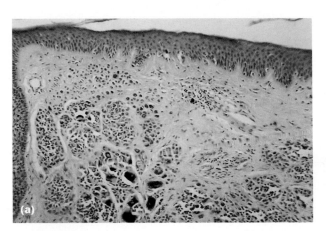
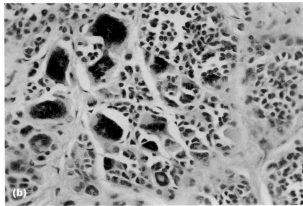

Figure 12.13 (a) Pathology of congenital melanocytic naevus showing packets or theques of naevus cells, some of which are 'naevus giant cells'. (b) Many large naevus giant cells.

Table 12.4 Differential diagnosis of an acquired naevus

Diagnosis	Comments
Acquired naevus (male)	Usually light brown, static
Seborrhoeic wart (keratosis, basal cell papilloma)	Brown, warty
Dermatofibroma (histiocytoma)	Firm, light brown
Malignant melanoma	Enlarging, irregular, variegate
Pigmented basal cell carcinoma	Smooth, pigmented nodule

some other pigmented lesion, or a malignant melanoma? The differential diagnosis for this situation is given in Table 12.4.

JUNCTIONAL NAEVI

These are flat, brown or black moles in which clumps of naevus cells can be observed at the dermoepidermal junction (Fig. 12.14) nestling in dermal papillae. It is presumed that this is the first stage in the 'life cycle' of the ordinary mole.

DERMAL CELLULAR NAEVI

Clumps of naevus cells are found within the upper dermis, accounting for the papular or nodular nature of these lesions. They are fawn or light brown or just skin coloured. They are common on the face and are often 'hairy', accounting for occasional episodes of pain, redness and swelling due to folliculitis. In some, there is a deep component with many spindle-shaped naevus cells that may superficially resemble the cellular component of a neurofibroma (see page 199). In the

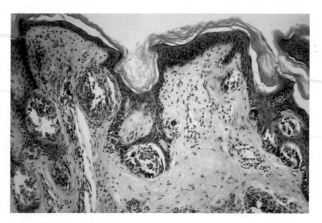

Figure 12.14 Many groups of naevus cells at the dermoepidermal junction in 'junctional naevus'.

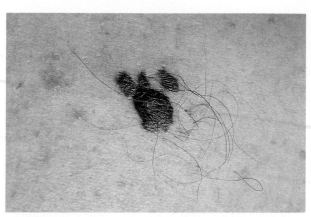

Figure 12.15 Blue naevus.

elderly when there is little pigment, they are often misdiagnosed as basal cell carcinomata.

COMPOUND NAEVI

These have the characteristics of a dermal cellular naevus, but there are areas of 'junctional activity' with foci of naevus cells at the dermoepidermal junction. It is presumed that these lesions are intermediary in development between the junctional naevus and the dermal cellular naevus.

Degenerative changes in naevi

Naevus cell naevi gradually become fewer during the ageing process and it is believed that moles develop involutional changes before disappearing. Some develop lipid vacuoles in their substance, others develop a type of foamy change, and others appear to calcify before finally disappearing.

BLUE NAEVI

In the ordinary *cellular blue naevus*, the melanin pigment and the bulk of the naevus cells are in the mid and deep dermis. The striking blue colour given by the pigment is due to the red wavelengths being filtered out by the superficial dermis and epidermis. This type of blue naevus is found over the scalp (Fig. 12.15) and the back of the hands or feet.

The *Mongolian spot* is a type of blue naevus commonly found in Asiatics. It occurs as a greyish discoloration over the sacral area in the newborn, becoming less prominent in later life.

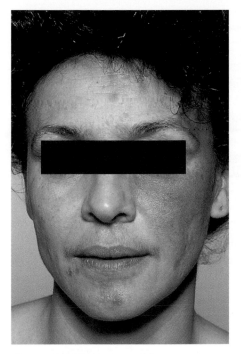

Figure 12.16 Naevus of Ota.

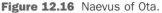

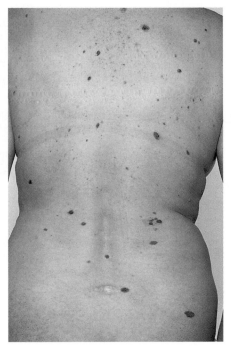

Figure 12.17 Multiple dysplastic moles with irregularity of shape and pigmentation.

The *naevus of Ota* and the *naevus of Ito* are due to spindle-shaped naevus cells over the upper face and lower face and neck, respectively (Fig. 12.16).

DYSPLASTIC NAEVUS SYNDROME (i.e. ATYPICAL MOLE SYNDROME)

Recognition of this syndrome is important because of the increased frequency of malignant melanoma associated with it. The condition may occur sporadically, but is also familial in many patients.

The lesions are variable in number and quite large compared to ordinary moles. They have irregular margins and irregular brown pigmentation, some having an orange-red hue (Fig. 12.17). It is said that the risk of a melanoma developing is approximately 1 per cent, but it is certainly much more than that in the familial form if one of the affected members of the family has had a melanoma – perhaps 10 per cent. It is even greater – possibly 100 per cent – if the individual has already had one melanoma.

These lesions often have what the dermatopathologists call a 'worrying appearance', meaning that many have one or more features suggesting melanoma. There may be a degree of cytological atypia and excessive mitoses.

JUVENILE MELANOMA

This is a quite uncommon, benign lesion of childhood and adolescence. Although usually solitary papules or small plaques, the lesions are occasionally multiple (Fig. 12.18). The individual lesions are pink or orange and may have a corrugated or *peau d'orange* surface. Their name derives from their histological appearance, which may look frighteningly like a melanoma to the uninitiated.

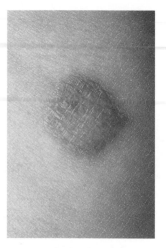

Figure 12.18 Juvenile melanoma: a red nodule on the arm of a 9-year-old boy.

Vascular malformations (angioma)/capillary naevi

STORK MARK

This is the popular name for the red discoloration at the back of the neck in a high proportion of newborns. It fades in later childhood and seems to be due to vasodilatation rather than to an excess of blood vessels.

PORT-WINE STAINS

These common vascular malformations may occur anywhere, but seem to be most common on the face and scalp. The deep crimson colour (or 'port wine') is distinctive and cosmetically very disfiguring (Fig. 12.19). The lesions contain many dilated blood vessels but no other obvious histological abnormality.

The surface of the lesion becomes more thickened and rugose with age and even develops polypoid outgrowths, adding to the grotesque appearance. When on a limb, deep vascular malformations may also be present, which can cause limb hypertrophy. Over the ophthalmic region, the obvious skin malformation of blood vessels may be associated with an underlying meningeal angiomatous malformation. When this combination of lesions is associated with epilepsy, the disorder is known as the Sturge–Weber syndrome.

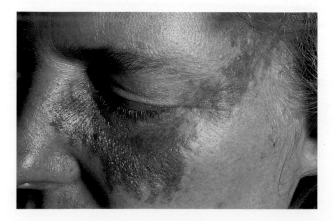

Figure 12.19 Typical port wine stain.

CAPILLARY ANGIOMA

The lesions are usually present at birth, but may develop in the first few months of life. They are raised, purplish nodules and plaques whose surface is often lobulated (supposedly like a strawberry) and show an enormous range of sizes. The smaller lesions have little functional significance (Fig. 12.20) and usually flatten or disappear at puberty. The larger lesions are very deforming and may cover quite a large area of skin (Fig. 12.21). The larger lesions, particularly, may ulcerate after minor trauma, presumably due to ischaemia of the overlying superficial dermis and overlying epidermis because of the shunting of blood between the larger, deeper vessels of the angioma. Any bleeding can be stopped with gentle pressure and the eroded area gradually heals with routine care. One other rare complication only occurs with the largest of capillary angiomas. Blood platelets become sequestered in the abnormal vascular channels of the angioma, creating a consumption coagulopathy and uncontrolled bleeding (Katzenbach–Merritt syndrome). The bleeding can be dealt with by administration of systemic steroids.

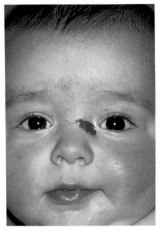

Figure 12.20 Small strawberry naevus on the left side of the nose.

CAVERNOUS HAEMANGIOMA

This is a soft, compressible, mauvish-blue swelling composed of large vascular spaces. This lesion shows little tendency to reduce in size in later life.

LYMPHANGIOMA CIRCUMSCRIPTUM

This lesion is a malformation of lymphatic channels, although there may also be an associated blood vessel anomaly. The lesions usually have a deep component, which it is almost impossible to eradicate surgically. Clinically, the malformation is recognized as a diffuse skin swelling with what appears to be a cluster of tense vesicles at the skin surface, with a frogspawn-like appearance (Fig. 12.22).

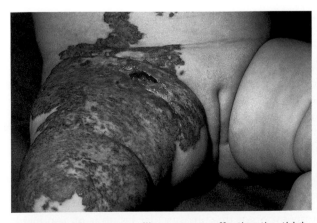

Figure 12.21 Large capillary naevus affecting the thigh and lower abdomen.

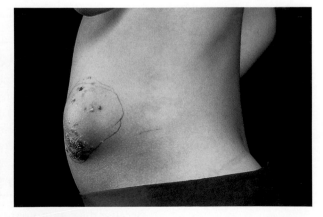

Figure 12.22 Lymphangioma circumscriptum affecting the abdomen. There is a deep component making eradication difficult.

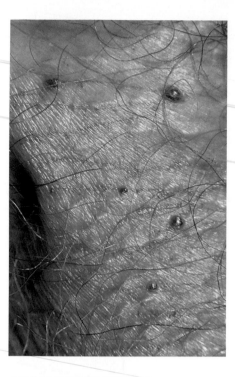

Figure 12.23 Angiokeratoma of the scrotum.

ANGIOKERATOMA

There are several types of angiokeratoma, which all consist of a small, subepidermal vascular malformation surmounted by a hyperkeratotic epidermis. They may occur as solitary red papules or, occasionally, as a crop of red spots over the scrotum (Fig. 12.23). When literally hundreds of tiny red papules develop over the trunk in young men, the possibility of the very rare inherited metabolic abnormality known as angiokeratoma corporis diffusum must be considered.

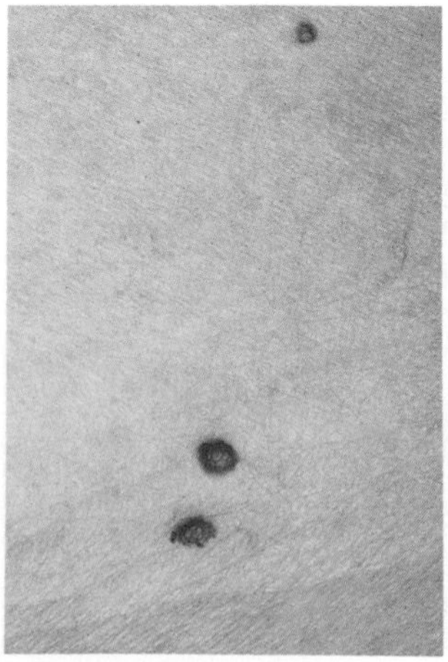

SENILE ANGIOMA (CAMPBELL DE MORGAN SPOT, CHERRY ANGIOMA)

As with seborrhoeic warts and skin tags, senile angioma is a frequent accompaniment of skin ageing. Histologically, it resembles the capillary angioma, but clinically its smooth-surfaced, dome-shaped, purplish or cherry-red appearance is quite characteristic (Fig. 12.24). Many lesions may appear over a period of some months, but apart from the distress that their appearance seems to cause, they have no special significance for general health.

Figure 12.24 Senile angioma on the trunk in a man aged 63 years.

CAPILLARY ANEURYSM

Because the commonest presentation of this tiny vascular lesion is of a suddenly appearing black pinhead spot, it is sometimes mistaken for an early malignant melanoma. If left, it gradually fades.

GLOMUS CELL TUMOUR

This benign vascular tumour arises from the glomus cells controlling tiny vascular shunts between arterial and venous capillaries at the periphery. The constituent cells have a characteristic cuboidal appearance and the lesion, which often occurs around the fingertips, is often quite painful.

PYOGENIC GRANULOMA

This odd lesion characteristically appears suddenly over a week or two and then disappears after several weeks. Typically, it is a red, dome-shaped papule with a glazed or eroded surface (Fig. 12.25), often on the fingers and toes. Histologically, it consists of a matrix of oedematous, glassy connective tissue in which there are numerous thin-walled vascular channels and a moderately dense, mixed cellular infiltrate. Its cause is unknown and it is certainly not due to 'pyogenic' micro-organisms.

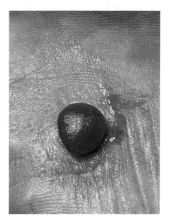

Figure 12.25 Dome-shaped, plum-red-coloured, shiny nodule of pyogenic granuloma.

Dermatofibroma (histiocytoma, sclerosing haemangioma)

There are no true 'fibromas' of dermal connective tissue and it is not certain whether the dermatofibroma is a benign neoplasm or some form of localized chronic inflammatory disorder. It certainly does contain many spindle-shaped and banana-shaped mononuclear cells, which may be fibroblast derived, and there is a variable amount of new collagenous dermal connective tissue. There are also many histiocytic cells present, which often contain lipid or iron pigment, both of which may derive from the large number of small blood vessels also contained in the lesion.

Clinically, dermatofibromas are firm or hard intracutaneous nodules. They are usually found on the limbs as solitary lesions, but sometimes two or three or even more are found in the same patient. Generally they are brownish in colour (from the haemosiderin pigment) and have a rough or warty surface because these dermal nodules have the propensity to thicken up the epidermis immediately above them (Fig. 12.26). The lesions have no serious clinical significance, but are sometimes mistaken for melanomas.

HYPERTROPHIC SCAR

A scar is a reparative response to injury of some kind, accidental or surgical, or tissue destruction from an inflammatory skin disorder, in which the tissue architecture cannot be entirely restored and the defect is made good with fibrous tissue.

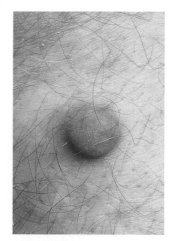

Figure 12.26 Dermatofibroma: brownish red, firm, intracutaneous nodules.

197

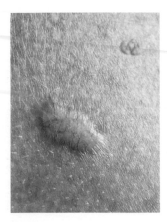

Figure 12.27 Hypertrophic scar.

A hypertrophic scar is usually pink, smooth and variably raised (Fig. 12.27). The excess scar tissue generally flattens after some months or can be encouraged to do so with topical corticosteroids and firm pressure bandaging.

KELOID SCAR

Like hypertrophic scar, this lesion arises in response to injury, but the response is inappropriate to the often minor degree of trauma. It tends to occur in young adults and adolescents, particularly women, and particularly around the shoulders, upper limbs and upper trunk. Some ethnic groups also appear more likely to develop these lesions, black-skinned individuals being particularly prone. Clinically, the lesions are raised and appear to send extensions into neighbouring skin (Fig. 12.28). They show little tendency to regress, and surgical treatment alone is usually insufficient, as they tend to recur in the scar. Corticosteroids, interferons, radiotherapy and topical retinoic acid have all been tried, with varying success. The use of silastic sheeting applied firmly to the affected area has been claimed to be effective. The histological appearance of keloid scar, with oedematous, pale connective tissue, suggests reversion to embryonic type of collagen.

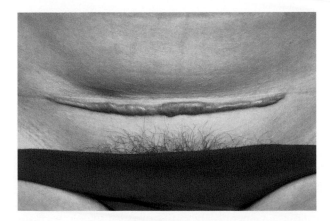

Figure 12.28 Keloid scar occurring at the site of a scar from a Caesarean section.

Leiomyoma

This is an uncommon benign tumour of plain muscle that arises either from arrector pilores muscle of hair follicles or from the smooth muscle of blood vessel walls. It is mostly smooth surfaced, oval and bluish red in colour, varying in size from 1 cm to 3 cm in length and 0.5 cm to 1.5 cm in breadth. It may be spontaneously painful, especially in the cold, and indeed can sometimes be seen to contract when cooled. It can be confused histologically because of its spindle-shaped and strap-shaped plain muscle cells, which may look like fibrous or neural tissue.

Neural tumours

These are, in fact, tumours of the connective tissue accompanying the neural elements.

NEUROFIBROMA AND VON RECKLINGHAUSEN'S DISEASE

The neurofibroma is mostly multiple and part of a, not uncommon, inherited syndrome known as neurofibromatosis or Von Recklinghausen's disease. The individual lesions are often quite large, soft, compressible and skin coloured (Fig. 12.29). Histologically, the typical picture is of a non-encapsulated dermal mass composed of interlacing bundles of spindle-shaped cells, often in a 'nerve-like' arrangement, set in a homogeneous matrix amidst which mast cells may be seen. Von Recklinghausen's syndrome is inherited as a dominant characteristic, but 30–50 per cent of patients do not give a family history, suggesting that there is a high rate of new gene mutation.

Neurofibromata start to appear in childhood and increase in numbers during adolescence. They are cosmetically very disabling and in the worst cases result in gross deformity. Ultimately, large numbers may be present. Some of these lesions become very large, soft, diffuse swellings; others become pedunculated and pendulous. Alongside the neurofibromata, light-brown, uniformly pigmented, irregular macular patches appear (*café au lait* patches) over the trunk and limbs (Fig. 12.30). A useful diagnostic point is the presence of small, pigmented macules

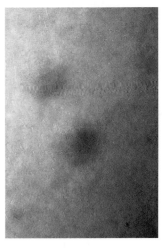

Figure 12.29 Soft mauve or pink, compressible lesions of neurofibroma.

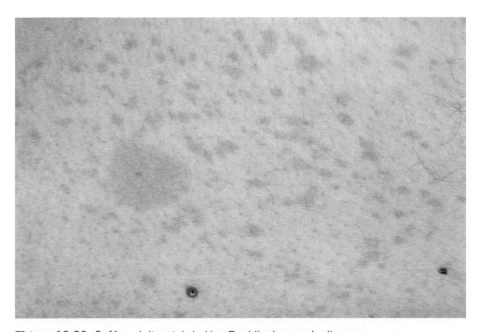

Figure 12.30 Café au lait patch in Von Recklinghausen's disease.

at the apices of the axillae. There is a greatly increased risk of tumours affecting the central and peripheral nervous systems as well as of tumours of sympathetic tissue such as phaeochromocytoma. Genetic counselling of affected individuals is of great importance.

NEURILEMMOMA

The neurilemmoma is an uncommon benign tumour of neural connective tissue. The lesions vary in size and occur anywhere on the skin surface. Microscopically, they consist of thin, spindle-shaped cells arranged in a stacked or 'storiform' manner.

NEUROMA

This rare, benign neural tumour is the most differentiated of all the neural connective tissue tumours and consists of well-formed nerve elements. It occurs at the site of nerve injury and occasionally seems to arise spontaneously.

Lipoma

Lipomata are common, solitary or sometimes multiple, benign tumours of fat. They may be enormous in size or only 1–2 cm in diameter and can occur anywhere. They are soft, skin-coloured and have poorly defined edges. Histologically, they consist of mature fat cells.

Collagen and elastic tissue naevi

These are rare intracutaneous plaques and nodules, often with a knobbly or corrugated skin surface. They are very difficult to identify histologically because they are composed of normal connective tissue. They may occur as 'shagreen patches' in tuberose sclerosis.

TUBEROUS SCLEROSIS (EPILOIA)

This recessively inherited syndrome is a neurocutaneous disorder. The cutaneous components include shagreen patches (see above), ash leaf-shaped hypopigmented patches on the trunk, subungual fibromata, which are fibrous nodules that develop beneath the toenails and fingernails, and adenoma sebaceum. Adenoma sebaceum occurs on the cheeks and the central part of the face of patients with tuberose

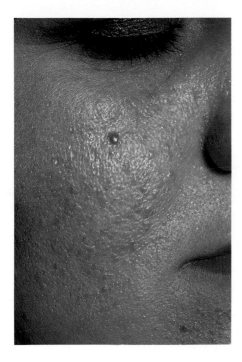

Figure 12.31 Pink nodules characterizing the disorder known as adenoma sebaceum.

sclerosis. Pink or red, firm papular lesions develop (Fig. 12.31) in which vascular fibrous tissue is found rather than an excess of sebaceous glands.

Mast cell naevus and mastocytosis

These lesions are characterized by an excess of mast cells that may or may not release histamine and occasionally heparin on stimulation.

MAST CELL NAEVUS (MASTOCYTOMA)

This lesion represents one, or occasionally several, localized collections of mast cells. It presents as a pink or red nodule, 1–3 cm in diameter in infants and young children, but usually disappears spontaneously later in childhood. Rubbing or heating it may result in it swelling and a red halo – Darier's sign.

MASTOCYTOSIS (URTICARIA PIGMENTOSA)

This term is used to describe a group of disorders in which there may be excess mast cells in many tissues, but which is mainly manifest in the skin. The term urticaria pigmentosa was formerly employed because it is not uncommon for the

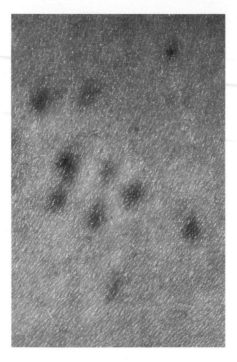

Figure 12.32 Red-brown papules of urticaria pigmentosa.

individual lesions to become pigmented. In the juvenile form, numerous pink or red-brown papules develop over the trunk and limbs (Fig. 12.32). In some young patients, the lesions are intensely itchy and they experience discomfort and erythema when bathing. Juvenile mastocytosis usually remits spontaneously during adolescence.

In the adult, the papular variety is somewhat like the juvenile form except that it persists. Another adult type is telangiectasia macularis eruptiva perstans of Parkes Weber. Clincially, in early adult life, pink or pink-brown telangiectatic macules start to appear, persist and increase in number over the years.

In all the generalized varieties of mastocytosis, studies have shown that there are deposits of mast cells in visceral structures such as liver, spleen and bone in an appreciable number of cases – up to 20 per cent in some series. They are mainly of importance if alcohol, opioids or other drugs cause histamine release. Special fixation (e.g. in alcohol) and special stains (e.g. toluidine blue) are necessary to show up the metachromatic granules of the mast cells.

Cysts

A cyst is an epithelium-lined cavity filled with fluid or semi-solid material. The distinguishing features of the commonly encountered cysts of the skin are summarized in Table 12.5.

Table 12.5 Differential diagnosis of common skin cysts

Cyst type	Body site	Clinical features
Epidermoid	Virtually anywhere	Smooth-walled, firm lesions may become inflamed if they leak; common
Milium	At sites of blistering, spontaneously on upper cheeks	Pinhead-sized, white, hard lesions
Pilar	Scalp and scrotum	May be inherited; often multiple; less common than epidermoid cysts; smooth walled but not as firm as epidermoid cysts
Sebocystoma multiplex	Anywhere, but especially the upper trunk	May be inherited; always multiple; usually small, smooth walled; contents less firm than other types; may become inflamed and develop acne-like lesions; uncommon
Dermoid	Face, particularly around the eyes	Deep set in skin; may be oval and less mobile than other cyst types

EPIDERMOID CYSTS

These lesions are lined by epidermis and produce stratum corneum. They are often surrounded by a tough, fibrous capsule, presumably stimulated by leakage of the cyst contents. If these cyst contents find their way into the dermis, considerable inflammation results. The horny content may eventually degenerate, forming a foul-smelling, semi-solid material. The fancied resemblance of this to sebum has mistakenly led to the term 'sebaceous cysts' for these lesions. Epidermoid cysts may occur anywhere, but are most common over the head, neck and upper trunk.

MILIA

Milia are tiny epidermoid cysts that occur at the sites of subepidermal blistering as in porphyria cutanea tarda (see page 259) or spontaneously over the upper cheeks and beneath the eyes. They are usually no larger than a pinhead and are white. They contain tiny accretions of horn, which can be expressed by slitting the thin epidermis over them with a needle tip.

PILAR CYSTS (TRICHOLEMMAL CYSTS)

The lining epithelium of these less common cysts is derived from a portion of the hair follicle neck and shows a quite characteristic type of keratinization in which there is abrupt formation of a glassy-appearing type of horn without a granular cell layer. Pilar cysts are usually multiple and are often genetically determined as an autosomal dominant trait. They occur on the scalp and on the scrotum in particular.

SEBOCYSTOMA MULTIPLEX (STEATOCYSTOMA MULTIPLEX)

These cystic malformations are formed from sebaceous gland tissue and other hair follicle-derived epithelium. They are always multiple, often being present in very large numbers. They are inherited as an autosomal dominant trait. Their content is sometimes pure sebum. Large numbers of small cysts are distributed over the body, but particularly over the upper trunk.

DERMOID CYSTS

Dermoid cysts are uncommon lesions that seem to contain embryonic epithelium capable of forming a wide spectrum of tissue types. They may occur anywhere, but are especially often found around the eyes as oval, firm, smooth-walled swellings.

FOLLICULAR RETENTION CYSTS

When large hair follicles develop a hard, immovable comedonal plug in the follicular neck or at the skin surface, the follicle distends because of the continuing secretion of sebum and production of horny material. Often, these cysts rupture, causing inflammation, but sometimes this does not happen and quite large swellings are produced. This seems to occur particularly frequently over the back in the elderly, when they are sometimes known as giant comedones.

Treatment of benign tumours, moles and birthmarks

It should be remembered that on many occasions it is the appearance of the lesion that is the predominant concern of the patient and it is not helpful, for example, to substitute a simple facial mole with an ugly surgical scar. One overriding principle is important to remember: if any form of surgical removal or destruction is planned, histological evidence of the nature of the lesion is required. Even the most experienced dermatologist is not more than 65–70 per cent accurate in the clinical diagnosis of non-typical pigmented lesions, and is only a little better with non-pigmented tumours.

Minimally scarring procedures such as curettage and cautery and shaving of small, benign, dome-shaped lesions flush with the skin may be adequate and prevent unpleasant scar formation. Cryotherapy may also be useful for some superficial lesions. Treatment by lasers requires specialized instrumentation and personnel with experience and skill.

Case 11

Mrs J.G. was quite confused. Here she was, at the age of 57, developing more moles on her back and abdomen! She already had ordinary acquired naevi on her face and arms, as well as a large, pigmented patch of 2 cm² diameter over her upper back that she had been born with and that had been termed 'a congenital mole'. The new brown, warty spots over her abdomen and back irritated and worried her and she didn't like the look of them. Her doctor told her that these new pigmented lesions were nothing to worry about, but were common seborrhoeic warts that could easily be removed by scraping them off – curettage under a local anaesthetic.

Summary

- Seborrhoeic warts are extremely common, benign epidermal tumours of ageing skin. They are usually brownish and warty and may occur in large numbers over the trunk. The differential diagnosis includes epidermal naevus, solar keratosis, viral wart and, most important of all, malignant melanoma.

- Epidermal naevus is a localized, warty nodule or a flat, brownish patch over the shoulder or buttock (Becker's naevus). Naevus sebaceous is another type of epidermal naevus, which contains sebaceous glands and maybe other adnexal structures.

- Benign tumours of sweat gland origin include syringoma, cylindroma, nodular hidradenoma and eccrine poroma.

- Calcifying epithelioma of Malherbe (pilomatrixoma) is a common, benign, hair follicle-derived tumour occurring over the head and neck in young adults, which eventually calcifies.

- Sebaceous gland hyperplasia is often seen in elderly facial skin as one or several yellowish nodules.

- Melanocytic naevi ('moles') are extremely common developmental anomalies that contain many immature melanocytes. Congenital naevi are present at birth. They are usually more than 1 cm² in diameter and dark brown in colour. Some, such as those that cover large areas of the shoulder or elsewhere on the trunk, are very deforming. A few of these develop malignant melanoma.

- Acquired naevi appear after birth and include junctional naevi, which are flat, brown lesions containing clumps of naevus cells at the dermoepidermal junction, dermal cellular naevi, with clumps of naevus cells in the dermis, and compound naevi, with clumps of naevus cells both within the dermis and at the junction.

- In blue naevi, the characteristic colour is due to the depth of the naevus cells in the dermis. In the dysplastic naevus syndrome, the naevi are irregular and odd looking and there is an increased risk of malignant melanoma. Juvenile melanoma occurs in children and adolescents and is so called because of the histological appearance, which can simulate malignant melanoma.

- Port-wine stains are crimson blotches in which there is marked capillary dilatation compared to a capillary angioma, which is a red nodule or plaque containing proliferating endothelial cells. The latter tend to flatten and disappear at puberty. Larger ones may cause problems from bleeding and/or erosion. Cavernous haemangiomata are larger and compressible, containing large vascular spaces.

- Lymphangioma circumscriptum contains dilated lymphatic channels. Senile angiomas (Campbell de Morgan spot) are bright-red papules on the trunk of the elderly, with a similar histological appearance to capillary angiomas. Glomus cell tumours develop from arteriovenous shunts at the fingertips and tend to be painful. Pyogenic granuloma suddenly arises as a moist, red papule and spontaneously subsides after a few weeks. It contains primitive connective tissue, inflammatory cells and thin-walled blood vessels.

- Dermatofibroma (histiocytoma) is a brownish, firm, Intracutaneous nodule containing fibroblasts, histiocytes and vascular channels, which may be inflammatory in origin. Several may develop simultaneously on the limbs. Keloid scars are unsightly scars, larger than the original injury, containing embryonic connective tissue and difficult to eradicate.

- Neurofibroma is a benign tumour of neural sheath, which is mostly seen as part of a dominantly inherited disorder (Von Recklinghausen's disease) in which multiple lesions occur alongside flat, brown macules (*café au lait* patches). Whorls of spindle cells are typical in this lesion. Neurilemmoma is another benign tumour of neural sheath.

- Connective tissue naevi are uncommon, but are of importance in the inherited disorder known as tuberose sclerosis, in which fibrovascular lesions occur on the face (adenoma sebaceum) alongside connective tissue naevi on the trunk (shagreen patches).

- Mastocytosis (urticaria pigmentosa) causes pigmented lesions in the skin which may urticate. Mast cells may also proliferate in other organs such as the marrow and the liver.

- Cysts are epithelial-lined cavities. Common epidermoid cysts have a lining epidermis that produces horn. Pilar cysts lined with hair-sheath epithelium produce a different type of horn. Cysts also develop from sebaceous gland tissue – known as sebocystoma multiplex. Dermoid cysts are congenital in origin and contain a mixture of tissues.

Malignant disease of the skin

Introduction

All forms of malignant disease of the skin are becoming more common. The reasons for this are:

- increased exposure to solar ultraviolet radiation (UVR)
- an increasingly 'elderly' population
- increasing exposure to an increasing number of carcinogenic substances
- an increasing number of people who are immunosuppressed.

Non-melanoma skin cancer

SOLAR KERATOSES (ACTINIC KERATOSES)

Definition

Solar keratoses are common, localized areas of epidermis due to chronic solar exposure in which epidermal growth and differentiation are irregular and abnormal.

Clinical features

The typical solar keratosis is a raised, pink or grey, scaling or warty hyperkeratotic plaque or papule (Fig. 13.1). Solar keratoses are usually 2–5 mm in diameter,

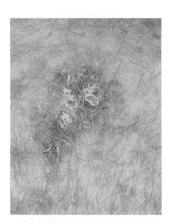

Figure 13.1 Typical solar keratosis.

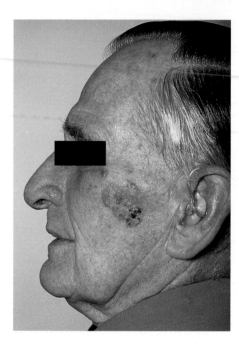

Figure 13.2 Large solar keratosis affecting the left cheek.

Table 13.1 Differential diagnosis of scaling and/or warty lesions on exposed sites

Diagnosis	Comments
Solar keratosis	Small, may be pink
Bowen's disease (intraepidermal epithelioma)	Often large, may be psoriasiform
Squamous cell carcinoma	History of recent growth, may ulcerate
Viral wart	Mostly in young, usually small
Seborrhoeic wart (keratosis, basal cell papilloma)	May be multiple, often brown
Epidermal naevus	Often linear, present from early age

but may be much larger (Fig. 13.2). They are found on the exposed areas of skin of elderly, fair-skinned subjects who show other signs of solar damage. Multiple lesions are the rule, and when a solitary solar keratosis is found, it may be assumed that there is widespread solar damage and that further solar keratoses will appear.

The differential diagnosis of small scaling or warty lesions of exposed skin sites is given in Table 13.1. The clinical diagnosis of solar keratosis may be difficult and with 'not quite typical' lesions, an accuracy of more than 65 per cent is good, even for experienced clinicians.

PATHOLOGY: AETIOPATHOGENESIS OF BOTH SOLAR KERATOSES AND NON-MELANOMA SKIN CANCER

Parakeratosis and/or hyperkeratosis surmount the variably thickened epidermis, which demonstrates heterogeneity of cell and nuclear size, shape and staining (epidermal dysplasia). The edges of the epidermal abnormality are usually quite distinct and sloped. Sweat ducts are conspicuously uninvolved. There is always a subepidermal inflammatory cell infiltrate of lymphocytes, which is occasionally a dense 'lichenoid band'.

Chronic exposure to solar UVR is the most important causative agency, although chronic heat damage, X-irradiation and chemical carcinogens (such as arsenic) may also be responsible in some subjects. The fact that solar keratoses occur alongside other forms of solar damage on light-exposed skin in fair-skinned subjects who have had much sun exposure, and similar lesions can be produced experimentally by UVR in mice, is persuasive evidence that solar UVR is of major importance.

It is thought that solar keratoses represent one pre-malignant phase on the path to squamous cell carcinoma, even though only a tiny proportion (perhaps 0.2 per cent) ever transform to malignant lesions.

The role of papillomaviruses in the causation of skin cancer has long been debated. Modern techniques (e.g. *in situ* hybridization) indicate that some antigenic types of human papillomavirus (HPV), e.g. HPV16 and HPV18, may provoke neoplasia. The high prevalence of non-melanoma skin cancer (NMSC) in renal transplant patients is believed to be due, at least in part, to papillomaviruses.

Immunological factors are also of importance in the development of solar keratoses and other forms of NMSC. As mentioned above, patients who have had renal transplants and who are immunosuppressed have a greatly increased incidence of solar keratosis and NMSC, depending on the length of time they have been immunosuppressed. Patients with acquired immune deficiency syndrome (AIDS) are also at increased risk of skin cancer (see page 97).

EPIDEMIOLOGY AND NATURAL HISTORY

In the subtropical parts of Australia, solar keratoses have been found in more than 50 per cent of the population over the age of 40 years. In the equable damp climate of South Wales, approximately 20 per cent of the population aged over 60 have been found to have these lesions. Solar keratoses gradually become more common after the age of 50 years. They are much more common in fair-skinned subjects, particularly those with reddish hair and blue eyes. Subjects with Celtic ancestry seem peculiarly sensitive to NMSC from solar exposure and, although their susceptibility is mostly due to their light complexions, it may be that they also have some metabolic abnormality akin to xeroderma pigmentosum (see page 218). No racial types are immune to solar keratoses or other forms of NMSC. For example, albino black-skinned Africans are prone to develop such lesions, and dark-skinned subjects from the Middle East develop NMSC if they are excessively exposed to the sun.

A small proportion of solar keratoses disappear spontaneously.

TREATMENT

Clearly, solitary lesions or small numbers of solar keratoses may be curetted off or removed by cryotherapy with liquid nitrogen.

Chemotherapy is sometimes appropriate when there are very large numbers of lesions present, for individuals who are seriously 'photodamaged', and three types are available. The first is topical 5-fluorouracil as a 5 per cent ointment (Efudix, Roche). This agent is applied daily or twice daily to the lesions over a 10-day or 14-day schedule. The lesions often become sore and inflamed, and the patient should be warned and given a topical corticosteroid to improve the symptoms. This treatment is effective in some 50 or 60 per cent of cases and often saves considerable inconvenience and discomfort for elderly patients. Topical diclofenac (Solaraze – Shire) also appears to be quite effective. Imiquimod – the immune response-modifying agent – may also be used for topical treatment.

Systemic retinoids (either acitretin or isotretinoin) may be used for patients with multiple solar keratoses or other types of NMSC of several sites for whom other types of therapy are unsuitable and who can tolerate the uncomfortable side effects (see page 140). They are given in the same doses as for disorders of keratinisation, for periods of between 3 and 6 months. They reduce the size and number of lesions and reduce the rate of appearance of new lesions. Topical retinoids are also employed and certainly have a prophylactic as well as a therapeutic effect when used over long periods.

Intralesional injections of alpha-2B interferon, two or three times weekly (1 000 000 units of alpha-2B on each occasion), for 3 or 4 weeks causes resolution in 70–100 per cent of lesions of solar keratoses or other types of NMSC. This treatment is only suitable for very large lesions for which surgical or other destructive types of therapy are unsuitable.

BOWEN'S DISEASE (INTRAEPIDERMAL EPITHELIOMA)

Definition

Bowen's disease is a localized area of epidermal neoplasia remaining within the confines of the epidermis.

Clinical features

The most typical type of lesion of Bowen's disease is a raised, red, scaling plaque, and lesions are often very psoriasiform in appearance. They are mostly present on light-exposed areas of skin and are often seen on the lower legs of women (Fig. 13.3), which receive both incident UVR and UVR reflected from the pavement.

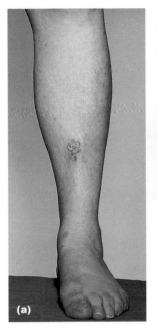

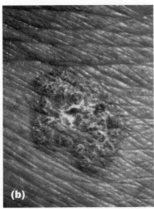

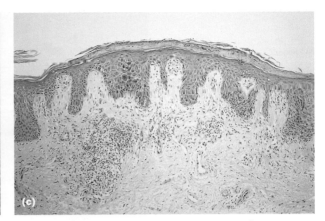

Figure 13.3 (a) Psoriasiform patch of Bowen's disease on the lower leg of an elderly woman. (b) Bowen's disease on the cheek. (c) Pathology of Bowen's disease showing irregular thickening of the epidermis and cellular irregularity.

Single lesions are most common, but multiple lesions may occur. Lesions on the trunk were common when arsenic was used as a treatment for psoriasis and other 'chronic ailments'. Individual lesions gradually enlarge and thicken and may eventually transform to squamous cell carcinoma.

Pathology and aetiopathogenesis

The histological appearance could be described as an exaggerated version of a solar keratosis in which there is marked thickening and marked heterogeneity of the epidermal cells (Fig. 13.3c). Bizarre, large keratinocytes (cellules monstreuses) complete the distinctive appearance. There is also parakeratosis and a superficial resemblance to psoriasis.

Erythroplasia of Queyrat

This is the term used for Bowen's disease affecting the glans penis. It presents as a red, velvety patch that slowly progresses, eventually transforming into a squamous cell carcinoma if left untreated. Surgical excision of the affected area is the best form of treatment.

SQUAMOUS CELL CARCINOMA/SQUAMOUS CELL EPITHELIOMA

Clinical features

The majority of lesions of squamous cell carcinoma are warty nodules or plaques that gradually or, in some cases, rapidly enlarge to form exophytic eroded nodules or

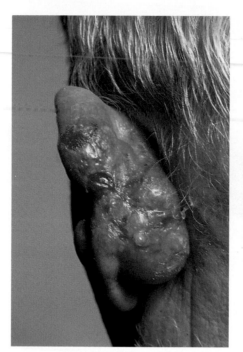

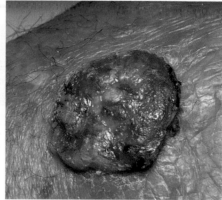

Figure 13.4 Irregular nodular plaque on the ear due to squamous cell carcinoma.

Figure 13.5 Eroded nodule of squamous cell carcinoma.

ulcerated plaques (Figs 13.4 and 13.5). The lesion is in most case solitary, although it often occurs against a background of solar damage with multiple solar keratoses.

Metastases occur if the primary lesions are left untreated, spreading to local lymph nodes, local skin sites and ultimately lungs, bone and brain.

The development of squamous cell carcinoma should be suspected in areas of:

- severe photodamage
- X-ray dermatitis
- chronic heat injury such as erythema ab igne
- chronic inflammatory skin disease such as chronic discoid lupus erythematosus and chronic hypertrophic lichen planus.

Pathology and aetiopathogenesis

There is marked epidermal thickening with cellular and nuclear heterogeneity and atypia and evidence of abnormal mitotic activity. There is also evidence of focal and inappropriate keratinization so that so-called 'horn pearls' are formed (Fig. 13.6). There is usually evidence of invasion of surrounding tissue by epithelial clumps and columns.

Squamous cell carcinoma has to be distinguished from the massive but benign epidermal thickening known as pseudoepitheliomatous hyperplasia seen in hypertrophic lichen planus, prurigo nodularis and lichen simplex chronicus.

The factors in the aetiology of squamous cell carcinoma are as follows.

- Chronic UVR damage from solar exposure.
- X-irradiation damage to the skin.

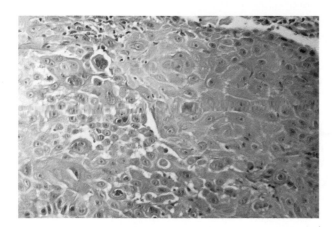

Figure 13.6 Pathology of squamous cell carcinoma showing a mass of abnormal epithelium with scattered areas of differentiation (horn pearls).

- Persistent heat injury to the skin (as in erythema ab igne).
- Chronic inflammatory and scarring disorders of the skin, such as discoid lupus erythematosus, hypertrophic lichen planus and dystrophic epidermolysis bullosa.
- Certain genodermatoses and localized congenital malformations, such as xeroderma pigmentosum, epidermodysplasia verruciformis and epidermal naevus.
- Papillomavirus infection – certain antigenic types (e.g. HPV5, HPV16 and HPV18) seem particularly likely to cause malignant transformation in immunosuppressed renal transplantation patients, in epidermodysplasia verruciformis and giant warty tumour of the genitalia.
- Exposure to chemical carcinogens, such as industrial contact with tars and pitch or systemic administration of arsenic.

Epidemiology and natural history

Squamous cell carcinoma predominantly occurs in the same population groups as described for solar keratosis. Regrettably, it is difficult to obtain accurate figures for the incidence of the disease, as reporting is not as complete as it should be. In one survey in subtropical Australia, approximately 2 per cent of the population over the age of 40 years had one squamous cell carcinoma when examined. Studies indicate that squamous cell carcinomas as well as other forms of NMSC are increasing in incidence.

Most squamous cell carcinomas are removed before they metastasize, but some patients die from the spread of their lesion.

Treatment

Excision, with an adequate margin to ensure inclusion of all neoplastic tissue and some healthy tissue all around the lesion, is sufficient for cure in more than 95 per cent of patients. For the very elderly with solitary, large, difficult to remove lesions, treatment by radiotherapy may be the kindest and most efficient method. Systemic retinoids may be appropriate when there are multiple solar keratoses and

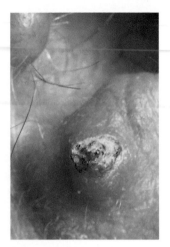

other signs of photodamage as well as the index lesion, and intralesional interferon may be suitable for large lesions.

KERATOACANTHOMA (MOLLUSCUM SEBACEUM)

This term describes a suddenly appearing epidermal tumour with some of the characteristics of a squamous cell carcinoma, but which resolves after a short period.

It usually appears within a week or two on light-exposed skin as a solitary crateriform nodule (Fig. 13.7). It then gradually enlarges for a few weeks and stays at that size for a variable period before finally remitting after a total of 3 or 4 months. Lesions that are more persistent should be suspected of being a squamous cell carcinoma. The most important differential diagnosis is squamous cell carcinoma. If left to resolve spontaneously, scarring often occurs.

Figure 13.7 Solitary crateriform nodule of keratoacanthoma.

Pathology and aetiopathogenesis

Keratoacanthoma has a characteristic, symmetrical, cup-shaped or flask-shaped structure (Fig. 13.8). There is a minor degree of epidermal dysplasia and little evidence of tissue invasion. It seems to be provoked by the same stimuli that cause solar keratoses, but is much less common. It has been suggested that keratoacanthomas develop from hair follicle epithelium.

Treatment

Excision or curettage and cautery may be employed.

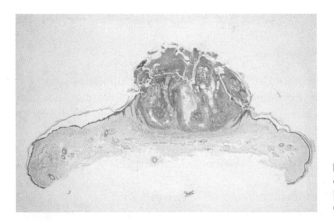

Figure 13.8 Pathology of keratoacanthoma. Note the cup-shaped epidermal invagination.

BASAL CELL CARCINOMA (BASAL CELL EPITHELIOMA)

Definition

Basal cell carcinoma is a locally invasive but rarely metastasizing malignant epithelial tumour of basaloid cells without the tendency to differentiate into horny structures.

Table 13.2 Clinical types of basal cell carcinoma

Clinical type	Comment
Nodulocystic	Solid or cystic nodule; commonest
Ulcerative	Usually a later stage of nodulocystic lesion; has a rolled margin; this type is known as rodent ulcer
Pigmented	Darkly pigmented nodule, may be confused with melanoma
Morphoeic	Flat, white, scar-like; often difficult to diagnose
Superficial	Flat, scaling, pink patch; often with a fine, hair-like margin

Clinical features

There are several clinical types (see Table 13.2).

- *Nodulocystic.* These are by far the commonest variety. Translucent or skin-coloured, dome-shaped nodules (0.5–1.5 cm in diameter) slowly appear on the skin and remain static for long periods, often for several years, before ulcerating (Fig. 13.9). They often have a telangiectatic overlying skin and may be flecked with pigment. They usually occur as solitary lesions on the exposed areas of the skin of the head and neck and are uncommon on the limbs. Some 20 per cent occur on the trunk. They must be distinguished from dermal cellular naevi, sebaceous gland hypertrophy and benign hair follicle tumours.
- *Ulcerative.* The nodulocystic type eventually breaks down to form an ulcer with raised everted edges (Fig. 13.10). This type is known colloquially as 'rodent ulcer'.
- *Pigmented.* Nodulocystic lesions may become quite darkly pigmented and are then quite often mistaken for melanomas (Fig. 13.11).

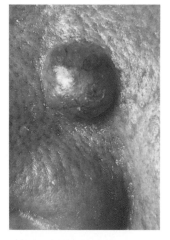

Figure 13.9 Typical nodulocystic basal cell carcinoma.

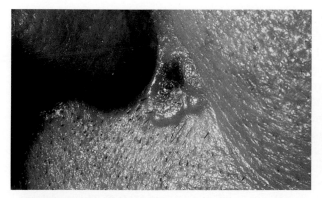

Figure 13.10 Ulcerated plaque of nodulocystic basal cell carcinoma (rodent ulcer).

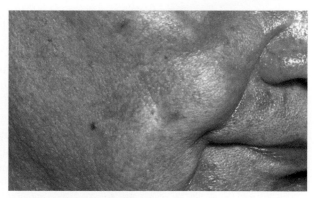

Figure 13.11 Several small, black nodules of pigmented basal cell carcinoma on the face of a patient with basal cell naevus syndrome.

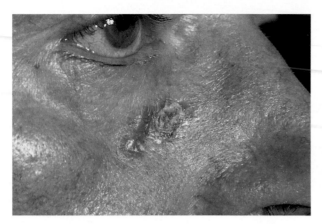

Figure 13.12 Eroded sclerotic plaque of morphoeic basal cell carcinoma.

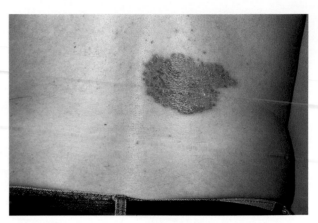

Figure 13.13 Large superficial basal cell carcinoma affecting the back. Note the psoriasiform appearance with the well-defined edge.

- *Morphoeic.* These are often whitish, scar-like, depressed, firm plaques, and are so named because of their supposed resemblance to localized scleroderma (Fig. 13.12).
- *Superficial.* These take the form of a variably sized, thin, pink, scaling plaques with a well-defined edge (Fig. 13.13). If the edge is examined with a hand lens, a fine, 'hair-like', raised margin can be discerned. They may be mistaken for Bowen's disease or even a patch of psoriasis. They often occur on the trunk and limbs.

All types of basal cell carcinoma gradually expand and invade and destroy local tissue structures such as the ear, nose and eye. They metastasize rarely, but it is difficult to know how often. However, when it is realized that basal cell carcinoma is one of the most common human tumours and that metastasis has been recorded in the literature only about 500 times, the proportion of lesions that do metastasize must be extremely small.

Pathology and aetiopathogenesis

Clumps of small basophilic epidermal cells occupy the upper dermis, the outermost cells often being more columnar than the rest and arranged in a neat palisade around the nodule (Fig. 13.14). Many mitotic figures may be seen amongst the mass of basal cells, as may many degenerate cells – it is thought that the slow rate of growth is explained by cell death keeping pace with cell proliferation in the tumour. In routine histological sections, it is common to find a gap between the clumps of tumour cells and the surrounding dermis, due to the dissolving out of soluble glycoprotein-like material.

Most lesions of basal cell carcinoma are due to chronic solar exposure and UVR damage, as they occur on light-exposed sites in photodamaged subjects. However, a larger proportion occurs in younger, non-light-exposed, non-photodamaged subjects than solar keratoses or other forms of NMSC. The explanation for this is uncertain, but it may be that some lesions arise from congenital malformations and are unrelated to UVR exposure.

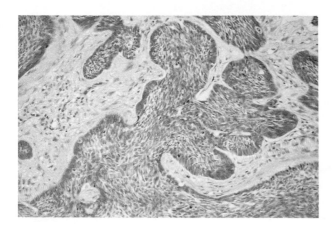

Figure 13.14 Pathology of basal cell carcinoma showing well-defined clumps of basaloid cells with peripheral palisading.

Epidemiology

The occurrence of basal cell carcinoma mirrors that of solar keratosis. As with squamous cell carcinoma and other forms of photodamage, basal cell carcinoma appears to be increasing in incidence.

Treatment

The majority of lesions can easily be excised. Smaller lesions can be curetted and the base cauterized. Both these surgical ablative techniques result in a 95 per cent cure. Larger lesions may be treated by radiotherapy after confirming the diagnosis by biopsy.

Case 12

Liam was a farmer. He had spent most of his 63 years on the land and loved it. Unfortunately, his skin did not. He had begun to notice lumps, bumps and scaly patches a few years before, but now they really needed treatment. On his bald scalp were multiple, scaling patches and small, warty lesions. These were diagnosed as solar keratoses and were treated by a combination of curettage, cryotherapy and topical 5-fluorouracil ointment. Of more significance were an ulcerated, pearly plaque on one nostril and a thick, warty patch on his left ear. The first was a basal cell carcinoma and the latter was a squamous cell carcinoma. Both received expert treatment from the local dermatologist, who was a 'dab hand' at removing such lesions.

BASAL CELL NAEVUS SYNDROME (GORLIN'S SYNDROME)

Definition

This is a rare, autosomally inherited condition in which multiple pigmented basal cell carcinoma lesions develop as part of a multi-system disorder.

Clinical features

Multiple basal cell carcinomas may start to develop in the second decade of life and erupt in large numbers in succeeding years. Less severely affected individuals start to develop them later in life and develop fewer lesions. The lesions are mostly pigmented and may occur anywhere on the skin surface. Small pits may be found on the palms, but otherwise there are no skin abnormalities.

A series of skeletal anomalies is also present in the majority of patients, including mandibular cysts and bifid ribs. In addition, patients have a high incidence of ovarian, central nervous system and spinal tumours.

In recent years, considerable progress has been made in identifying the gene responsible for this disorder.

Treatment

Individual lesions should be removed as necessary. When there are large numbers present and new lesions are continuing to appear, the administration of systemic retinoids will reduce the numbers of lesions and the rate of appearance of new basal cell carcinomas (see page 140).

XERODERMA PIGMENTOSUM

Definition

Xeroderma pigmentosum is the name given to a group of rare, inherited disorders in which there is faulty repair of damaged DNA and the development of numerous skin cancers.

Clinical features

The phenotypic expression depends on the particular genetic abnormality responsible, but in all types, pre-neoplastic and neoplastic lesions including solar keratoses, squamous cell carcinomas, basal cell carcinomas and melanomas develop from childhood, and in the worst cases cause death in later adolescence or early adult life. The development of skin cancers is accompanied by severe photodamage, resulting in a characteristic and pitiful appearance (Fig. 13.15). In one severe recessive variety known as the de Sanctis–Caccione syndrome, there are also crippling neurological defects, including cerebellar ataxia and intellectual impairment.

Epidemiology and natural history

It has been estimated that, overall, the incidence of xeroderma pigmentosum is 1 in 250 000, but in some areas, such as parts of the Middle East, the condition is unusually common.

Treatment

Management is directed to genetic counselling, removal of neoplastic lesions as they occur and prevention of further photodamage by advice and sunscreens.

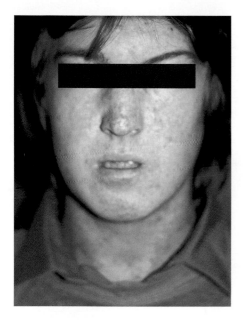

Figure 13.15 A patient with xeroderma pigmentosum. (Reproduced with thanks to Dr Dafydd Roberts.)

Recently, the use of systemic retinoids has been shown to reduce the rate of development of new cancers and is now an important aspect of the management of these patients.

Melanoma skin cancer

LENTIGO MALIGNA (HUTCHINSON'S FRECKLE)

Lentigo maligna is a slowly progressive, pre-neoplastic disorder of melanocytes, which develops insidiously on exposed areas of skin, particularly the skin of the face. The lesion itself is a pigmented macule with a well-defined, rounded or polycyclic edge, which may be up to 5 cm in diameter or even larger (Fig. 13.16). A characteristic feature is the varying shades of brown and black contained within the lesion – a feature known as variegation. The differential diagnosis includes seborrhoeic wart, simple senile lentigo and pigmented solar keratosis (see Table 13.3).

The disorder is usually slowly progressive over a period that may be in excess of 20 years. If left untreated, a true malignant melanoma develops within the lentigo maligna, which then has the characteristics of a typical malignant melanoma (see below).

Pathology

There are many abnormal, often spindle-shaped, melanocytic clear cells at the base of the epidermis and clumps of melanin pigment in the upper part of the dermis. As the disease progresses, clumps of abnormal melanocytes appear, projecting into the dermis, and a dense infiltrate of mononuclear cells develops.

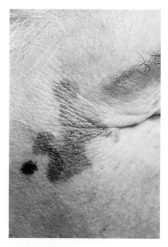

Figure 13.16 Lentigo maligna. Note the variegated pigmentation and irregular margin.

Table 13.3 Differential diagnosis of melanoma

Type of lesion	Main differentials	Comment
Lentigo maligna	Seborrhoeic wart, senile lentigo, pigmented solar keratosis	Seborrhoeic wart tends to be warty; senile lentigo is not variegated; solar keratosis tends to be scaly and pink/brown
Superficial spreading malignant melanoma	Seborrhoeic wart, pigmented basal cell carcinoma, vascular malformation, melanocytic naevus	Seborrhoeic wart tends to be warty; basal cell carcinoma has a pearly look; vascular lesion may blanch if not thrombosed; melanocytic naevus is less variegated
Acral lentiginous melanoma	Melanocytic naevus, vascular malformation	Melanocytic naevus is less variegated; malformation may blanch if not thrombosed
Malignant melanoma growing vertically downwards	Seborrhoeic wart, pigmented basal cell carcinoma, vascular malformation, melanocytic naevus, pyogenic granuloma	Seborrhoeic wart tends to be warty; basal cell carcinoma has a pearly look; vascular lesion may blanch if not thrombosed; melanocytic naevus is less variegated; pyogenic granuloma tends to be redder and smaller than malignant melanoma

Treatment

This is dictated by the size and exact site of the lesions. Often, they are of size and site precluding surgical removal. In these instances, other locally destructive measures have been used, including curettage and cautery and radiotherapy. Careful follow-up is required to detect the earliest signs of development of a frank melanoma.

MALIGNANT MELANOMA

Malignant melanoma is an invasive, neoplastic disorder of melanocytes in which the tendency is for invasion either horizontally and upwards into the epidermis (superficial spreading malignant melanoma, SSMM) or vertically downwards (nodular malignant melanoma, NMM).

Clinical features

Some 50 per cent of lesions of malignant melanoma develop from a pre-existing melanocytic naevus and the other 50 per cent develop *de novo* on any part of the

Table 13.4 Clinical features of malignant melanoma

Recent
  Growth in size, or appearance of new pigmented lesion
  Change in colour (mostly increased pigmentation)
  Change in shape (development of irregular margin)
Development of itchiness in lesion
Irregularity of margin/pigmentation
Erosion and/or crusting
Appearance of satellite nodules (late)
Enlargement of regional lymph nodes (very late)

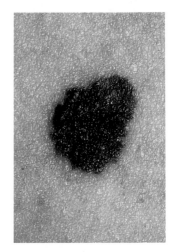

Figure 13.17 Nodular malignant melanoma. This lesion enlarged and darkened over a period of 3 months.

skin surface. Any pigmented lesion that suddenly develops or any change in the size, shape or colour of a pre-existing lesion should be suspected of being a malignant melanoma. Particular signs that are valuable in the recognition of these lesions are irregularity in the margin or in the degree of pigmentation, and erosion or crusting of the skin surface (Fig. 13.17, Table 13.4). Itchiness of the lesion is a not uncommon symptom in malignant melanoma.

One way in which this lesion may present is as a rapidly growing, non-pigmented nodule with an eroded surface, looking somewhat like a pyogenic granuloma (Fig. 13.18).

Another unusual variety of malignant melanoma is the acral lentiginous melanoma, which develops around the fingers or toes and sometimes subungually. This form has a particularly poor prognosis.

Late local signs are the development of satellite pigmented nodules and enlargement of the regional lymph nodes. Redness and other signs of inflammation may be present, but benign compound moles may also become inflamed and inflammatory change *by itself* is not common in malignant melanoma.

Although this is a potentially fatal disorder, the early stages are easily curable and it is vitally important that every physician learns the signs of malignant melanoma. Pigmented lesions can be very difficult to diagnose and there is no shame in requesting another opinion.

The differential diagnosis includes melanocytic naevus (see page 188), pigmented basal cell carcinoma (see page 214), histiocytoma (see page 197) and vascular malformation (see page 194).

The rate of progress of the disease seems largely determined by the inherent biology of the malignant melanoma. When the lesion spreads horizontally (SSMM), it tends to be noted and treated earlier than when the predominant direction of growth is vertically downwards (NMM). It is therefore not surprising that the overall prognosis is much better for SSMM than for NMM. The single most important determinant of prognosis appears to be depth of invasion into the dermis (see below). Thus, patients with small lesions of less than 1 mm invasion into the dermis have an expectancy of a 5-year survival rate in excess of 95 per cent. Because of the significance for prognosis of the depth of invasion into the dermis,

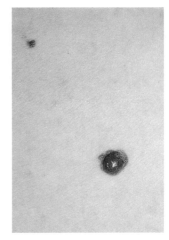

Figure 13.18 Red, shiny nodule due to malignant melanoma that was initially diagnosed as a pyogenic granuloma.

various classifications based on microscope measurements have been developed. The two most common are the Breslow's thickness technique and the Clark staging method. In the Breslow technique, three categories are recognized: less than 1.5 mm, 1.5–3.5 mm, and more than 3.5 mm. Clark's staging method recognizes five stages dependent on where the tumour reaches: stage 1 being confined to the epidermis, and stage 5 where there is infiltration of the subcutaneous fat. Stages 2, 3 and 4 describe progressively deeper levels within the dermis.

Spread of malignant melanoma is local, regional and distant. Distant metastases occur by haematogenous spread. Haematogenous metastases may occur anywhere, but quite commonly they develop in the lungs, liver and brain. Regional spread is via the lymphatics to regional lymph nodes. When regional lymph node metastases have been found, the 5-year survival rate is less than 25 per cent, and when distant metastases have occurred the comparable figure is around 5 per cent.

Secondary satellite lesions develop around the primary malignant melanoma in many instances. When metastases are widespread, the production of melanin pigment and its subsequent release into the circulation may be sufficiently great to result in a generalized darkening of the skin and even excretion of melanin in the urine (melaninuria), although this is quite rare. Occasionally, regression of part of the lesion occurs and, rarely, the entire lesion and metastases may undergo spontaneous resolution.

Overall, men have a worse prognosis than women. Back lesions in men and leg lesions in women have the least favourable prognoses.

Pathology and aetiopathogenesis

Typically, there are clumps of abnormal melanocytes at the dermoepidermal junction. In SSMM, abnormal melanocytes tend to invade upward into the epidermis and horizontally along the epidermis. In NMM, there are groups of abnormal cells invading vertically downwards (Fig. 13.19). There is usually some accompanying inflammatory cell infiltrate. It has to be said that the histological diagnosis of melanoma may be difficult and should be left to the expert.

Solar UVR is believed to be the single most important causative factor, but, as up to 50 per cent of lesions of malignant melanoma occur on non-sun-exposed sites, other factors may play a role. The propensity for patients with the dysplastic mole syndrome (see page 193) and large congenital melanocytic naevi to develop this condition suggests that developmental factors may also be involved in some instances. There is some evidence that episodes of intense sun exposure over short periods, with sunburn, may be very harmful. This could explain why malignant melanoma is relatively common on areas of skin that are only occasionally exposed to the sun.

Epidemiology

Malignant melanoma is rare before puberty, but can occur at any age after that. It is seen in all racial types, but is more common in fair-skinned, Caucasian types. Acral lentiginous melanoma seems most frequent in black-skinned individuals and subjects of Japanese or other Asian descent. The incidence has increased in all countries that keep accurate figures and increases have been noted since records

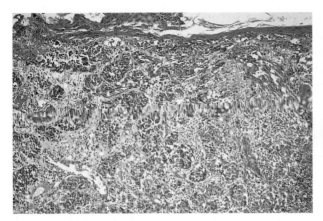

Figure 13.19 Pathology of malignant melanoma. Note the irregular clumps of abnormal naevus cells throughout the upper dermis.

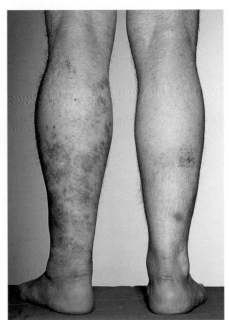

Figure 13.20 Classical Kaposi's sarcoma with brown macules and mauve plaques on the lower legs.

first began. The rate of increase seems to be of the order of 7 per cent per annum. The incidence is greatest in Queensland, Australia, and tends to be high in the hot, sunny areas that have a large fair-skinned population of European descent.

Treatment

The treatment of choice is excision with a generous margin of normal skin. There is debate concerning the width of the margin, but it should be at least 2 cm around the lesion for a malignant melanoma of 1 cm diameter. There is also debate as to whether or not regional lymph nodes should be removed prophylactically. The balance of opinion suggests not, provided that there is no clinical evidence of spread.

Metastatic disease responds poorly, if at all, to chemotherapy, but some decrease in the size of metastatic deposits and occasional temporary remission have been noted with combinations of antimetabolites and other anticancer drugs as well as with retinoids, interferons and interleukin-2.

NEOPLASTIC DISORDERS OF MESENCHYMAL ELEMENTS

Kaposi's sarcoma (idiopathic haemorrhagic sarcoma)

Kaposi's sarcoma is a rare, multi-focal, malignant vascular tumour of skin and other organs, which occurs either as an endemic, slowly progressive disease or as a rapidly progressive disorder in the immunosuppressed.

The endemic type occurs predominantly in elderly males of either Jewish origin from central Europe or of Italian origin from around the Po valley. Mauve or purplish-red nodules and plaques and brownish macules (Fig. 13.20) develop over the dorsa of the feet and the lower legs. These lesions are usually accompanied by swelling of the lower legs. They are slowly progressive and may not appear in other sites for many years. It has been estimated that the mean survival time after the appearance of the first lesions is approximately 12 years. Eventually, lesions disseminate to other parts of the skin and to the viscera.

The rapidly progressive type occurs in patients with AIDS, particularly male homosexuals, renal transplant patients and in areas of Africa notably Uganda. The clinical manifestations are similar to those of endemic Kaposi's sarcoma, but are much more extensive and much more rapidly progressive.

Pathology and pathogenesis
The lesions consist of abnormal, slit-like vascular channels lined with spindle-shaped cells, a mixed inflammatory cell infiltrate, haemorrhage and fibrosis. It is believed that a herpes-type virus is involved in the causation.

Treatment
As the disorder appears to be multi-focal, cure does not appear possible at the moment. However, radiotherapy keeps localized areas in check and systemic interferon produces partial regression and remission in many patients. A new topical retinoid, alretin, has also been shown to be effective.

Dematofibromasarcoma

This is a slowly progressive neoplastic disorder of fibroblasts. It looks quite similar to a histiocytoma histologically and is an intracutaneous form of plaque clinically. Treatment is excision.

Lymphomas of skin (cutaneous T-cell lymphoma)

MYCOSIS FUNGOIDES

Mycosis fungoides is a multi-focal, neoplastic disorder of T-lymphocytes that primarily affects the skin.

This uncommon disorder starts off as a series of red macules and scaly patches over the trunk and upper limbs, which gradually extend and become more prolific, but at first only cause inconvenience because of their appearance and mild pruritus (Fig. 13.21). The red patches persist, although they may fluctuate in intensity, and eventually start to thicken and become plaques and, later still, eroded tumours (Fig. 13.22). The ringworm-like appearance of some of the early patches and the fungating plaques in the late stages were presumably responsible for the term mycosis fungoides. In the later stages of the disorder, lymph node enlargement, hepatosplenomegaly and infiltration of other viscera occur. At the time of writing, the disorder is inevitably fatal, although the rate of progress is quite variable, with survival ranging from 2 or 3 years in some patients to 20 years in others.

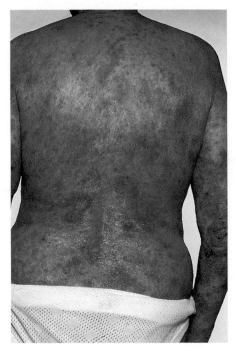

Figure 13.21 Multiple infiltrated, red plaques on the trunk of a patient with mycosis fungoides.

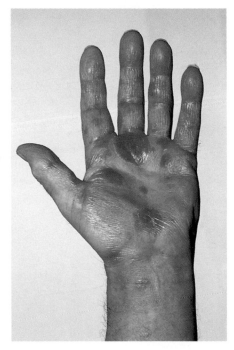

Figure 13.22 Eroded nodules on the palm of a patient with terminal mycosis fungoides.

The above sequence is the 'classical' type of mycosis fungoides, and other less common variants are occasionally seen.

SÉZARY SYNDROME

This is marked by an erythroderma that has a particular intense erythematous colour, a picture sometimes referred to as *l'homme rouge*. It is accompanied by thickening of the tissues of the face, neck and palms. It is also characterized by the appearance of abnormal mononuclear cells circulating in the peripheral blood. These cells, which are identified in the 'buffy coat', are large and have a large, dense, reniform nucleus.

OTHER FORMS OF T-CELL LYMPHOMA

In addition to the above declared forms of cutaneous T-cell lymphoma, there are a number of uncommon precursor disorders which were known collectively (and inappropriately) as *parapsoriasis*. These by no means always progress to T-cell lymphoma, and their true nature is uncertain. In addition, they are not well characterized clinically.

Summary

- Solar keratoses are localized areas of disorderly epidermal growth and differentiation due to chronic solar exposure. Typically, they are small, pink or grey, warty or scaling lesions on the exposed skin of fair-skinned, elderly subjects.

- Solar UVR, heat, X-rays HPV infection, chronic arsenic poisoning and immunosuppression are all factors that may be involved in the causation of solar keratoses. These lesions may be regarded as pre-malignant, although they rarely progress and often spontaneously remit.

- Solar keratoses often respond to topical 5-fluorouracil, diclofenac or imiquimod. Systemic retinoids and intralesional interferons have also been employed.

- Bowen's disease is a localized area of epidermal neoplasia remaining within the epidermis, with even greater cellular irregularity than a solar keratosis. Red, scaling psoriasiform plaques on the legs are typical. These plaques enlarge and thicken, eventually transforming to squamous cell carcinoma. Erythroplasia of Queyrat is Bowen's disease of the glans penis.

- Squamous cell carcinoma is usually a warty nodule or plaque that eventually ulcerates, invades local structures, but metastasizes late. Histologically, there is marked epidermal thickening and irregularity, with cellular heterogeneity and focal dyskeratosis. Solar UVR, heat, X-rays, HPV infection, chemical carcinogens and chronic inflammation may be involved in the aetiology.

- Keratoacanthoma arises suddenly as a solitary, horn-filled crateriform nodule consisting of an invaginated epidermal cup. It remits spontaneously after 3–4 months.

- Basal cell carcinoma is a very common, locally invasive epithelial tumour of basaloid cells. Nodulocystic types form pearly papules or plaques, which eventually ulcerate. Some may be pigmented. Superficial basal cell carcinoma spreads very slowly as well-defined psoriasiform plaques. Morphoeic basal cell carcinomas form firm plaques as the cells evoke a fibrotic reaction. Histologically, areas of mucoid degeneration amongst the basophilic basal cell clumps are common.

- Basal cell naevus syndrome is a rare genodermatosis in which there are multiple developmental anomalies, multiple pigmented basal cell carcinomas, bifid ribs and palmar pits. Xeroderma pigmentosum is another rare genodermatosis in which there is a deficiency in the ability to repair DNA damaged by UVR. This results in skin cancers of various types.

- Lentigo maligna (Hutchinson's freckle) is a slowly progressive, pre-malignant lesion of melanocytes on exposed skin. Characteristically, it is a large macule with varying shades of pigmentation. If left untreated, a malignant melanoma often develops within the lesion.

- Some 50 per cent of malignant melanomas develop from a pre-existing melanocytic naevus. The rest develop de novo. Sudden enlargement, irregularity of pigmentation and margin, erosion, crusting and itching are important signs of melanoma. The early stages are curable and the diagnosis should be considered in any pigmented lesion. Malignant melanoma must be distinguished from seborrhoeic wart, pigmented basal cell carcinoma, pigmented mole, histiocytoma and vascular malformations.

- Lesions of superficial malignant melanoma with lateral spread have a better prognosis than the nodular lesions. The depth of invasion into the dermis is a major prognostic indicator – less than 1 mm invasion and there is a better than 95 per cent 5-year survival. Metastases of malignant melanoma may occur early. With lymph node metastases, there is less than 25 per cent 5-year survival. With blood-borne metastases (liver, lung, brain), the survival rate is less than 5 per cent.

- Kaposi's sarcoma is a rare, multi-focal, malignant vascular tumour of skin, which may occur as a slowly progressive endemic disease or as a rapidly progressive disorder in AIDS and other immuno-suppressed states. Affected individuals develop mauve/purple patches, nodules and plaques in the legs and elsewhere on the skin and in the viscera.

- Mycosis fungoides is a rare, multi-focal, neoplastic disorder of T-lymphocytes, characterized by the appearance of red, sometimes psoriasiform, plaques over the skin, which is ultimately fatal. Sézary syndrome is a similar disorder, but differs in that the whole of the skin is affected.

Skin problems in infancy and old age

Infancy

FUNCTIONAL DIFFERENCES

In the neonatal period and early infancy, the skin's defences are not yet fully developed, and it is much more vulnerable to chemical, physical and microbial attack. Apart from the depressed skin defences, the surface area to weight ratio is higher than at other times and there is a greater hazard from increased absorption of topically applied medicaments. For example, serious systemic toxicity can result from the application of corticosteroids or a salicylic acid preparation. There is also a greater rate of transepidermal water loss through intact, non-sweating skin in the newborn compared to the adult, indicating immaturity of the skin's barrier function. This is easily confirmed by the use of a special water-sensor device known as the evaporimeter.

During the early weeks of life, newborns possess the blood levels of hormones found in the mother at birth. This may be of special significance for the sebaceous glands, which react to circulating androgenic compounds by enlargement and increased sebum secretion.

MANAGEMENT PROBLEMS IN INFANCY

Medicaments are absorbed from infants far more easily and are more likely to cause systemic toxicity. Topical agents that are well tolerated by adults may cause quite severe reactions in infancy because of the lack of maturity of the barrier.

The ability to scratch does not seem to develop until around the age of 6 months and, when it does, the rash may alter substantially because of the excoriations and

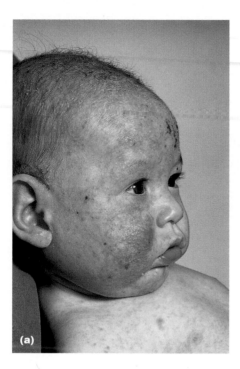

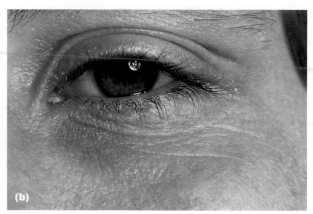

Figure 14.1 (a) Atopic dermatitis of the face at age 4 months. There is marked inflammation but no excoriations. (b) Lichenification around the eyes in an older child due to rubbing.

the physical effects of persistent scratching on the skin (lichenification) as well as the presence of infective lesions (Fig. 14.1). The inability of the infant to complain of discomfort and irritation leads to general irritability and persistent crying. When this continues for long periods, the parents cannot sleep and the intrafamilial emotional tension spirals upwards within the family home, necessitating attention to all those involved.

Widespread rashes may lead rapidly to dehydration in infancy because of the greatly increased rate of water loss through the abnormal skin. The same is true of heat loss from the inflamed skin. Hypothermia can develop very rapidly in young infants who have a widespread inflammatory skin disorder and, like dehydration, is a dangerous complication. These two complications, dehydration and hypothermia, may be prevented by:

- anticipation and monitoring water loss with an evaporimeter and monitoring body temperature by taking the rectal temperature
- nursing infants with severe widespread skin disease in an incubator or supplying the necessary extra heat and fluid.

NAPKIN RASH

Several different skin disorders localize to the napkin area, which is perhaps not surprising when the physical assault that the wearing of napkins provides is considered.

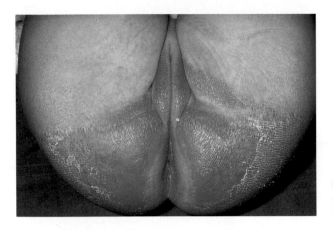

Figure 14.2 Erosive napkin dermatitis. Note sparing in the flexures.

Erosive napkin dermatitis

This is the commonest type of napkin dermatitis. Red, glazed, fissured and even eroded areas develop on the skin at sites in contact with the napkin (Fig. 14.2). The flexures are mostly spared, with the worst areas appearing on the convexities. There is often a strong ammoniacal smell when the napkin is removed. This is due to the release of ammonia from the action of the urease released from the faecal bacteria on the urea in the urine.

The condition responds to nursing without napkins for 2 or 3 days, but if this is not possible, more frequent napkin changes, the use of soft muslin napkins and avoidance of abrasive towelling napkins help, as do efficient disposables that leave the skin surface dry. An emollient washing agent and an emollient used 2 or 3 times per day also help. Topical 1 per cent hydrocortisone ointment twice daily could be used if the condition proves resistant.

Case 13

Casey was the first child born to June. At the age of 4½ months, a nasty, bright-red rash developed on the convexities of her buttocks. This erosive napkin dermatitis healed quite rapidly when June followed the advice she was given to use only either good-quality, disposable napkins or soft, muslin napkins and to change them more frequently. The use of an emollient also seemed to help.

Seborrhoeic dermatitis

Scaling, red areas develop, mainly in the folds of the skin, although the eruption 'overflows' on to other areas in the napkin area. When the condition is severe and 'angry', other sites such as the scalp, face and neck may be affected (Fig. 14.3). The involved sites may also crack and become exudative. The same kind of care of the napkin area as outlined above for erosive napkin dermatitis should be advised.

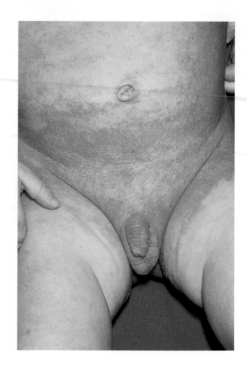

Figure 14.3 Napkin dermatitis of seborrhoeic dermatitis type.

In addition, the use of a weak topical corticosteroid in combination with broad-spectrum antimicrobial compounds such as an imidazole (e.g. miconazole or clotrimazole) should be used twice daily. The involvement of the yeast *Candida albicans* in this form of napkin dermatitis has been claimed but not confirmed.

Napkin psoriasis

This is an uncommon, odd, psoriasis-like eruption that develops in the napkin area and may spread to the skin outside (Fig. 14.4). Treatment should once again be directed to better hygiene. Weak topical corticosteroids and emollients used as indicated above usually improve the condition quite quickly.

ATOPIC DERMATITIS (see also Chapter 8)

The condition rarely starts before 4–6 weeks of age and usually begins between the ages of 2 and 3 months. It may first show itself on the face, but spreads quite quickly to other areas, although the napkin area is conspicuously spared – presumably as a result of the area being kept moist. The ability to scratch develops after about 6 months of age and the appearance of the disorder alters accordingly, with excoriations and lichenification. At this time, the predominantly flexural distribution of the disorder begins, with thickened, red, scaly and excoriated (and sometimes crusted and infected) areas in the popliteal and antecubital fossae. Emollients are important in management and mothers should be carefully instructed on their benefit and how to use them. Similarly, bathing should be quick 'dunks' in

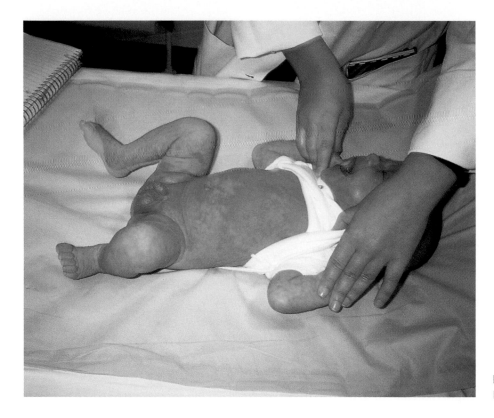

Figure 14.4 Napkin psoriasis.

lukewarm water, with patting dry, rather than long-lasting hot scrubs with vigorous towelling afterwards. Weak topical corticosteroids only should be used – 1 per cent hydrocortisone and 0.1 per cent clobetasone butyrate are appropriate. Preparations of 1 per cent hydrocortisone containing urea are helpful.

CRADLECAP

The newborn often develop yellowish scale over the scalp with very little other abnormality apparent. This has no special significance and usually disappears after a few weeks. Application of olive oil or arachis oil with 2 per cent salicylic acid and shampooing with 'baby shampoos' hasten its removal.

INFANTILE ACNE

It is not uncommon for infants a few months old to develop seborrhoea, comedones, superficial papules and pustules on the face (Fig. 14.5). This infantile acne has no special significance, other than that maternal androgens have caused the infant's sebaceous glands to enlarge and become more active. When the disorder develops in later infancy and is severe, the possibility of virilization due to an

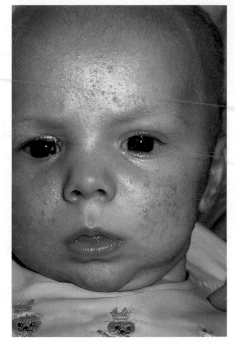

Figure 14.5 Infantile acne showing numerous acne spots affecting the cheeks and forehead.

endocrine tumour or adrenocortical hyperplasia has to be considered. Other signs of androgen over-activity, such as precocious muscle development and male distribution of facial and body hair, should be sought.

Although the disorder usually subsides within a few weeks, it can be unpleasantly persistent. Rarely, deep nodules and even cysts develop.

Treatment with mild topical agents is usually sufficient, e.g. 0.05 per cent tretinoin gel or 5 per cent benzoyl peroxide gel.

TOXIC EPIDERMAL NECROLYSIS (STAPHYLOCOCCAL SCALDED SKIN SYNDROME)

There are two different severe disorders that share some features as well as the name *toxic epidermal necrolysis*. The first is covered in Chapter 6 and is a reaction to certain drugs. The other, which is seen in early infancy and is better termed the staphylococcal scalded skin syndrome, is described here. It affects infants in the first few weeks of life, but can occur in older children. There is a widespread erythematous eruption with striking desquamation of large areas of skin, as in a scald or burn. There may be a slight fever and some systemic disturbance, but usually the children are not severely ill, although there is a 2–3 per cent mortality. The disorder is due to a particular phage type of *Staphylococcus aureus* (phage type II), which releases an erythematogenic exotoxin. This toxin can be shown experimentally to cause shedding of the most superficial part of the epidermis and stratum corneum in the skin of the newborn.

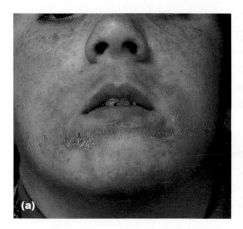
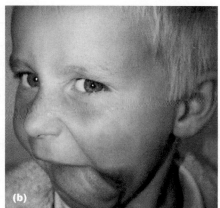

Figure 14.6 (a) and (b) Lip-licking cheilitis.

Treatment should be with an appropriate systemic antibiotic such as flucloxacillin. The skin should be managed as for a burn, and concern over heat loss, dehydration and severe infection is necessary.

LIP-LICKING CHEILITIS

Children aged 4–8 years develop an area around the mouth which becomes sore, red, scaly and cracked (Fig. 14.6). It is due to licking the lips and the skin around the lips, which become irritated and dry and are then licked to moisten them, making the situation worse. The treatment is to explain patiently the nature of the problem to mother and child and to use an emollient on the affected area.

JUVENILE PLANTAR DERMATOSIS

This disorder has apparently become more common in recent years, affecting children aged 6–12 years predominantly. It is a type of eczema that affects the soles of the forefeet and the toes. The affected skin becomes 'glazed', scaly and cracked, and the condition tends to be very persistent. Treatment with emollients, topical corticosteroids and weak tar preparations is recommended, but the disorder tends to resist treatment and eventually remits spontaneously.

Old age

There is a growing acreage of elderly skin because of the staggering increase in the proportion of the population over the age of 60 years. The increase in longevity since the beginning of the twentieth century is approximately equal to that seen in the human race in the previous 5000 years. We certainly need to know more about the ageing process and its effects on the skin.

THE AGEING PROCESS

Very little is known as to why tissues age. Generally, we distinguish between intrinsic ageing and extrinsic ageing. The latter is not true ageing, i.e. the effects of the passage of time alone on the tissues, but the results of cumulated environmental trauma. As far as the skin is concerned, the most significant environmental trauma stems from solar radiation in the form of ultraviolet radiation (UVR: see page 27).

There are many hypotheses to account for intrinsic ageing, which range from a kind of built-in obsolescence within the DNA molecule itself to the cumulated results of metabolic damage from active oxygen species and free radicals. Whatever the explanation, at present there is very little that can be done to stem the tide of the passing years, other than carefully choosing long-lived parents! Another inexplicable aspect of ageing is its variability. There are enormous variations in the rates at which different individuals age, as well as major differences in the rates at which individual organs and systems age within one individual.

SKIN CHANGES IN THE ELDERLY

Structural changes

Both the epidermis and the dermis become thinner on non-light-exposed sites with the passing of the years. The degree of thinning is variable, but, between the ages of 20 and 80, dermal thickness on the flexor aspect of the forearm changes in men from a mean of 1.1 mm to 0.8 mm. The epidermis thins from four to five cells thick at age 20 to approximately three cells thick at age 80. The individual keratinocytes also shrink with age, although the horn cells at the surface inexplicably increase in area. Interestingly, the stratum corneum does not appear to change substantially in thickness during ageing.

Blood vessels decrease in number with age, but thicken. Adnexal structures also decrease in size and number with increasing age. This applies also to the hair (see page 268), but not always to the sebaceous glands, as on the face they may, paradoxically, enlarge, which is sometimes clinically evident in the condition of sebaceous gland hyperplasia (see page 188).

The dermal connective tissue loses much of its proteoglycan ground substance and the collagen fibres become mainly tough, insoluble and heavily cross-linked biochemically. Pigment cells become fewer in number and smaller, and Langerhans cells are also less in evidence in the skin of the elderly.

Functional changes

Wound healing is slower and may be less complete in the elderly. The aged also respond less vigorously to chemical and physical trauma – the erythema and swelling are less marked and slower to develop. Delayed hypersensitivity is depressed and this also applies to other components of the immune response.

The activity of the pigment cells is depressed, and non-exposed areas of skin are in general paler in the elderly than in young and mature subjects. On exposed areas of skin, melanocytes show irregular increases in pigmentation.

Sweat gland responses to heating decrease, and the rate of sebum secretion also decreases, although this is less marked than many other functions in the elderly.

Sensory discrimination decreases in the elderly, but, unfortunately, not the sensations of itch or pain!

SKIN DISEASE IN THE ELDERLY

There are very few skin disorders that are specific to the elderly. However, there are many disorders that are more common in the aged, and others that have a different natural history and appearance.

Dry and itchy skin

As the skin ages, it becomes drier and tends to become itchier. This tendency is heightened by:

- low relative humidity
- frequent hot bathing and vigorous towelling
- low ambient temperature.

The itchiness can be disabling and it is important to try to reduce the desiccating stimuli to which the skin is exposed. The generous use of emollients as topical applications as cleansing agents and of bath additives is mandatory.

Although itchiness due to dry skin in the elderly is quite common, it has to be remembered that scabies and the other causes of generalized pruritus also occur in this age group and should be diligently sought.

Eczema

Eczema is a common problem in one form or another in the elderly. It is dealt with in Chapter 8, but some points are worth emphasizing here. In most cases, no cause is found for the development of eczema, particularly in elderly people, in whom it can spread rapidly and become extremely disabling.

Atopic dermatitis is uncommon in the elderly and is as trying and uncomfortable as at other times of life when it does occur.

Discoid eczema is a form of constitutional eczema that is more common in the elderly.

Eczema craquelée is an eczematous disorder that is virtually specific to the skin of the elderly, occurring against a background of generalized xerosis, or drying of the skin surface.

Photosensitive eczema is more common in elderly men and is often very persistent, causing great difficulties in its management.

Minor degrees of *seborrhoeic dermatitis* are very common in the elderly and occasionally the disorder can spread to become generalized.

Treatment

The treatment of eczema in the elderly is similar to that in other age groups. However, emollients are even more important and there should be greater readiness to use systemic remedies, including cyclosporin, azathioprine and corticosteroids.

Case 14

William was 83 and lived by himself. His winter bronchitis worsened one day and he developed pneumonia. After being in hospital for 4 days, his chest improved with the use of antibiotics, but he began to develop an odd, itchy, 'crazy paving' pattern of rash on his shins. This eczema craquelée was due to the increased washing and decreased humidity in the hospital. It responded to reduced rubbing and scrubbing and the use of emollients.

Skin tumours

Skin tumours are a frequent reason for the elderly consulting a physician. Seborrhoeic warts are found in virtually everyone over the age of 60 years and, although benign, often result in minor symptoms and some cosmetic embarrassment. They can easily be removed by curettage and cautery, but when present in large numbers, can present an insoluble problem. Solar keratoses are another frequent cause of presentation – some 4 per cent of all new patient consultations in the dermatology department of the University Hospital of Wales were for solar keratoses. Although very few progress to squamous cell cancer, they indicate that serious solar damage has occurred and that more significant lesions may develop. They are uncommon below the age of 45 years and very common over the age of 60 years. As with seborrhoeic warts, solar keratoses may also cause minor symptoms and some cosmetic problems.

Basal cell carcinomas (see page 214) are almost as common as solar keratoses. Because of their capacity for local invasion and tissue destruction, they cause considerable morbidity. Squamous cell carcinomas (see page 211) are much less common, but can metastasize as well as cause local tissue destruction. Malignant melanoma (see page 219) is slightly more common in the elderly compared to young age groups, but lentigo maligna (see page 219) is virtually restricted to the elderly.

Management of skin disorders in the elderly

Through no fault of their own, the elderly are often physically, socially and economically deprived. Their housing, hygiene, nutrition, clothing and means of heating may all be deficient, and this should be taken into account when designing treatments. If they live alone, as is often the case, they may well be unable to find anyone to help with the application of ointments to body parts they cannot reach themselves or to assist with bandages because of lack of mobility.

It must be remembered that the elderly may also have difficulty in hearing, understanding and/or remembering instructions, especially if these are complex and involve more than one medicament. If possible, instructions on the medications should also be given to an accompanying relative or legibly written out.

The above potential difficulties need to be taken into account when trying to help an elderly patient with a skin problem.

Summary

- Neonatal skin is not mature functionally, so that excess water loss may occur, leading to dehydration. Similarly, the barrier of infants' skin is less efficient than in adult life, permitting greater amounts of topically applied agents to be absorbed. Infant skin is also less able to withstand infection.

- Rashes in the napkin area may be due to 'erosive dermatitis' on the convexities from persistent skin contact with faeces and urine or due to seborrhoeic dermatitis where the rash is mainly in the flexures. It may also be psoriasiform in type, although the relationship of this to adult psoriasis is uncertain. Frequent changes of nappies and the use of softer materials, together with the use of emollients and emollient cleaners and, if required, hydrocortisone, will rapidly improve most affected infants.

- Atopic dermatitis starts at 2–4 months, with rash on the face at first. The ability to scratch does not develop before 6 months of age, when the distribution and appearance of the rash change. Flexural lesions and excoriations start to develop. Advice on bathing and the frequent use of emollients and weak corticosteroids should help.

- Infantile acne with seborrhoea, comedones, papules and pustules is not uncommon and may be persistent. If it develops late in infancy, look for other signs of virilization (such as muscle growth).

- The staphylococcal scalded skin syndrome occurs in young infants and is a type of toxic epidermal necrolysis. It is caused by the erythematogenic toxin of a particular phage type of *Staphylococcus aureus* (phase type II). The rash is red and peeling and is accompanied by mild fever and some systemic disturbance.

- Lip-licking cheilitis is a perioral rash caused by licking the skin around the mouth. Juvenile plantar dermatosis is an eczematous rash of 6–12-year-old children affecting the forefeet.

- Apart from the intrinsic ageing process which all tissues undergo, the skin also experiences cumulative damage from the environment, particularly solar UVR, which we incorrectly identify as due to ageing. Intrinsic ageing is of unknown cause and is variable in rate and severity.

- Both the epidermis and dermis thin with age, losing about one-third of their thickness by the age of 80. Blood vessels, adnexae and pigment cells are all reduced in ageing. In addition, wound healing slows and the immune defences diminish.

- Dry, itchy skin is common in the elderly. Eczema craquelée, photosensitive eczema and discoid eczema are more common in this age group. Seborrhoeic dermatitis is also common in the elderly.

- Seborrhoeic warts are very common in the elderly and may be present in large numbers. Solar keratoses also increase with age. Basal cell carcinoma, squamous cell carcinoma and melanoma are all more common in the elderly (see Chapter 13). The elderly often have difficulty coping with instructions given for treatment.

Pregnancy and the skin

Physiological changes in the skin during pregnancy

PIGMENTATION

Most women develop a generalized increased pigmentation of the skin notable in the midline of the abdomen, converting the linea alba into the linea nigra. The areolae of the breasts change in colour from pink to brown and the skin of the external genitalia also darkens.

In addition, dark areas appear symmetrically across the cheeks, around the eyes and over the forehead, giving a mask-like appearance (Fig. 15.1). This is known as melasma (or chloasma) and seems much more common and troublesome in darker, Mediterranean and Asian skin types. The same problem is sometimes seen in non-pregnant women and it is claimed that the contraceptive pill is responsible. Some 60 per cent of pregnant women develop some melasma, and 30 per cent of women on the pill do so.

The commonest type of melasma is centrofacial (about 65 per cent). The 'malar' type, with pigmentation on the cheeks, and the mandibular pattern, with pigmentation along the lower jaw, are less common.

The increase in blood levels of melanocyte-stimulating hormone and the consequent stimulation of melanocyte activity or the increase in oestrogen and progesterone may be involved in the cause.

Pigmented moles also darken during pregnancy and new moles may appear – both causing concern.

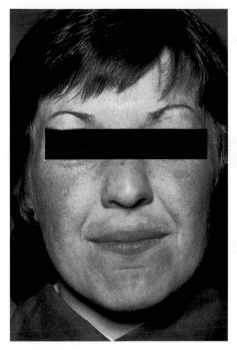

Figure 15.1 'Mask of pregnancy', also known as melasma or chloasma.

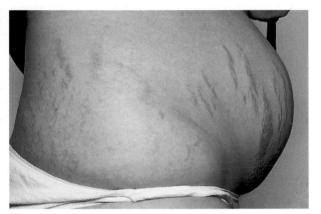

Figure 15.2 'Stretch marks', or striae distensae, on the abdomen 6 months postpartum.

STRIAE GRAVIDARUM

Striae distensae (or stretch marks) are linear areas of apparent atrophy of the skin due to disruption of dermal connective tissue fibres (Fig. 15.2) as a result of ruptured dermal elastic fibres. They occur at sites of skin stretching when there is excess glucocorticoid activity. They occur normally in early adolescence, in Cushing's syndrome after both systemic and topical corticoid therapy, and in pregnancy, when they are called striae gravidarum.

Striae gravidarum occur predominantly over the lower abdomen and over the breasts during the third trimester and are of major cosmetic concern.

CUTANEOUS VASCULARITY

One of the oddest of phenomena that occur in pregnant women is the appearance of small vascular malformations known as spider naevi (Fig. 15.3). These only develop on the face, upper trunk and arms, i.e. the area of drainage of the superior vena cava. As with liver disease, in which these lesions also occur, it may be that in pregnancy there is a relative excess of oestrogenic activity that provokes these vascular anomalies. Also, the palms in pregnancy become redder and feel warmer, as in liver disease. Both the spider naevi and the palmar changes fade following delivery.

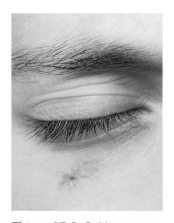

Figure 15.3 Spider naevus.

PRURITUS IN PREGNANCY

Generalized itching is sometimes a problem for pregnant women. In some instances, there appears to be intrahepatic cholestasis leading to biliary retention in the last trimester. There is little that can be done concerning this problem, other than using emollients and mentholated oily calamine preparations.

Effects of pregnancy on intercurrent skin disease

Common inflammatory skin disorders such as psoriasis and atopic dermatitis often improve during pregnancy, but this is by no means invariable. Systemic lupus erythematosus is reputed to worsen. Great care must be taken with systemic medication during pregnancy. Systemic retinoids are very teratogenic and should not be given to women in the reproductive age group unless they take reliable contraception. Other drugs such as antibiotics and hormones should also be avoided.

Topical treatments must also be assessed for their teratogenic potential. Most topically applied materials are absorbed to a greater or lesser extent and, at least theoretically, could constitute a risk to the fetus. The possibility that topical tretinoin could be responsible for fetal malformations after usage for acne has been extensively investigated, but discounted because insufficient is absorbed through the skin. Fortunately, this applies to most of the routine topical agents used for psoriasis, eczema and acne – providing the affected area does not amount to 10 per cent or more of the body surface area.

Effects of intercurrent maternal disease on the fetus

The fetus is occasionally affected by skin disorders in the mother.

THE INHERITED GENODERMATOSES

Genetic faults may be passed on and phenotypically expressed in the child. This is obvious with dominant disorders such as some of the ichthyoses (see page 246).

IMMUNOLOGICALLY MEDIATED DISEASES

In some disorders, pathogenetic antibodies cross the placenta and cause disease in the fetus. This may be the case in lupus erythematosus and, in one rare variety of this condition, congenital heart block can be induced in the child. It may also occur in the rare blistering condition of pemphigus. In most of these cases, the fetal skin disorders only last as long as the transplacentally transmitted antibodies in the newborn child's circulation.

INFECTIONS

These are of most concern now with regard to human immunodeficiency virus (HIV) infection, and frighteningly high rates of HIV positivity have been found in pregnant women in some communities. Syphilis may still be a problem if undiagnosed and then transmitted congenitally. Other infective skin disorders that may be passed from mother to fetus include chickenpox, herpes simplex, candidiasis and warts, although the last two are better classified as 'intranatal' infections, as they are caught from the birth passages.

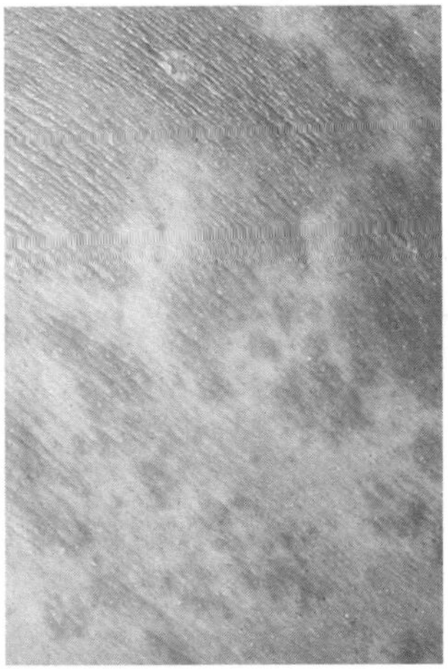

Skin disorders occurring in pregnancy

ITCHY RASHES IN THE LAST TRIMESTER

Several patterns of itchy, erythematous rash occur in the last trimester of pregnancy. Their causes are unknown, they are transient, remitting spontaneously before delivery or, at worst, shortly afterwards, and they produce much discomfort. In some cases, they are associated with pre-eclamptic toxaemia.

The rash mostly occurs over the abdomen and flanks, but also appears on the upper limbs. The lesions are mainly micropapules, but in some patients red, urticaria-like plaques develop (Fig. 15.4). Annular and odd figurate lesions may also occur. Treatment is symptomatic, with emollient or weak topical corticosteroids.

Figure 15.4 Common itchy erythematous eruption of pregnancy.

Case 15

Charlotte, aged 24, is 7 months pregnant with her first child and has suddenly developed an itching, red rash on her abdomen, buttocks and thighs. Apart from striae and midline pigmentation, there are only a few nondescript papules to see. This is the common maculopapular rash of pregnancy, which will quickly subside when she has been delivered and will obtain some relief from simple emollients.

HERPES GESTATIONIS (PEMPHIGOID GESTATIONIS)

This is an uncommon, extremely irritant, blistering rash, occurring in the last trimester of pregnancy. The eruption starts on the flanks or over the abdomen with itchy urticarial papules and vesicles and blisters (Fig. 15.5). The blistering is subepidermal and is quite similar to that seen in senile pemphigoid (see page 88). There is often a circulating antibody directed to the dermoepidermal junctional area, although this is present in 'low titre'.

The rash usually remits shortly after birth, but may recur in subsequent pregnancies or even after taking oral contraceptives. Treatment should be confined to topical applications in the first instance. If this does not help, dapsone may be tried for short periods.

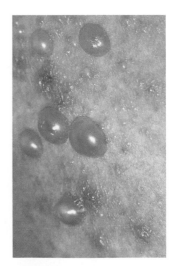

Figure 15.5 Blistering rash due to pemphigoid gestationis.

Summary

- The breast areolae, the midline of the abdomen, the external genitalia and areas on the face become hyperpigmented during pregnancy. The facial changes, known as melasma, occur in 60 per cent of pregnant women.

- Striae distensae (or stretch marks) occur in Cushing's syndrome, during treatment with corticosteroids, in pregnancy (striae gravidarum) and in normal adolescence.

- Spider naevi may develop during pregnancy. Generalized itching may occur during the third trimester due to intrahepatic cholestasis.

- Inflammatory dermatoses may either improve or worsen during pregnancy. Great care should be taken to ensure that the developing fetus is not exposed to potentially teratogenic drugs, whether administered systemically or topically to the pregnant woman.

- The fetus may be affected by genodermatoses, by immunodermatoses because of transplacental carriage of pathogenic antibodies (e.g. pemphigus) or infection from transplacental spread of infection such as HIV, syphilis and chickenpox, or from intranatal contamination, e.g. wart virus.

- Various transient, itchy rashes occur in the last trimester of pregnancy. In addition, a very itchy, blistering rash occurs in the last trimester associated with a circulating antibody, which remits after delivery but may recur in subsequent pregnancies.

Disorders of keratinization and other genodermatoses

Introduction

EPIDERMAL DIFFERENTIATION

The differentiation process in which basal epidermal cells gradually mature and transform into stratum corneum cells is known as keratinization. In this process, which takes about 14 days, plump, cuboidal or spheroidal, hydrated, highly metabolically active cells gradually become tough, hardened, biochemically inactive, thin, shield-like structures that are programmed to desquamate off the skin surface (Fig. 16.1). This process is biochemically complex and it is not surprising that it is subject to genetically determined errors. During keratinization, a tough, chemically resistant, cross-linked protein band is laid down just inside the plasma membrane and the whole cell flattens to a thin disc (corneocyte, Fig. 16.2). The corneocyte's water content is reduced from the usual 70 per cent to 30 per cent and most of the cellular organelles, including its nucleus, are eliminated. The keratinous tonofilaments become organized in bundles and are spatially orientated. A further characteristic feature of the normal stratum corneum is the presence of an intercellular cement material that contains non-polar lipid and glycoprotein.

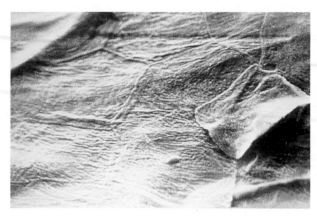

Figure 16.1 Corneocyte desquamating from the skin surface as seen by scanning electron microscopy.

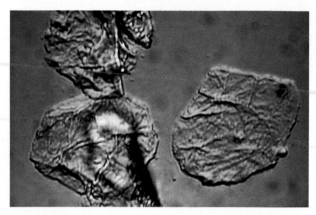

Figure 16.2 Single corneocytes as seen by phase contrast microscopy.

STRATUM CORNEUM FUNCTION

The stratum corneum is the major barrier to water loss from the skin and to the penetration of chemical agents that come into contact with the skin. It also provides some mechanical protection and prevents penetration by microbes.

SCALING

A scale is merely an aggregate of horn cells that have failed to separate from each other in desquamation, and the condition of hyperkeratosis is an exaggeration of this problem. Thus, regardless of the particular metabolic fault ultimately responsible, the final common pathogenetic pathway is a failure in the normal loss of intercorneocyte binding forces (cohesion) in the superficial portion of the stratum corneum.

ICHTHYOSIS

The term ichthyosis (meaning fish) is unfortunate, as the scale of 'modern' fish is, in fact, mesodermal rather than ectodermal in origin. The term ichthyosis is used to describe generalized, non-inflammatory disorders of keratinization and implies a congenital origin. However, there are many exceptions!

DISABILITY IN DISORDERS OF KERATINIZATION

Contrary to popular (both lay and medical) belief, skin diseases can be very disabling. There is a primitive revulsion at a disordered skin surface, which results in significant isolation and social and emotional deprivation. Patients with chronic skin disorders often become severely depressed. Also, it is not often appreciated just how severely physically disabled some patients with skin disease are. The abnormal scaling and hyperkeratotic skin does not have the normally excellent extensibility and compliance, so that movements are limited.

Xeroderma

Xeroderma does not represent a single disease process. The term derives from the Greek *xeros*, meaning dry, and xeroderma just means dry skin. In fact, xeroderma is used to describe scaliness rather than water content. Because the appearance of scaling transiently disappears if the abnormal skin is hydrated, it has mistakenly been believed that scaling is the manifestation of water deficiency.

CAUSES

There are some normal individuals who tend to have a 'dry' skin and they are more susceptible to stimuli that provoke scaling of the skin surface. Ageing tends to make the surface of the skin feel 'drier' and this seems to be associated with pruritus in susceptible individuals. A low relative humidity aggravates the problem, as does repeated vigorous washing, especially in hot water with some soaps and cleansing agents. Presumably, the toilet procedures leach out important substances that are vital to the integrity of the stratum corneum. Xeroderma tends to be worse in the wintertime and, when accompanied by itching, is known, logically enough, as 'winter itch'. This is particularly a problem in the north-eastern USA because of the low relative humidity.

Xeroderma is seen in many patients with atopic dermatitis. It has been suggested that this is a manifestation of ichthyosis, but there is more evidence in favour of the disorder being the result of the eczematous process itself. Xeroderma is also seen during the course of severe wasting diseases such as carcinomatosis, intestinal malabsorption and chronic renal failure, but should not be confused with acquired ichthyosis (Table 16.1).

Table 16.1 Precipitating causes of acquired ichthyosis

Precipitating cause	Comment
Hodgkin's disease and other reticuloses	Rarely, other neoplastic diseases
Essential fatty acid deficiency	Due to dietary deficiency, blind loop syndrome, or intestinal bypass operation
Serum lipid-lowering drugs	For example, nicotinamide, butyrophenones
Leprosy	Usually subsequent to treatment
AIDS	Accompanied by severe pruritus

KERATOSIS PILARIS

Horny plugs occur in the hair follicles of the outer aspect of the upper arms, forming sheets of pink, horny papules (Fig. 16.3), and occasionally on the thighs. It is seen in 'ordinary xeroderma', in autosomal dominant ichthyosis, and sometimes in normal young women for no apparent reason.

TREATMENT

Patients should be instructed to shower rather than bathe, to use lukewarm water rather than hot water, to use emollient cleansing agents rather than ordinary soaps, and to pat dry rather than vigorously towelling after bathing. If the patient lives in centrally heated rooms, humidifiers should be employed to raise the relative humidity. Emollients are a mainstay of treatment (see page 306). These act by supplying an oily film on the skin surface to prevent evaporation of water and encourage a build-up of this in the skin. Emollients act for a short time only – up to 2–3 hours at most – and need to be frequently applied. Their action can be supplemented by bath oils, which deposit a film of lipid on the skin surface.

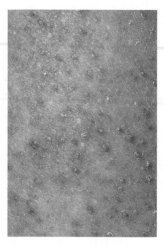

Figure 16.3 Keratosis pilaris. Horny red papules on the upper arms.

Autosomal dominant ichthyosis

DEFINITION

This is a common disorder of keratinization, characterized by mild generalized scaliness clinically and reduction of the granular cell layer histologically, which is inherited in an autosomal dominant manner.

CLINICAL FEATURES

There is widespread fine scaling over the skin surface, which tends to be worse in the wintertime when the humidity is low. It spares the flexures and is most noticeable over the extensor aspects of the limbs and trunk, being most noticeable over the back, the lateral aspects of the upper arms, the anterolateral thighs and particularly the shins (Fig. 16.4). Keratosis pilaris may be seen over the outer aspects of the upper arms in a few subjects. The condition is hardly noticeable in most people, but is quite marked and disabling in a few. In the worst affected, large, polygonal, dark scales form on the shins. The disorder is lifelong, but may worsen in old age.

PATHOLOGY AND AETIOPATHOGENESIS

The condition is inherited as an autosomal dominant disorder, but the biochemical basis is unclear. It has been estimated that the gene occurs with a frequency of

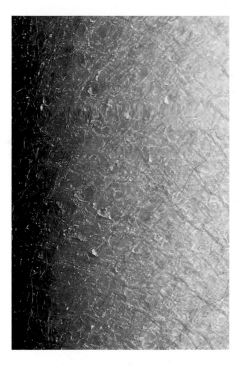

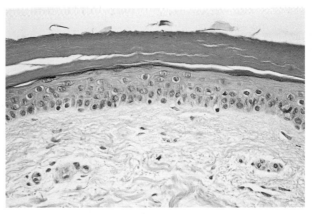

Figure 16.4 Moderately severe scaling in autosomal dominant ichthyosis.

Figure 16.5 Pathology of autosomal dominant ichthyosis. Note the virtual absence of granular cell layer.

1 in 500. Histologically, the only abnormality detectable is a much diminished granular cell layer (Fig. 16.5).

Ultrastructurally and biochemically, there is decreased content of a basic histidine-rich protein known as filaggrin, which is important in the orientation of the keratin tonofilaments.

TREATMENT

Generally, little is required in the way of treatment other than emollients. Patients who have very severe scaling may be helped by the use of topical keratolytic agents, including preparations containing urea (10–15 per cent) and salicylic acid (1–6 per cent). The latter is particularly effective in encouraging desquamation, but may not be used on large body areas for any length of time, as salicylic acid preparations when applied to abnormal skin may cause salicylate intoxication (salicylism). Concentrations of more than 2 per cent may also irritate the skin.

Sex-linked ichthyosis

DEFINITION

This is an uncommon, moderately severe disorder of keratinization that is inherited as a sex-linked characteristic in which the underlying metabolic fault is deficiency of steroid sulphatase.

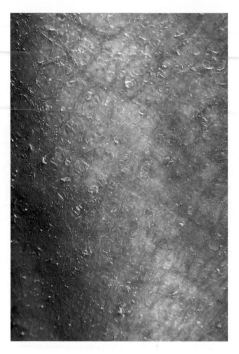

Figure 16.6 Skin scaling in sex-linked ichthyosis.

CLINICAL FEATURES

The male children who are born with this disorder are often the products of post-mature pregnancies and difficult labours. The reason for this appears to be a placental deficiency of the steroid sulphatase and a consequent failure of the usual splitting of circulating maternal oestrone sulphate in the last trimester of pregnancy. The free oestrone is thought to have a role in priming the uterus to oxytoxic stimuli.

The scaling is usually more severe than in autosomal dominant ichthyosis (Fig. 16.6). It is also more marked over the extensor aspects of the body surface, but does not always spare the flexures and often affects the sides of the neck and even the face. The scales are often quite large, particularly over the shins and have a dark-brownish discoloration. Patients with sex-linked ichthyosis may be significantly disabled by their disorder.

ASSOCIATED DISORDERS

There is an association with cryptorchidism and, rarely, even with testicular cancer on the basis of this. There is also an association with a form of cataract.

PATHOLOGY AND AETIOPATHOGENESIS

The trait is carried on an X chromosome and is recessive, so that it is not manifest in women (XX) who become carriers, but it is in male offspring (XY). In fact, the carrier female may demonstrate patchy scaling that is consistent with the 'random deletion' (or Lyon) hypothesis. The disorder is quite uncommon, having a gene frequency of approximately 1 in 6000.

Histologically, there is a minor degree of epidermal thickening and mild hypergranulosis. Biochemically, affected male subjects show a steroid sulphatase deficiency, but for diagnostic purposes, fibroblast, lymphocyte or epidermal cell cultures are tested. The steroid sulphatase abnormality results in excess quantities of cholesterol sulphate in the stratum corneum with diminished free cholesterol. This has been used as the basis of a diagnostic test and has been suggested as the underlying basis for the abnormal scaling.

TREATMENT

Treatment is as for autosomal dominant ichthyosis, but some patients may need oral retinoids.

Case 16

J.S. presented at the age of 17 with generalized scaling, 'dry' skin. He had had it since birth, although it didn't start to be a problem until he reached the age of 11. He complained of itchiness – especially in the wintertime, when, in addition to the itch, the skin of his hands became sore and 'cracked' in places. He had a brother who was affected and his maternal grandfather also had the disease. Close questioning of his mother revealed that J.S. was born 2 weeks late after a difficult delivery. It was clear that he had sex-linked ichthyosis, which could be expected to persist, but the symptoms of which should be helped by emollients.

Non-bullous ichthyosiform erythroderma

Non-bullous ichthyosiform erythroderma (NBIE) is inherited as a rare, autosomal recessive disorder. It is probably heterogeneous, as, although the skin abnormality is similar in all patients, there are associations with abnormalities in other organ systems in some groups of patients.

CLINICAL FEATURES

Characteristically, there is generalized erythema and fine scaling (Fig. 16.7). There is a history of a collodion membrane (see page 252) in a few patients. Ectropion, deformities of the ears and sparsity of scalp hair are common accompaniments. Neurological and immunological abnormalities occur in some patients. The condition persists throughout life, although the erythema tends to decrease.

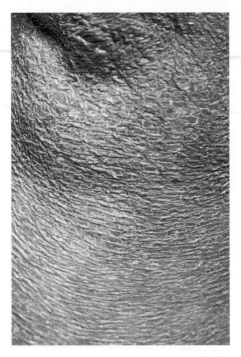

Figure 16.7 Non-bullous ichthyosiform erythroderma.

Histologically, there is a psoriasiform hyperplasia and parakeratosis. As in psoriasis, there appears to be a rapid rate of epidermal cell production. The biochemical basis for this ichthyotic disorder is unknown.

TREATMENT

Topical treatments with emollients and keratolytics as for patients with autosomal dominant ichthyosis may be sufficient.

Severely affected patients may benefit from the use of long-term oral retinoid drugs. The agent usually used is acitretin, but isotretinoin has been used for some patients. The dose of these drugs is 0.3–0.7 mg/kg body weight per day, given in two divided doses daily with food. The disorder starts to improve after 2–4 weeks, but full improvement may not take place before 6 weeks.

The oral retinoids appear to affect the process of keratinization rather than any particular component of NBIE. Although there is often considerable improvement, evidence of the underlying problem is always present, and the condition always relapses when treatment is stopped. The oral retinoids have major and minor toxicities (see page 140) and are markedly teratogenic, so that fertile women *must* use effective contraception. Patients must be regularly monitored for hepatotoxicity, hyperlipidaemia and bone toxicity. Most patients notice drying of the mucosae – of the lips particularly – and some an increase in the rate of hair loss.

Bullous ichthyosiform erythroderma (epidermolytic hyperkeratosis)

Epidermolytic hyperkeratosis is a rare, autosomal dominant disorder of keratinization. As in NBIE, there is generalized erythema and the disorder is presaged by a collodion membrane at birth in some patients (see page 252). The condition is characterized by the tendency to blister or develop erosions at the sites of trauma (Figs 16.8 and 16.9). The erythema and blistering improve with age. Scaling and hyperkeratosis are characteristically ridged or corrugated at flexures.

Patients often present a pathetic picture because of their severe hyperkeratosis, which causes physical disability and discomfort as well as a socially unacceptable appearance. In addition, the hyperkeratotic areas often become infected and smell unpleasant. Ectropion and deformed ('crumpled') ears are common.

The pathognomonic histological feature of epidermolytic hyerkeratosis is a reticulate degenerative change in the epidermis (Fig. 16.10). As in NBIE, there is a high rate of epidermal cell production. In recent years, mutations in certain keratin genes have been identified in this disorder.

Topical emollients and keratolytics are not often very helpful. The oral retinoids may improve the appearance considerably, although the dose has to be

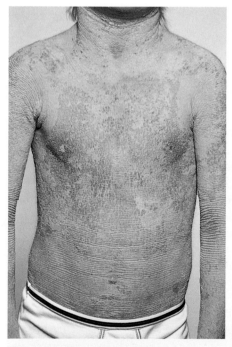

Figure 16.8 Epidermolytic hyperkeratosis showing typical severe hyperkeratosis and scaling.

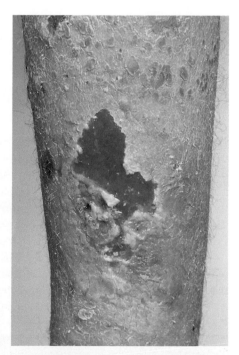

Figure 16.9 Erosion in epidermolytic hyperkeratosis following minor injury to this area.

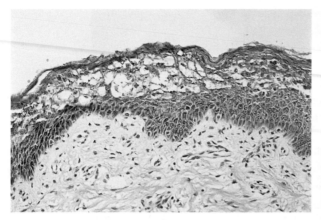

Figure 16.10 Pathology of epidermolytic hyperkeratosis with reticulate degenerative change.

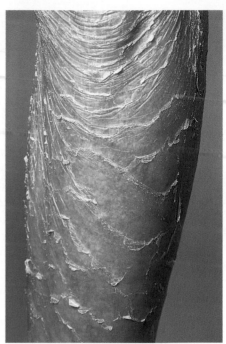

Figure 16.11 Lamellar ichthyosis, with marked hyperkeratosis and scaling.

carefully regulated, as these drugs may temporarily increase the blistering as well as decreasing the hyperkeratosis!

Lamellar ichthyosis

This is a rare, autosomal recessive disorder of keratinization, characterized by a striking degree of hyperkeratosis but not much erythema. As with NBIE and epidermolytic hyerkeratosis, some patients develop the condition after being born in a collodion membrane. The hyperkeratosis may be discoloured brown, for reasons that are unclear (Fig. 16.11). As with the other severe disorders of keratinization, there may be marked ectropion and ear deformities (Fig. 16.12).

Histologically, there is marked hyperkeratosis and hypergranulosis.

Treatment is similar to that for NBIE and epidermolytic hyperkeratosis, with oral retinoid drugs being the only available agents that can produce any substantial improvement.

Collodion baby

This is an odd condition in which babies are born covered by a shiny, transparent membrane (Fig. 16.13). This gradually peels off after a week or so, the peel looking

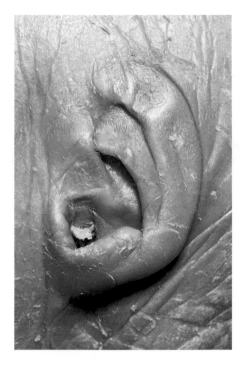

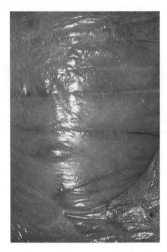

Figure 16.12 'Crumpled ear', seen in many severe disorders of keratinization.

Figure 16.13 Shiny membrane covering the skin in a collodion baby.

like 'collodion' – hence the name. Ultimately, the child may develop normally or may develop one of the severe disorders of keratinization discussed above.

Nothing is known of the cause. Collodion babies need to be carefully nursed, as their skin barrier function may be abnormal, so that they lose much water and become dehydrated.

HARLEQUIN FETUS

This is a rare and mostly fatal disorder in which the child is born encased in thick, abnormal, fissured, hyperkeratotic skin. This disorder is also due to abnormalities of keratin synthesis. Survival of a few of these unfortunate children has been reported with the use of oral retinoids.

REFSUM'S SYNDROME (HEREDOPATHIA ATACTICA NEURITISFORMIS)

This is a very rare, autosomal recessive, metabolic disorder in which there is, in all tissues, accumulation of phytanic acid. This fatty acid substitutes for other fatty acids in membrane lipids, which is probably responsible for many of the clinical manifestations of the disorder. These manifestations include cerebellar ataxia, polyneuritis, retinitis pigmentosa, nerve deafness and generalized ichthyosiform scaling.

ACQUIRED ICHTHYOSIS

Generalized skin scaling without accompanying inflammation develops in adult life in this disorder. The most important cause of acquired ichthyosis is underlying malignant disease – particularly lymphoma – such as Hodgkin's disease (see Table 16.1).

Other disorders of keratinization

DARIER'S DISEASE (KERATOSIS FOLLICULITIS)

Darier's disease is an uncommon disorder that appears to be inherited as an autosomal dominant disorder, but also occurs sporadically.

A characteristic feature is the appearance of groups of brownish, horny papules over the central trunk, shoulders, face and also elsewhere (Figs 16.14 and 16.15). These papules easily become irritated and/or infected and become exudative and crusted. Other features include the presence of tiny pits on the palms and a nail dystrophy in which there is a vertical ridge starting at an indentation at the nail-free border.

There is a curious loss of cohesion between keratinocytes above the basal layer – a little like the acantholysis seen in pemphigus (see page 91). The suprabasilar

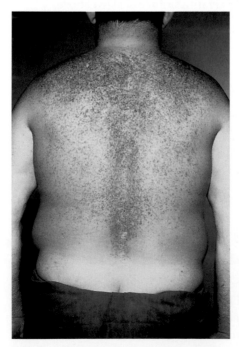

Figure 16.14 Brown keratotic papules on the trunk in Darier's disease.

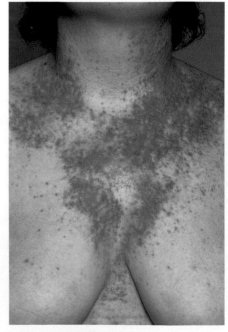

Figure 16.15 Red exudative papules on the chest in Darier's disease.

clefting that results is accompanied by an odd form of premature keratinization in which eosinophilic bodies (corps ronds) and small, dense basophilic bodies (grains) are formed, to be carried upwards by the epidermis.

Topical treatment with mild keratolytics such as 2 per cent salicylic acid or 0.025–0.05 per cent tretinoin may be helpful. Oral retinoids are often of considerable assistance.

HAILEY–HAILEY DISEASE (CHRONIC BENIGN FAMILIAL PEMPHIGUS)

This is a rare, familial disorder with some similarities to Darier's disease. Fissured, exudative, infected lesions develop in the groins, the axillae and around the neck in particular. It does not usually start before early adult life and is much worse in summertime.

TYLOSIS

This term describes a group of disorders in which there is marked thickening of palmar and plantar skin due to some localized abnormality of keratinization (Fig. 16.16). The disorder is clearly heterogeneous, with autosomal dominant, autosomal recessive and sex-linked recessive types being described. There is also a wide range of clinical features, with involvement of the dorsa of the hands and feet in some patients and an odd 'punctate' palmar pattern in others.

In one inherited variety, there is a close association with the development of carcinoma of the oesophagus.

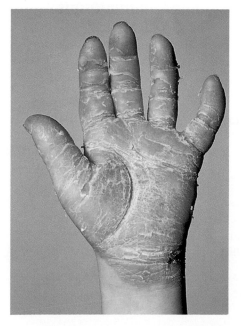

Figure 16.16 Massive palmar hyperkeratosis in one variety of tylosis.

255

Fortunately, most patients are not as disabled as may be thought from the clinical appearance. As long as they keep their skin surface flexible and smooth with emollients and keratolytics, they can manage everyday activities quite well.

PACHYONYCHIA CONGENITAL

This is a rare, autosomal recessively inherited disorder in which there is striking thickening of the nails. There are also hyperkeratotic areas over the palms and sometimes elsewhere.

Other genodermatoses

TUBEROUS SCLEROSIS

Tuberous sclerosis is a rare, autosomal dominantly inherited disorder in which defects occur in many organ systems.

Major skin abnormalities include the appearance of pink-red papules around the nose and cheeks, which increase in number during adolescence and are known, inappropriately, as adenoma sebaceum. Firm, whitish plaques (shagreen patches) with a cobblestone surface, depigmented leaf-shaped macules and subungual fibromata are other skin signs. Cerebral malformations often result in epilepsy. Renal hamartomas occur in 50 per cent of patients. Mental deficiency is seen in many patients with this disease.

VON RECKLINGHAUSEN'S DISEASE (NEUROFIBROMATOSIS)

This is a not uncommon, autosomal dominant disorder, but a high frequency of new gene mutations and variable expression of the disorder make its occurrence difficult to predict.

THE MAIN FEATURES ARE AS FOLLOWS

- Brown macules appear, varying in size and aptly described as *café au lait* patches, characterized by the presence of giant melanosomes. The appearance of such freckle-like lesions in the axillae is diagnostic of the disorder.
- Skin-coloured to pink-mauve compressible, soft skin tumours develop, some of which are pedunculated (Fig. 16.17). These are neurofibromata and may be present in large numbers, causing a considerable cosmetic disability.
- Larger tumours of the limbs occur. These are plexiform neuromas.

The numbers of lesions increase with age. Patients are also subject to the development of a wide range of neoplastic lesions, including acoustic neuroma, phaeochromocytoma and fibrosarcoma.

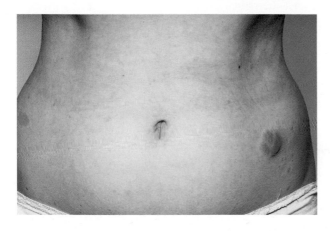

Figure 16.17 A mildly affected patient with neurofibromatosis. There is a neurofibroma on the abdomen.

ANHIDROTIC ECTODERMAL DYSPLASIA

In this rare disorder, there are characteristic frontal bosses on the skull as well as a saddle deformity of the nose. There are no eccrine sweat glands present, so that individuals are subject to hyperpyrexia in hot weather. The hair may be sparse and fine and there are multiple abnormalities of the teeth.

Summary

- Keratinization involves the transformation of epidermal cells into tough, thin, shield-like corneocytes, which make up the stratum corneum barrier.
- Scaling is the result of failure of the final stage of keratinization in which corneocytes separate individually. Thus, a scale is an aggregate of unseparated corneocytes and occurs in any disturbance of keratinization – congenital or acquired.
- Scaling may cause considerable disability, both physical and psychological. Xeroderma just means 'dry skin' – which is, in fact, scaling skin and due to a wide variety of disturbances of keratinization. Xeroderma is common in the elderly and in atopic eczema and is worse in low relative humidity such as in wintertime.
- Treatment of xeroderma is focused on the frequent use of emollients and emollient cleansers as well as on gentle showering rather than bathing.
- Autosomal dominant ichthyosis is characterized by generalized fine scaling that is worse on the extensor surfaces. It may be accompanied by keratosis pilaris, in which there are horny plugs in the hair follicle canals. Its frequency is 1 in 500. Its biochemical basis is uncertain. Emollients and, if necessary, keratolytics may help some patients who need them.
- The scaling in sex-linked ichthyosis is more pronounced. Affected males are often born post-mature and with difficulty. The metabolic basis is steroid sulphatase deficiency, which can be detected in fibroblast, epidermal or lymphocyte culture. Women are carriers of this sex-linked, recessive gene, which has an overall frequency of 1 in 6000.
- Non-bullous ichthyosiform erythroderma is a rare, autosomal recessive condition, characterized by generalized erythema and fine scaling. Oral acitretin helps some patients, although there may be severe adverse side effects.
- In the rare bullous ichthyosiform erythroderma (also known as epidermolytic hyperkeratosis), there is generalized erythema, corrugated hyperkeratosis

and the tendency to blister. There is a characteristic reticulate degenerative change in the upper epidermis. The disorder is dominantly inherited and due to certain keratin gene mutations. Oral retinoids may improve the appearance, but at the same time may increase the blistering.

- Lamellar ichthyosis is a rare, autosomal recessive disorder marked by hyperkeratosis and scaling.
- Patients with non-bullous ichthyosiform erythroderma, epidermolytic hyperkeratosis and lamellar ichthyosis may be born in a collodion membrane. This shiny, transparent membrane peels off after a week or so. It may also rarely occur in normal infants. Its presence signifies compromised barrier function and affected children need careful nursing.
- Acquired ichthyosis may occur in reticulosis, human immunodeficiency virus (HIV) disease, leprosy, essential fatty acid deficiency and with the use of some lipid-lowering drugs.
- Darier's disease is an uncommon disorder, occurring either as a autosomal dominant condition or sporadically. Typically, brownish, crusted papules occur over the face and upper trunk alongside palmar pits and a nail dystrophy. Histologically, suprabasilar clefting and premature keratinization are evident.
- Tuberous sclerosis is a rare, autosomal dominant condition in which many abnormalities occur. The presence of pink-red papules around the nose and cheeks is characteristic.
- Von Recklinghausen's disease (neurofibromatosis) is a not uncommon, autosomal dominant disorder in which large numbers of pinkish, compressible, soft skin tumours develop. Brown macular *café au lait* patches accompany the condition.

Metabolic disorders and reticulohistiocytic proliferative disorders

Porphyrias

The porphyrias are a group of disorders of metabolism of the haem molecule. Acute, intermittent porphyria has no skin manifestations. Porphyrias that demonstrate skin disorder as a component are summarized in Table 17.1.

PORPHYRIA CUTANEA TARDA

Porphyria cutanea tarda (PCT) is a so-called hepatic porphyria. There is a genetic component to the disorder, although it has not been completely characterized. It is much more common in those with alcoholic liver disease, but has also been seen in patients with liver tumours and those with hexachlorbenzene poisoning.

Metabolic basis

There appears to be a defect in the action of the enzyme uroporphyrinogen decarboxylase, resulting in the accumulation of uroporphyrins and coproporphyrins in the blood, stools and urine.

Clinical features

When associated with alcoholic liver disease, the disorder is more often seen in middle-aged men. The characteristic features are seen in the light-exposed areas. In the early stages of the disease, blistering and fragility of the skin on the face and backs of the hands are noted (Fig. 17.1). The affected areas also develop an odd

Table 17.1 Enzyme defects in porphyrias with cutaneous manifestations

Disorder	Enzyme affected	Inheritance
Porphyria cutanea tarda (cutaneous hepatic porphyria)	Uroporphyrinogen decarboxylase	Autosomal dominant/ acquired
Variegate porphyria	Protoporphyrinogen oxidase	Autosomal dominant
Erythropoietic porphyria (Gunther's disease)	Uroporphyrinogen cosynthetase	Autosomal recessive
Erythropoietic protoporphyria	Ferrochelatase	Autosomal dominant

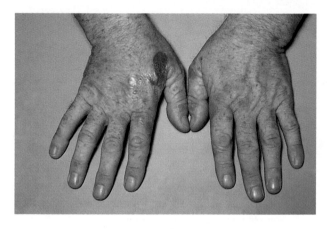

Figure 17.1 Porphyria cutanea tarda. Note the eroded areas in the light-exposed skin of the backs of the hands.

pigmented and mauve, suffused appearance (Fig. 17.2). Later, increased hair growth occurs on the involved skin and a sclerodermiform thickening of the skin develops. The diagnosis is made by finding increased uroporphyrins and coproporphyrins in the stools and urine. If available, monochromatic testing (to irradiate the skin with very narrow wavelength bands of light or ultraviolet radiation) will reveal photosensitivity at 404 nm.

Pathology and pathogenesis

The enzyme defect results in abnormal amounts of the metabolites uroporphyrin III and coproporphyrin III accumulating in the tissues. These substances are responsible for the photosensitization. Iron overload is also a frequent accompanying feature. Histologically, the blistering is subepidermal and, in the long-standing case, fibrosis develops and deposits of immunoglobulin are found perivascularly.

Treatment

The objective is to reduce the circulating levels of porphyrins. This is achieved by regular venesection – removing a pint of blood at a time – every 2 or 3 weeks, or by the use of chloroquine orally, resulting in the secretion of large amounts of porphyrins in the urine.

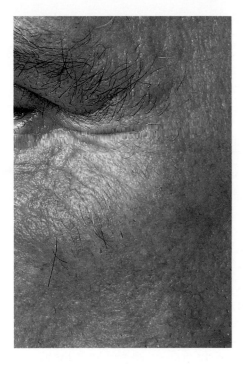

Figure 17.2 Suffused, slightly pigmented and hairy area on the upper cheek and the area lateral to the orbit in a patient with porphyria cutanea tarda.

PORPHYRIA VARIEGATA

This is a very rare combination of PCT and acute intermittent porphyria. The latter is caused by a deficiency of delta-aminolaevulinic acid synthetase and is precipitated by certain drugs and anaesthesia, amongst other things.

ERYTHROPOIETIC PROTOPORPHYRIA

Erythropoietic protoporphyria is a very rare, autosomal dominant disorder in which excess protoporphyrins are produced. These protoporphyrins are detectable in the blood and this forms the basis of diagnostic tests. Clinically, the disorder often presents in childhood as episodes of skin soreness and extreme discomfort when exposed to the sun. Swelling, redness and urticarial lesions may develop in exposed skin. Later, fine, pitted scarring is found on exposed sites. Pigment gallstones may develop.

ERYTHROPOIETIC PORPHYRIA (GUNTHER'S DISEASE)

This is another very rare abnormality of porphyrin metabolism, inherited as an autosomal recessive disorder. Affected individuals are extremely photosensitive and shun the light. They develop dreadful facial scarring, with hirsutes. This combination of clinical features has suggested to some that these patients provoked the fable of 'werewolves'.

HAEMOCHROMATOSIS (BRONZED DIABETES)

There are primary and symptomatic forms of this disorder. In the primary form, there is excessive gastrointestinal absorption of iron, resulting in iron deposition in the liver, testes, skin and pancreas. Involvement of the skin causes a brown-grey pigmentation due to both the iron and increased melanin in the skin. There is diabetes due to deposition of iron in the pancreas, and cirrhosis from liver involvement. The condition seems to be inherited as a recessive characteristic, but is much more common in men.

Secondary forms are found in conditions necessitating repeated blood transfusion and in conditions in which there is chronic haemolysis (e.g. sickle cell disease).

AMYLOIDOSIS

Amyloidosis is the term used for a group of disorders in which an abnormal protein is deposited in tissues. Generalized amyloidosis is divided into primary and secondary forms. The latter develops after long-standing inflammatory disease, including infections such as chronic tuberculosis and chronic osteomyelitis. It may also occur in patients with long-standing severe rheumatoid arthritis. There are no skin manifestations in secondary amyloidosis. In primary amyloidosis, the abnormal protein components are synthesized by clones of abnormal plasma cells and the condition is sometimes associated with multiple myeloma. In primary amyloid disease amyloid is deposited in various organs as well as in the skin. In the skin, it is deposited in and around the dermal capillary blood vessels, which become fragile and leaky. Swollen mauve-purple areas develop around the eyes and around the flexures.

There are also 'amyloid' disorders that are restricted to the skin. In the rare macular amyloid, itchy, 'rippled', brown macular areas appear over the trunk (Fig. 17.3). It seems to be more common in women and in patients of Asian origin. Histologically, the deposits of amyloid are detectable subepidermally. Lichen amyloidosis is another rare cutaneous form of amyloid in which lichen planus-like lesions occur.

Amyloid can be detected in tissue using various histochemical tests, including birefringence with Congo red stain and fluorescence with thioflavine T, as well as by immunocytochemical tests.

XANTHOMATA

Xanthomata are deposits of lipid in histiocytes in skin and may be associated with normal levels of lipids in the blood (normolipaemia) or with elevated levels of serum lipids (hyperlipidaemia). The lipidized histiocytes have a characteristic 'foamy' appearance. The main hyperlipidaemic conditions are given in Table 17.2.

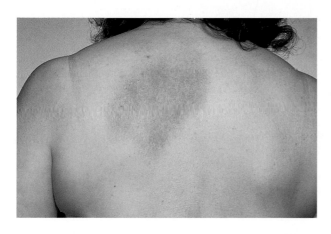

Figure 17.3 Pigmented area on the back in macular amyloid.

Table 17.2 The hyperlipidaemias (World Health Organization classification)

Type	Plasma cholesterol	Plasma triglycerides	Lipoproteins elevated	Inheritance	Skin lesions	Systemic manifestations
I	N↑	↑↑↑	Chylomicrons	Autosomal recessive (Burger–Grütz disease	Eruptive xanthomata	Pancreatitis Hepatosplenomegaly Lipaemic retinalis
II	↑↑ ↑↑	N ↑	LDL LDL, VLDL	Autosomal dominant (familial hypercholesteraemia)	Xanthelasma Tendon/ tuberous xanthoma	Corneal arcus Accelerated atherosclerosis
III	↑↑	↑↑	Chylomicron Remnants LDL	Uncertain	Planar xanthoma Eruptive and tendon xanthoma	Accelerated atherosclerosis
IV	N↑	↑↑	VLDL	Uncertain	Eruptive xanthoma	Accelerated atherosclerosis Glucose intolerance Hyeruricaemia
V	N↑	↑↑↑	VLDL Chylomicrons	Uncertain	Eruptive xanthoma	Pancreatis Hepatosplenomegaly Sensory neuropathy Lipaemia retinalis Hyperuricaemia Glucose intolerance

LDL = low density lipoproteins; VLDL = very low density lipoproteins.

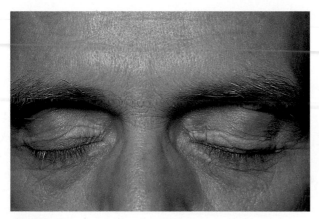

Figure 17.4 Yellowish plaques on the eyelids in xanthelasma.

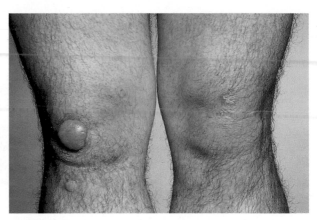

Figure 17.5 Xanthoma tuberosum affecting the knee.

Xanthelasma

Xanthelasma is a common form of xanthoma in which lesions appear as arcuate or linear plaques around the eyes (Fig. 17.4). The condition is not associated with hyperlipidaemia in 60–70 per cent of patients. The lesions can be removed by excision or by topical treatment with trichloracetic acid if the patient finds them a cosmetic nuisance. The latter can produce serious burns if it is used incorrectly. The area around the lesion should be protected with Vaseline and the surface of the lesion lightly wiped with a cotton-wool swab moistened with the acid. In a few seconds, the treated area turns white and later a scale or crust forms.

Xanthoma tuberosum

The lesions of xanthoma tuberosum are large nodules containing lipidized histiocytes and giant cells. The nodules develop around the tendons and extensor aspects of the joints in familial hyperlipidaemia (see Table 17.2), particularly over the Achilles' tendon, the knees and elbows (Fig. 17.5).

Eruptive xanthomata

These mostly develop in diabetes, but are also seen in congenital deficiencies of lipoprotein lipase (Burger–Grütz disease: see Table 17.2). Large numbers of yellowish-pink papules develop rapidly over the skin surface (Fig. 17.6).

Treatment

The treatment of these xanthomatous disorders is based on treatment of any underlying disease, diet and the use of lipid-lowering agents.

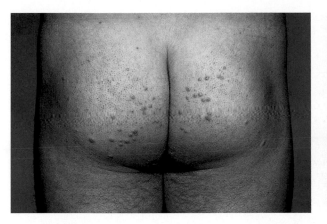

Figure 17.6 Yellowish pink papules on the buttocks in eruptive xanthoma.

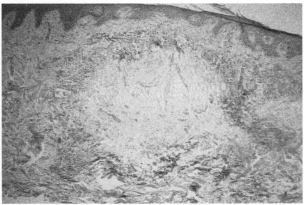

Figure 17.7 Pathology of granuloma annulare demonstrating a central necrobiotic area surrounded by inflammatory cells.

Necrobiotic disorders

The term 'necrobiosis' is applied to a particular histological change in which there are foci of damage making the dermal structure 'blurred' and more eosinophilic than usual. The foci are surrounded by inflammatory cells – lymphocytes, histiocytes and occasional giant cells (Fig. 17.7)

GRANULOMA ANNULARE

This, not uncommon, inflammatory disorder, often seen in children and young adults, is characterized by papules and plaques that adopt a ring-like pattern (Fig. 17.8). Lesions develop on the extensor aspects of the fingers, dorsa of the feet, hands and wrists.

Granuloma annulare tends to last for a few months and then disappears as mysteriously as it came. Treatment is generally not indicated.

A less common type, known as generalized superficial granuloma annulare, is characterized by macular, dull-red or mauve areas rather than rings (Fig. 17.9), which have a necrobiotic structure histologically. Diabetes is more common in this group of patients.

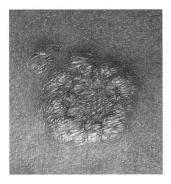

Figure 17.8 A typical ring of pale-pink papules in granuloma annulare.

Case 17

Annie, aged 11, was brought to the surgery because of several pink plaques that had developed in the previous 3 months on her ankles and the backs of the hands. The plaques were static and did not trouble her. They were clinically typical of granuloma annulare and this was confirmed by the finding of necrobiotic and granulomatous foci histologically. They resolved without treatment after a further 6 months.

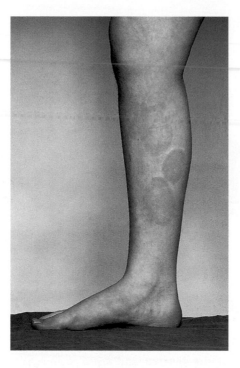

Figure 17.9 Flat, pink patches due to diffuse granuloma annulare. This patient also had diabetes.

NECROBIOSIS LIPOIDICA DIABETICORUM

This condition is seen in 0.3 per cent of diabetics and is strongly associated with the diabetic state. It occurs mainly on the lower legs as yellowish-pink plaques, which persist and become atrophic. It is characterized by necrobiotic foci histologically.

Reticulohistiocytic proliferative disorders

There is a group of poorly understood disorders that includes Letterer–Siwe disease (LSD), Hand–Schüller–Christian disease (HSCD), eosinophilic granuloma (EG), xanthoma disseminatum (XD) and juvenile xanthogranuloma (JX). LSD, HSCD and EG seem to belong to the same 'family of diseases', in which there appears to be a reactive proliferation of Langerhans cells.

LSD is an uncommon disorder of infants and young children, characterized by a papular and scaling eruption of flexures, trunk and scalp, with some resemblance to seborrhoeic dermatitis. There is a dense infiltrate of cells having the ultrastructural and immunocytochemical characteristics of Langerhans cells. There may be severe malaise and hepatosplenomegaly and some patients succumb. Treatment with corticosteroids and cytotoxic agents may be required.

In HSCD, abnormal Langerhans cell deposits occur mostly in the lung, pituitary, bone and orbit. In EG, the deposits are, for the most part, limited to the bony skeleton.

XD and JX do not belong to the same 'Langerhans cell' group of disorders, but are characterized by the presence of lipidized histiocytes, giant cells and an admixture of other cell types. In JX, isolated or limited numbers of yellowish-pink nodules occur in young infants, which eventually disappear. In XD, many papular lesions develop on the skin, and sometimes mucosae, which often persist for long periods without serious consequences.

Summary

- The porphyrias are disorders of haem molecule metabolism. In porphyria cutanea tarda, there is a defect in uroporphyrinogen decarboxylase, causing uroporphyrins and copirorphyrins to accumulate in the blood, stools and urine. PCT is associated with liver disease; its genetic basis is uncertain. Mauvish discoloration, blistering and hirsutes occur in light-exposed sites.

- Treatment is by regular venesection or by administration of chloroquine, both of which reduce levels of abnormal circulating porphyrins.

- Porphyria variegata is a very rare, dominant combination of PCT and acute intermittent porphyria. Erythropoietic protoporphyria is another rare, dominantly inherited disorder with photosensitivity.

- In primary haemochromatosis, there is excessive gastrointestinal absorption of iron, with its subsequent deposition in the viscera – particularly in the skin, causing pigmentation, and in the liver and pancreas, causing cirrhosis and diabetes, respectively. Secondary haemochromatosis occurs as a result of chronic haemolysis or repeated blood transfusion.

- Amyloidosis describes a group of disorders in which there is deposition of an abnormal protein. Primary generalized amyloidosis is the result of an abnormal clone of plasma cells and results in amyloid deposition perivascularly in skin and various organs. Secondary amyloidosis from long-standing infection (e.g. tuberculosis) or rheumatoid arthritis has no skin manifestations. Macular amyloid causes rippled pigmentation of the skin and is caused by subepidermal amyloid deposits.

- Xanthomata are deposits of lipid in histiocytes in skin. In xanthelasma, lipid deposits occur around the eyes without hyperlipidaemia in 70 per cent of cases. In xanthoma tuberosum, nodular deposits occur around tendons as a result of familial hypercholesterolaemia. In eruptive xanthoma, many small, pink-yellow papules develop in the course of diabetes or Burger–Grütz disease.

- Granuloma annulare is a not uncommon, self-limiting disorder, characterized by papules and annular plaques in which there is a characteristic histological picture of damaged connective tissue ('necrobiosis') and surrounding granulomatous inflammation. In necrobiosis lipoidica diabeticorum, large, yellowish pink plaques occur preferentially on the legs.

- Letterer–Siwe disease is a sometimes fatal disorder seen in infants and is marked by a papular and scaling rash in the flexures and scalp. There is an infiltrate of Langerhans cells in the skin and viscera. Xanthoma disseminatum and juvenile xanthogranuloma are in a different category and are characterized by deposits of lipidized histiocytes and other inflammatory cells focally in skin.

CHAPTER
18
Disorders of hair and nails

Both hair and nails are epidermal structures that arise from invaginations of the epidermis into the skin (Figs 18.1 and 18.2). Hair and nails may develop signs of disorder such as psoriasis or lichen planus in the absence of obvious skin disease. In addition, there are disorders that are confined to either the hair or the nails.

Disorders of hair (Table 18.1)

HAIR LOSS (ALOPECIA)

Hair loss may be diffuse over the scalp or localized to one or several sites on the scalp. The process may also be destructive and cause scarring or may be non-scarring in nature.

Congenital alopecia

Congenital alopecia may occur in isolation or with other congenital disorders. Rarely, scalp hair growth is very slow and hair shaft density is low (*congenital hypotrichosis*). A patch of scarring over the vertex with hair loss is another, uncommon, type of congenital alopecia.

Pattern alopecia

Definition
This is a common, dominantly inherited, progressive form of alopecia, which is mostly seen in men, develops symmetrically at certain specific sites on the scalp and eventually causes almost complete scalp hair loss in some patients.

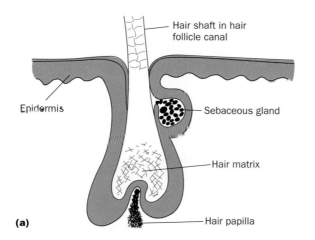

Hair shaft in hair follicle canal

Epidermis

Sebaceous gland

Hair matrix

Hair papilla

(a)

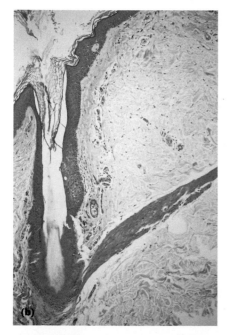

(b)

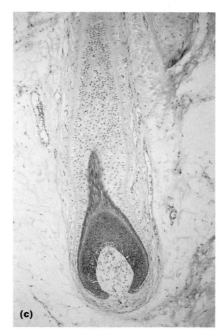

(c)

Figure 18.1 (a) Diagram of a hair follicle showing the relationship between the hair shaft, follicular epithelium and sebaceous glands. (b) Photomicrograph to show a hair follicle on the scalp with arrectores pilorum muscles. (c) Photomicrograph to show a hair follicle on the scalp with prominent hair matrix and hair papillae.

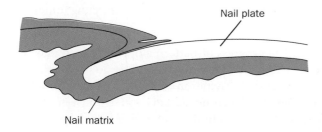

Nail plate

Nail matrix

Figure 18.2 Diagram to show the nail plate and the nail matrix tissue that forms it.

269

Table 18.1 Overview of hair disorders

Hair loss (alopecia)	Non scarring	Diffuse	Ageing Telogen effluvium Drug induced
		Localized	Male pattern alopecia areata Mechanical causes
	Scarring		Trauma Lupus erythematosus Lichen planus
Increased hair growth (hirsutes)			Constitutional Androgenization Drug induced

Clinical features

Loss of hair starts in both temporal regions. Shortly after this bitemporal recession, thinning of the hair and then alopecia develop over the vertex. The bald area over the vertex expands to meet the triangular temporal bald areas until, in the worst cases, almost complete loss of hair results. A general reduction in the density of hair follicles also occurs and this may be the main feature of the disorder in women, in whom bitemporal recession and some vertical thinning occur less commonly than in men.

The condition may start as early as in the late teens, but generally declares its presence in the third decade. Its rate of progress varies and seems uninfluenced by environmental factors.

Pattern alopecia causes an enormous amount of psychological distress and patients will go to extraordinary lengths to attempt to arrest and reverse the process and/or to disguise its presence. The condition is firmly embedded in popular mythology with regard to its supposed causes, which range from dietary deficiencies to sexual excesses.

Pathology and pathogenesis

The hair follicles in the affected areas become smaller and sparser and eventually disappear. Finally, true atrophy of the skin occurs at the involved sites. The disorder is dominantly inherited, but requires androgenic stimulus in the form of testosterone and the passing of the years for full phenotypic expression. The disorder can be precipitated by the administering of testosterone to female patients and is also a sign of masculinization in patients with a testosterone-secreting tumour.

Treatment

There is no effective treatment. The progress of pattern alopecia in men may be halted by castration, but there are few patients who would undergo the operation for this purpose. In women, 'chemical castration' with the use of an anti-androgen–prostagen combination (cyproterone acetate and ethinylestranol – Dianette) has been tried and some reduction in the rate of hair loss claimed. The antihypertensive vasodilator minoxidil has also been used topically, as increased hair growth was noted as a side effect from its oral use. Although the drug may increase hair growth in 20–30 per cent of patients, the hair is lost again when treatment stops, and the extent to which hair regrowth occurs is modest. More recently, the drug finasteride has been used (this is a 5-alpha-reductase inhibitor) in women, with good results claimed.

Case 18

Joan, aged 53, noticed that she was losing a lot of scalp hair. On examination, there was some overall thinning, but the hair loss was more marked over the vertex and at either temple. Joan remembered that her mother had also had some hair loss. It was thought that she had pattern alopecia and she was put on treatment with Dianette. After 6 months of treatment she thought the rate of hair loss was less.

Pattern hair loss in men may be disguised in a number of ways, including:

- wigs and toupées and hair weaving, in which the remaining hair is woven to cover the defect
- surgical manoeuvres, in which plugs of hair-containing skin from the scalp periphery are transplanted to holes made in the bald area or flaps of skin are advanced over bald areas.

Alopecia areata

Definition
Alopecia areata is an autoimmune disorder of hair follicles causing loss of hair in sharply defined areas of skin.

Clinical features
Alopecia areata often starts quite suddenly as one or more rounded patches from which the hair is lost (Fig. 18.3). The hair loss continues for days or weeks, until

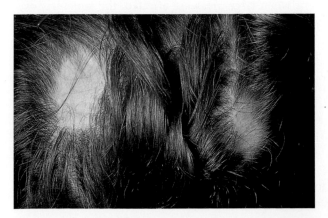

Figure 18.3 Small, discrete areas of hair loss in alopecia areata.

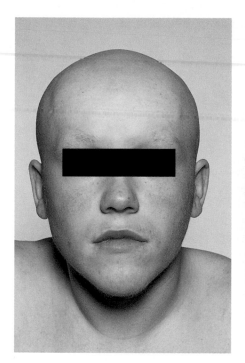

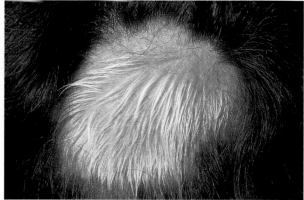

Figure 18.4 Alopecia totalis: there is loss of eyebrows too.

Figure 18.5 A large patch of alopecia areata showing regrowth of non-pigmented hair.

all the hair from the affected sites has fallen. The individual areas vary in size from $1\,cm^2$ to involvement of the entire scalp (alopecia totalis); rarely, the eyelashes and eyebrows (Fig. 18.4) and all body hair are lost as well.

Affected areas may extend outwards and disease activity can be recognized by the appearance of so-called 'exclamation mark' hairs at the margin of the lesions. The condition occurs over a wide age range, but seems particularly common between the ages of 15 and 30 years.

Regrowth of alopecia areata patches occur in most patients if the affected areas are small, limited in number, and the affected individual is 15 years old or less. When regrowth occurs, the new hair is fine and non-pigmented (Fig. 18.5). The outlook for regrowth worsens when large areas are affected, the patient is over 30 years old and also has atopic dermatitis.

Pathology and pathogenesis

The disorder is positively associated with autoimmune disorders, including vitiligo and thyrotoxicosis, and it has been assumed that an immune attack is launched against components of the hair follicle. When biopsies are taken from an actively extending patch, a dense 'bee swarm'-like cluster of lymphocytes can be seen around the follicles.

Differential diagnosis

Patches of baldness due to hair pulling (trichotillomania) are bizarrely shaped, not as well demarcated as alopecia areata, and have no exclamation mark hairs at the edge. Tinea capitis is marked by broken hairs and by a degree of redness and scaling of the scalp skin. Disorders that inflame the skin and destroy hair follicles can usually be easily differentiated by the scarring they cause.

Treatment

Patients with a solitary patch or few patches usually do not need treatment. When the patches coalesce to become a problem cosmetically or when there is alopecia totalis, treatment is often demanded by patients, but is not often effective. The following treatments have been used: potent topical steroids or systemic steroids; photochemotherapy with long-wave ultraviolet irradiation (PUVA); dithranol; allergic sensitization with diphencyprone; and topical minoxidil has been claimed to be partially successful. All of the above have inconvenient side effects and usually work only while they are being given.

Allergic sensitization with 1 per cent diphencyprone causes an eczematous response and 'kicks' the follicles back to life in about half the patients and is quite often used.

Many patients, having experienced the side effects and frustration of the lack of efficacy of the treatments, decide to cut their losses and disguise their disability with a wig. Sympathy and support are the most useful applications for this depressing disorder.

Diffuse hair loss

This is predominantly a problem for middle-aged and elderly women. It is not a single entity and the causes include pattern alopecia, virilization, hypothyroidism, systemic illness such as systemic lupus erythematosus, and drug administration (particularly the anticancer drugs and the systemic retinoids). Diffuse hair loss is also caused by telogen effluvium (see below). Ageing also results in a lesser density of hair follicles, which is more obvious in some subjects than in others.

Having considered the above possible causes, there are still some patients with obvious diffuse hair loss for whom there is no adequate explanation. Various deficiency states (particularly iron) have been incriminated, but in the majority of instances the supposed deficiency appears to have no other sequel and attempts at its rectification fail to improve the clinical state.

If there is no obvious cause for diffuse hair loss, the only medical treatment available is topical minoxidil, but this is unlikely to give substantial benefit.

Telogen effluvium

The human hair cycle (Fig. 18.6) is asynchronous, but can be precipitated into synchrony by childbirth or a sudden severe systemic illness such as pneumonia or massive blood loss. The stimulus causes all the scalp hair follicles to revert to the telogen, or resting, phase. There is a sudden and significant loss of terminal scalp hair some 3 months after the precipitating event, which continues for a few weeks but then spontaneously stops. Hair regrowth gradually restores the scalp hair to its original state.

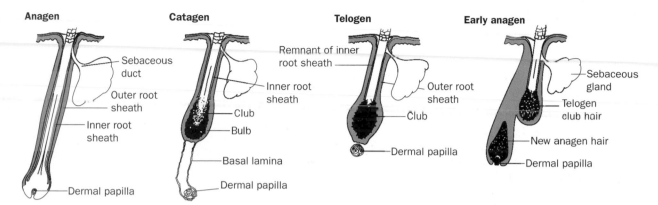

| Anagen | Catagen | Telogen | Early anagen |

Sebaceous duct
Outer root sheath
Inner root sheath
Dermal papilla

Remnant of inner root sheath
Inner root sheath
Club
Bulb
Basal lamina
Dermal papilla

Outer root sheath
Club
Dermal papilla

Sebaceous gland
Telogen club hair
New anagen hair
Dermal papilla

Figure 18.6 Diagram showing the various stages of the human hair cycle.

Traction alopecia

Repeated tugging and pulling on the hair shaft may produce loss of hair in the affected areas, such as occurs when hair rollers are used (Fig. 18.7). It can also develop in young children when they continually rub their scalp on their pillow. Youngsters sometimes tug at their hair, producing the same effect in a bizarre distribution over the scalp (trichitillomania, Fig. 18.8). The motivation for this strange behaviour usually remains obscure. The main differential diagnosis is alopecia areata.

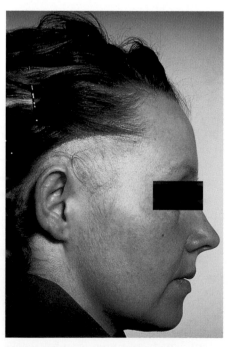

Figure 18.7 Traction alopecia due to the use of rollers.

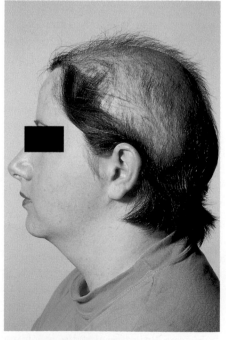

Figure 18.8 Trichotillomania: a bizarre pattern of hair loss from the scalp due to constant tugging of the hair.

Scarring alopecia

Any inflammatory process on the scalp sufficient to cause loss of follicles and scar formation will result in permanent loss of hair in the affected area. Mechanical trauma, burns, bacterial infections and severe inflammatory ringworm of the scalp can produce sufficient damage to cause scarring and permanent hair loss.

In discoid lupus erythematosus (see page 79) and lichen planus (see page 144), the scalp skin may be characteristically affected by the dermatosis concerned, but it may be difficult to distinguish these two conditions, even after biopsy. Usually, the affected area is scarred and there is loss of follicular orifices – the few remaining being distorted and dilated and containing tufts of hair (Fig. 18.9). An odd and unexplained type of scalp scarring known as *pseudopelade* is characterized by small, rounded patches of scarring alopecia without any inflammation.

Hair shaft disorders

Hair shaft abnormalities may be either congenital or acquired. Acquired abnormalities are more often seen. All long hairs tend to become 'weathered' at their ends due to climatic exposure and the usual washing and combing routines.

Twisting hairs between the fingers, and other obsessive manipulation of hair, results in a specific type of damage to the hair shafts known as *trichorrhexis nodosa*, in which expansions of the shaft (nodes) can be seen by routine light microscopy and scanning electron microscopy. These nodes rupture and leave frayed, 'paintbrush'-like ends (Fig. 18.10). This deformity leads to broken hairs and even to the complaint of loss of hair.

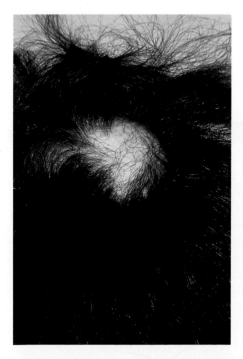

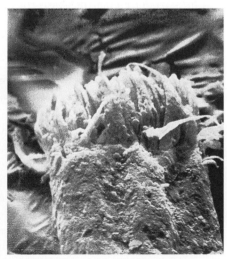

Figure 18.9 Scarring alopecia due to discoid lupus erythematosus.

Figure 18.10 Scanning electron micrograph of fractured hair shaft and paintbrush-like end in trichorrhexis nodosa.

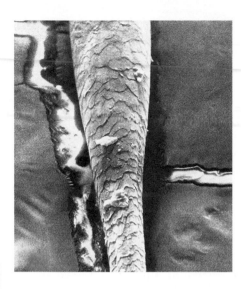

Figure 18.11 Hair shaft in monilethrix showing alternate fusiform expansions and thinning of the hair shaft in this congenital disorder.

Isolated congenital hair shaft disorders include the condition of *monilethrix*, in which there are spindle-like expansions of the hair shaft at regular intervals (Fig. 18.11), causing weakness and breaking of the scalp hair.

HIRSUTES

This is the name given to the complaint of excessive hair growth in women. When the hair growth is on the chin and upper lip, it causes considerable cosmetic embarrassment, even though in most cases it is normal. When hair growth is marked on the trunk and limbs, is accompanied by acne, early pattern alopecia and menstrual irregularities, tests for masculinization and polycystic ovarian syndrome should be performed. Removal of facial hair is usually by depilatories, waxing or electrolysis.

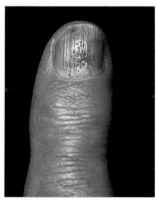

Figure 18.12 Thimble pitting of the fingernail in psoriasis. There is also an area of onycholysis.

Disorders of the nails

Psoriasis, lichen planus and eczema may all affect the nails, causing characteristic clinical appearances. Psoriasis characteristically causes 'thimble pitting' of the fingernails (Fig. 18.12). It also causes well-defined pink/brown areas and onycholysis (separation of the nail plate from the nail bed: Fig. 18.13). The toenails rarely show these changes, but the nail plates may be thickened, with a yellowish brown discoloration and subungual debris often making it difficult to distinguish from ringworm of the nails. In lichen planus, the nail plate may develop longitudinal ridging (Fig. 18.14), which, in the worst cases, may penetrate the whole nail. The process may even destroy the nail matrix and cause permanent loss of the nail. Eczema affecting the fingers may cause irregular deformities of the fingernails and even marked horizontal ridging.

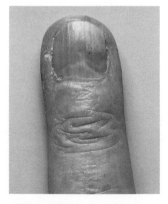

Figure 18.13 Fingernail in psoriasis showing marked onycholysis and some deformity of the nail plate.

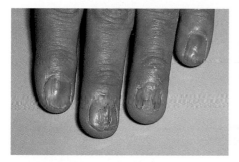

Figure 18.14 Longitudinally ridged fingernails in lichen planus.

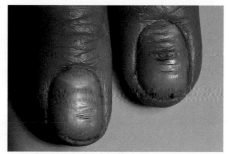

Figure 18.15 Irregular, discoloured nail plate seen in chronic paronychia.

PARONYCHIA

This term is applied to inflammation of the tissues at the sides of the nail. In the common form of chronic paronychia, the paronychial skin is thickened and reddened. It is often tender, and pus may be expressed from the space between the nail fold and the nail plate. The eponychium disappears and the nail plate is often discoloured and deformed (Fig. 18.15) and may demonstrate onycholysis (see below). There is a deep recess between the nail fold and the nail plate, containing debris and micro-organisms, which it is difficult to keep dry. The condition mostly occurs in women whose occupation involves frequent hand washing or other 'wet' activities (e.g. cooks, cleaners, barmaids), and it seems likely that the inability of this group of individuals to keep their hands dry contributes substantially to the condition's chronicity.

Candida micro-organisms may contribute to the recurrent inflammation to which the affected fingers are subject, but they are not the cause of the disorder. The cause is compounded from mechanical trauma and over-hydration resulting in microbial overgrowth in the nooks and crannies of the nail fold.

Treatment

The major goals in management are keeping the fingers completely dry and the avoidance of manual work. Antimicrobial preparations in aqueous or alcoholic vehicles are also useful (e.g. povidone-iodine or an imidazole lotion). Acute exacerbations may need to be treated with systemic antibiotics.

Providing the advice is taken and the treatment used, patients usually gradually improve.

ONYCHOLYSIS

Onycholysis is a physical sign in which the terminal nail plate separates from the underlying nail bed. It is observed in psoriasis, eczema, chronic paronychia, the 'yellow nail syndrome' (see below), thyrotoxicosis, as a result of repeated mechanical trauma and for no known reason.

> **Case 19**
>
> Pauline, aged 30, worked in a mobile phone factory and noticed that she was finding it difficult to pick up small articles from the bench because her nails showed some separation from the nailbeds. The dermatologist told her that this was called onycholysis and was due to her psoriasis.

BRITTLE NAILS AND ONYCHORRHEXIS

In older women, the nails may break easily and separate into horizontal strata (onychorrhexis). Probably the single most important factor causing this problem is repeated hydration and drying, as in housework, as well as mechanical and chemical trauma.

THE NAILS IN SYSTEMIC DISEASE

Onycholysis due to thyrotoxicosis has already been mentioned. In hypoalbuminaemia (as in severe liver disease), the lunulae may be lost and the nail plate turns a milky white. Beau's lines are horizontal ridges due to a sudden severe illness, trauma and/or blood loss and presumably have the same significance as telogen effluvium. They grow outwards and are eventually lost.

BROWN-BLACK PIGMENTATION

Pigmented linear bands along the length of the nail may be due to a mole or, if of recent onset, may be caused by a malignant melanoma. Brown-black areas may be due to melanin or haemosiderin from trauma, and the two may be very difficult to tell apart (Fig. 18.16). Uncommonly, *Pseudomonas* infection of the nail plate produces a diffuse black or black-green pigmentation. A blackish, yellow-green discoloration is also seen in the *yellow nail syndrome* (Fig. 18.17). In this rare disease, nail growth is greatly slowed and the nails are yellowish green, thickened and show increased curvature. In addition, ankle and facial oedema, sinusitis and pleural effusion often accompany this condition, which is of unknown cause.

RINGWORM OF THE NAILS (TINEA UNGUIUM)

Ringworm of the toenails is quite common, but much less common in the fingernails. The affected nails are thickened and crumbly and are discoloured yellow or yellowish white or black (Fig. 18.18). Subungual debris is often present. The differential diagnosis includes psoriasis and paronychia as well as the rare yellow nail syndrome.

Treatment

Treatment is dealt with on page 315.

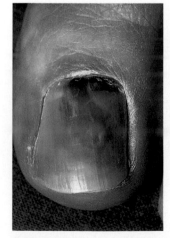

Figure 18.16 Subungual haematoma.

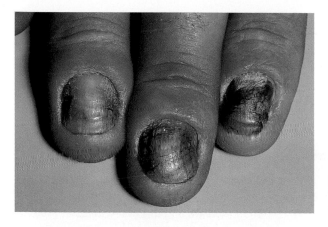

Figure 18.17 Nails in the yellow nail syndrome. The nails are discoloured a yellowish green and show increased curvature. There is also loss of eponychium.

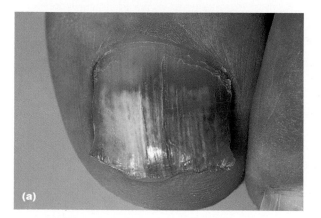

(a)

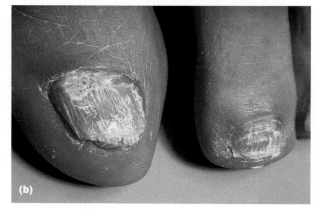

(b)

Figure 18.18 (a) Deformity, discoloration and subungual debris in a big toenail due to ringworm infection (tinea unguium). (b) Here, the second toe is also affected.

Summary

- Hair loss may be non-scarring or scarring. Pattern alopecia is a common, dominantly inherited, progressive, non-scarring alopecia. Starting in the temporal regions and on the vertex, it gradually spreads, even involving the entire scalp. The follicles become smaller in the affected area and then disappear. Although it is heritable, the androgenic stimulus of testosterone is needed for expression of the disorder. There is no effective treatment for men other than surgical transplant techniques. In women, the anti-androgen cyproterone acetate with ethinyl oestranol (Dianette) has been used, as has the 5-alpha-reductase inhibitor finasteride. Minoxidil (the antihypertensive) has been used topically to stimulate hair growth, but is only marginally effective.

- In alopecia areata, hair follicle growth is arrested in well-defined areas of variable size due to an autoimmune process. Regrowth usually occurs in young patients, but when the condition is extensive, affecting eyebrows and body hair, it may persist.

- Solitary or a few small patches usually do not require treatment. When extensive, topical or even systemic steroids or allergic sensitization with 1 per cent diphencyprone causing an eczema stimulates hair growth in a proportion of cases.

- Diffuse hair loss in mature and elderly women is caused by hypothyroidism, systemic illness, telogen effluvium and ageing, but is unexplained in many cases.
- Tologen effluvium is caused by sudden synchronization of many hair follicles so that they revert to the telogen phase because of sudden illness or blood loss. Hair loss occurs some 3 months after the event and the hair then regrows. Hair loss occurs focally due to hair pulling (trichitillomania) or other form of pulling (e.g. from rollers).
- Alopecia due to scarring occurs after trauma, infection or diseases such as discoid lupus erythematosus and lichen planus.
- Hair shaft abnormalities leading to broken hairs occur in trichorrhexis nodosa, characterized by nodular swellings along the hair shaft due to twisting and manipulation, and the congenital disorder monilethrix, in which fusiform swellings occur along the hair shaft.
- Pitting of the nail plate is commonly observed in psoriasis, with separation of the distal nail plate from the nail bed (onycholysis) and discolorations. Ridging and irregularities are observed in other inflammatory skin disorders.
- Paronychia is inflammation of the tissues at the side of the nail plate. The chronic form causes recurrent inflammation of the paronychial tissues and is due to trauma and maceration of the tissues between the nail plate and the skin. The most important part of the treatment is to keep the nail dry.
- Nails affected by ringworm (tinea unguium) are thickened and crumbly and discoloured yellowish white or brown-black.

Systemic disease and the skin

Skin markers of malignant disease

Some skin disorders are precipitated by an underlying malignancy and others almost always indicate a visceral neoplasm. Early recognition may assist detection of the underlying neoplastic disease (Table 19.1).

DISORDERS WITH A STRONG ASSOCIATION WITH UNDERLYING MALIGNANCY

Necrolytic migratory erythema

This is usually caused by a tumour of the pancreatic islet alpha cells that secrete glucagon, but it is sometimes caused by hyperplasia or benign adenomatosis of these cells. Rarely, no underlying abnormality can be found. Areas of erythema, which become eroded and crusted (Fig. 19.1), develop around the groins, on the lower trunk, around the flexures and at the sides of the mouth. They may temporarily remit at one site, to appear elsewhere. The skin disorder responds to removal of the underlying tumour, but usually complete removal is not possible.

Table 19.1 Skin markers of malignant disease

Disorder	Comment
Acquired ichthyosis	Distinguish from the mild xerosis caused by reticulosis, lipid lowering drugs, leprosy and AIDS
Acanthosis nigricans	Distinguish from pseudo-acanthosis nigricans; mostly associated with gastrointestinal adenocarcinoma
Dermatomyositis	Associated with several neoplastic diseases, but particularly of the genital system in women over 40
Erythema gyratum repens	Very rare; strong association with underlying carcinoma
Necrolytic migratory erythema	Strong association with pancreatic alpha-cell tumour; diabetes and low plasma amino acids accompany
Bullous pemphigoid	May be weak association with malignancy, but not certain
Skin metastases	6 per cent of all metastases; metastases from carcinomas of lung, prostate, breast, kidney and stomach

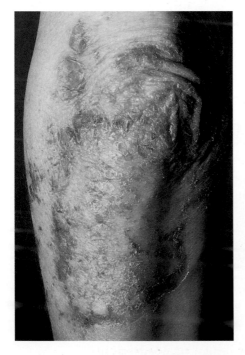

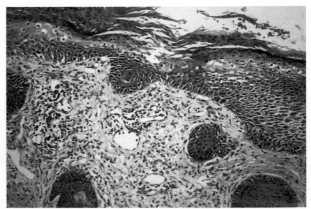

Figure 19.1 Necrolytic migratory erythema: an area of erythema and erosion on the forearm.

Figure 19.2 Pathology of necrolytic migratory erythema showing degenerative change in the upper epidermis with crusting and parakeratosis.

Characteristically, there is degenerative change in the upper epidermis (Fig. 19.2). Blood tests reveal increased circulating glucagon, hyperglycaemia and hypoaminoacidaemia and it is the last of these that may be responsible for this curious skin disorder.

Figure 19.3 Acanthosis nigricans: increased pigmentation and rugosity with skin tags in the axilla.

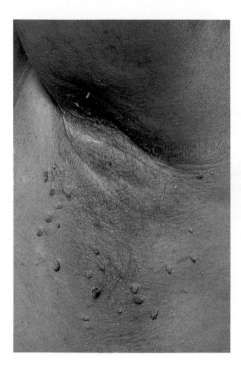

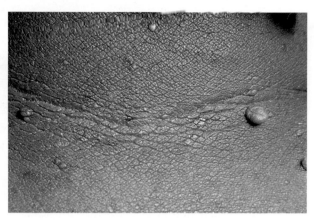

Figure 19.4 Acanthosis nigricans: increased pigmentation, rugosity and skin tags around the neck.

Acanthosis nigricans

Acanthosis nigricans may occur in association with endocrine disease and also, rarely, accompanies lipodystrophies. An identical clinical picture accompanies obesity and is then known as pseudoacanthosis nigricans. When the condition occurs in an adult unaccompanied by obesity or endocrine disease, an underlying neoplasm is usually the cause. The neoplasm involved is often a gastrointestinal adenocarcinoma.

There is a velvety thickening and increased rugosity of the skin of the flexures – the axillae and groins in particular (Fig. 19.3). The sides and back of the neck and the sides of the mouth are also affected.

The thickened areas are also pigmented and bear skin tags and seborrhoeic warts (Fig. 19.4). There may also be some generalized increase in pigmentation, as well as thickening and increased rugosity of the buccal mucosa and the palmar skin.

There is overall hypertrophy of all components of the skin of the affected areas. Insulin-like growth factors may be involved.

Erythema gyratum repens

This is probably the rarest of the specific skin markers of visceral malignancy. This odd disorder is almost always a marker of a neoplasm, often carcinoma of the bronchus.

Large rings composed of reddened polycyclic bands are seen; the rings contain concentric rings, giving a wood-grain effect (Fig. 19.5). The rings gradually enlarge and change shape. Rarely, other less dramatic types of annular erythema may be signs of an internal malignancy.

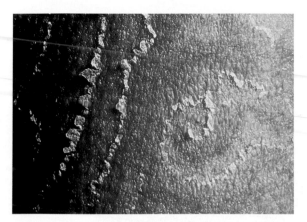

Figure 19.5 Erythema gyratum repens in a patient with carcinoma of the lung. Note the concentric areas of scaling.

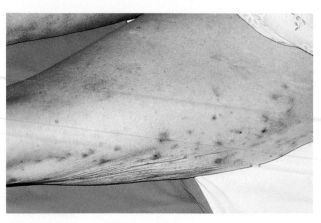

Figure 19.6 Numerous small metastases from carcinoma of the vulva.

Skin metastases

Carcinomas of the breast, bronchus, stomach, kidney and prostate are the most common visceral neoplasms to metastasize to the skin. Secondary deposits on the skin may be the first sign of the underlying visceral cancer. The lesions themselves are usually smooth nodules, which are pink or skin coloured (Fig. 19.6), but may be pigmented in deposits of melanoma.

Acquired ichthyosis

When generalized scaling without erythema begins in adult life, it is quite likely that there is an underlying neoplasm, particularly a reticulosis. This has to be distinguished from mild dryness of the skin and the slight irritation seen in many chronic disorders, known as xeroderma.

Other causes of acquired ichthyosis include acquired immune deficiency syndrome (AIDS), sarcoidosis and leprosy, but if these can be excluded, a neoplastic cause is the most likely explanation (Fig. 19.7).

DISORDERS THAT ARE SOMETIMES ASSOCIATED WITH UNDERLYING MALIGNANT DISEASE

Bullous pemphigoid

This subepidermal blistering disorder occurs mainly in those over 60 years of age, who are anyway more likely to be affected by a neoplasm. Nonetheless, there are a few patients with pemphigoid in whom the skin disorder is provoked by the malignancy and remits after the neoplasm has been removed.

Dermatomyositis

Women over the age of 40 years with dermatomyositis may have 50 per cent chance of a malignant tumour of the genitourinary tract, but infants with the

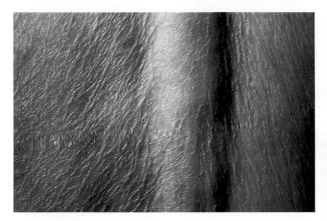

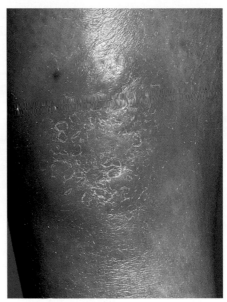

Figure 19.7 This woman suddenly developed 'dry and itchy' skin. On investigation, she was found to have Hodgkin's disease.

Figure 19.8 Plaque of pretibial myxoedema.

disease have no greater risk than a control group. Overall, even in adults, the association is not common and most cases of dermatomyositis occur without an identifiable cause. There is an impression that dermatomyositis provoked by malignant disease is more severe.

Figurate erythemas

Rarely, annular erythema and erythema multiforme (see page 75) seem to be caused by underlying malignant disease.

Endocrine disease, diabetes and the skin

THYROID DISEASE

Pretibial myxoedema is characterized by reddened, elevated plaques, often with a *peau d'orange* appearance on the surface (Fig. 19.8). Histologically, there is a cellular connective tissue with deposition of mucinous material. The serum from such patients contains substances that stimulate the growth and activity of fibroblasts.

The condition is almost always a sign of thyrotoxicosis and is accompanied by exophthalmos. It occurs in 5 per cent of patients with thyrotoxicosis. It is persistent and difficult to treat, although treatment with PUVA is sometimes successful. Rarely, there is diffuse infiltration with similar mucinous connective tissue of the hands and feet and finger clubbing in the condition of *thyroid acropachy*. Patients with thyrotoxicosis have warm, sweaty skin and a proportion complain of pruritus.

In myxoedema, the skin often feels dry and rough and may have a yellowish orange tint, as carotenaemia may accompany the disorder. In addition, there may be coarsening of the scalp hair, hair loss, loss of the outer third of the eyebrows, pinkish cheeks but a yellowish background colour – the so-called peaches and cream complexion.

SKIN MANIFESTATION OF DIABETES

Necrobiosis lipoidica

The skin manifestations of diabetes are summarized in Table 19.2. The most specific is necrobiosis lipoidica. More than 50 per cent of individuals who present with this disorder will already have insulin-dependent diabetes. Many of those who do not have diabetes when they present will develop diabetes or have a first-degree relative with diabetes.

Typically, irregular yellowish pink plaques occur on the lower legs and around the ankles (Fig. 19.9). Uncommonly, lesions may occur elsewhere and there may be areas of atrophy and ulceration. These plaques are persistent and quite resistant to treatment.

Histologically, there is a central area of altered and damaged collagen in the mid-dermis, surrounded by inflammatory cells, including giant cells.

Case 20

Julie, aged 19, reported to her GP that she was micturating much more often than usual and was also feeling abnormally thirsty. When she was examined, the doctor found an elevated, irregular, yellowish pink patch measuring 2.5 by 4.0 cm on her left shin. There was also a smaller, similar patch on her right lower leg. These patches had been present for 6 months. They had originally enlarged in size, but were now static. It was thought that Julie had diabetes and that the leg patches were due to necrobiosis lipoidica diabeticorum. It was explained to her that, unfortunately, there was no certain cure for the disorder.

Table 19.2 Skin manifestations of diabetes

Skin manifestation	Comment
Necrobiosis lipoidica	Majority of patients with this disorder eventually have diabetes
Diffuse granuloma annulare	Rare type of granuloma annulare with strong association with diabetes
Xanthomas	Eruptive xanthomata seen in uncontrolled diabetes
Neuropathic ulceration	Due to neuropathy; perforating ulcers may occur on sole of foot
Ischaemic changes and infection	Increased incidence and severity of atherosclerosis and microvascular disease may lead to ischaemic necrosis and increased incidence of skin infection

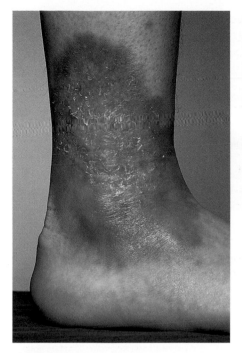

Figure 19.9 Necrobiosis lipoidica on the ankle.

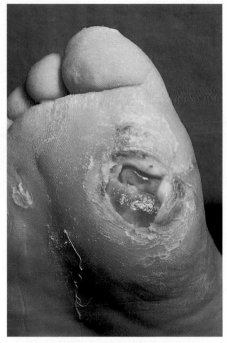

Figure 19.10 Perforating ulcer on the sole of a patient with diabetes.

Granuloma annulare

This disorder has some superficial resemblance to necrobiosis lipoidica, both clinically and histologically, but in its common form has no association with diabetes. However, there is a rare, generalized and 'diffuse' form that is strongly related to diabetes.

Ulceration of the skin in diabetes

The neuropathy of diabetes can result in neuropathic ulceration due to failure of the so-called nociceptive reflex, in which the limb is rapidly withdrawn from a painful stimulus. Deep 'perforating ulcers' may develop on the soles and elsewhere around the feet (Fig. 19.10).

Atherosclerotic vascular disease is more common in diabetics and the resulting ischaemia may also contribute substantially to the ulceration of the feet or legs. There is also a depressed ability to cope with infections, and infection of the ulcerated area usually complicates such lesions in diabetics. The resulting ulcerating areas tend to be moist, contain slough and be purulent. Wounds in diabetics also tend to heal more slowly, turning any minor injury of the foot into a serious health risk.

Xanthomata

Xanthomata are due to deposits of lipid within dermal histiocytes. Their clinical appearance and lipid composition depend on the type of lipid abnormality.

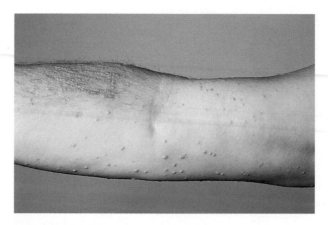

Figure 19.11 Numerous yellow-pink papules due to eruptive xanthoma in a patient with diabetes.

In diabetes, there is usually a mixed hyperlipidaemia in which both cholesterol and triglycerides are elevated. When the lipid levels are very elevated, eruptive xanthomata may develop in which numerous, small, yellow-pink papules appear anywhere, but especially on extensor surfaces (Fig. 19.11).

Skin infection and pruritus

As mentioned above, diabetics appear particularly susceptible to skin infections. Monilial infection is a particular problem and monilial vulvovaginitis and balanoposthitis are common. These are 'itchy disorders' and it may be that this is how it came to be believed that diabetics can develop generalized itch. In fact, there is little evidence that diabetes is responsible for generalized itch.

CUSHING'S SYNDROME

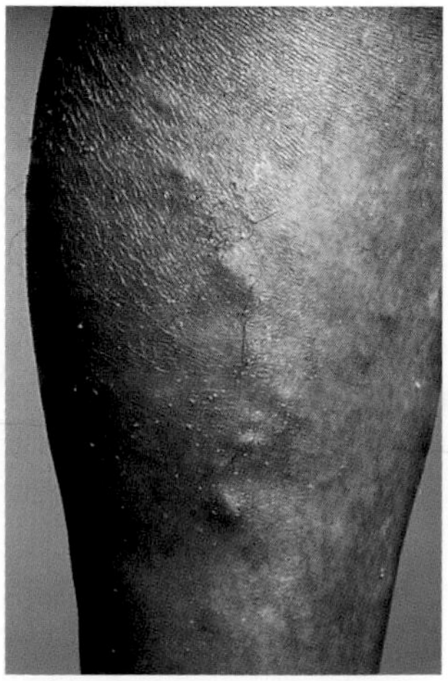

The cutaneous signs of Cushing's syndrome are the same regardless of whether they are caused by an adrenal tumour, hyperplasia or the administration of corticoids.

Clinical features

- The most consistent clinical feature is skin thinning. The underlying veins can be easily seen and the skin has a 'transparent' quality (Fig. 19.12). The thinning is due to the suppressive action of glucocorticoids on the growth and synthetic activity of dermal fibroblasts and the epidermis.
- The dermal thinning also results in rupture of the elastic fibres and striae distensae (Fig. 19.13). These are band-like atrophic areas that develop in areas of maximal stress on the skin. A certain number are found on the upper arm, the anterior axillary fold, the lower back and occasionally elsewhere in normal adolescents. They also occur in most pregnant women on the thighs, breasts,

Figure 19.12 Skin thinning in Cushing's syndrome.

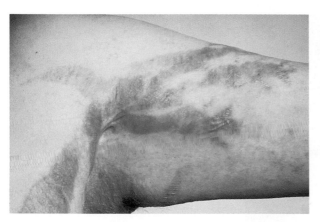

Figure 19.13 Striae distensae of the anterior axillary fold in iatrogenic Cushing's syndrome.

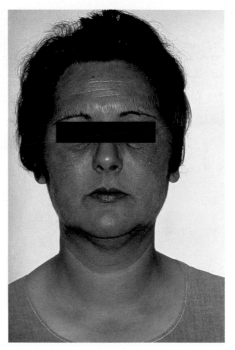

Figure 19.14 Hyperpigmentation of facial skin in Addison's syndrome.

anterior axillary folds and lower abdomen. It is thought that both tissue tension and the level of circulating glucocorticoids are important in the production of striae.

- Acne papules occur on the chest, back and face in most patients with Cushing's syndrome. Steroid acne lesions are more uniform in appearance than adolescent acne and consist predominantly of small papules with few comedones. This type of acne is more resistant to treatment than ordinary acne.
- Skin infections are also more common and more severe in patients with Cushing's syndrome. Pityriasis versicolor is often present and often very extensive.

ADDISON'S DISEASE

This disorder, due to destruction of the adrenal cortex from autoimmune influences, tuberculosis and amyloidosis of metastatic neoplastic disease, results in weakness, hypotension and generalized hyperpigmentation (Fig. 19.14). The increased pigmentation may be particularly evident on the buccal mucosa and in the palmar creases.

Androgenization (virilization)

This disorder of women is due to androgen-secreting tumours of the ovaries or the adrenal cortex, but is usually due to polycystic ovaries in which there is an

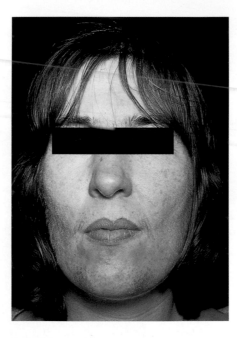

Figure 19.15 Hirsutes due to androgenization.

abnormality of steroid metabolism leading to an accumulation of androgens. Patients present with acne and increased greasiness of the skin.

Increased hair growth is also a major complaint of patients with androgenization. Vellus hair on forearms, thighs and trunk is transformed to pigmented, thick, terminal hairs. A masculine distribution of body and limb hair develops.

The appearance of beard hair is usually the reason for patients attending the clinic (Fig. 19.15). In clinical practice, the most common problem is to distinguish hirsutes due to androgenization from hirsutes due to non-endocrine causes. It is not generally recognized that the presence of some terminal hair on the face or limbs of some otherwise healthy women is normal. This is particularly the case in dark-complexioned women of Arab, Asian or Mediterranean descent. The tendency for 'excess hair' is also familial. Thinning of the scalp hair and pattern alopecia are also quite common and very distressing to women with virilization.

In authentic virilization, the following features help distinguish the condition from 'non-endrocrine' hirsutes:

- the excess hair is recent in onset and progressively becoming more noticeable
- the hirsutes is accompanied by other physical signs including acne and seborrhoea
- there is significant menstrual disturbance.

In most cases, extensive investigation is not appropriate and plasma testosterone and abdominal ultrasound are all that are required.

Nutrition and the skin

VITAMIN A (RETINOL)

Retinol is a vital, lipid-soluble vitamin found in dairy produce and liver and is also obtainable in the form of beta-carotene from carrots, tomatoes and other vegetables. It is essential for growth and development, resistance to infection, reproduction and visual function. In deficiency states, it causes follicular hyperkeratosis and roughening of the skin (phrynoderma). When excessive amounts are ingested, pruritus, widespread erythema and peeling of the palms and soles occur. These symptoms and signs are similar to those of retinoid toxicity.

NICOTINIC ACID

This is a water-soluble B vitamin found in grains and vegetables. Deficiency causes the condition of pellagra, resulting in diarrhoea, dementia and a photosensitivity dermatitis. The photosensitivity dermatitis develops a characteristic post-inflammatory hyperpigmentation and is often very marked around the neck.

VITAMIN C (ASCORBIC ACID)

Vitamin C is a water-soluble vitamin found in fruit and vegetables. Deficiency results in scurvy, which causes a clotting defect and poor wound healing. A characteristic rash seen in patients with scurvy consists of numerous tiny haemorrhages around hair follicles.

KWASHIORKOR

This is due to severe protein deficiency in children and is seen in the poorer, underprivileged parts of the world, including areas of Africa and India. Generalized oedema develops and the degree of skin pigmentation decreases. In addition, the hair becomes reddish during the time of the deficiency – the so-called flag sign.

SENILE OSTEOPOROSIS

In this disorder of faulty bone mineralization due to vitamin D deficiency, bone thinning and multiple fractures, the skin becomes 'thinner' and is almost transparent, with the veins being abnormally prominent (Fig. 19.16). The thinning can be demonstrated by ultrasound.

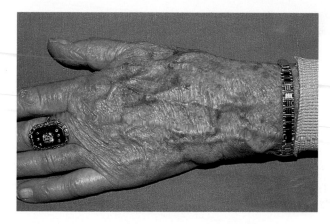

Figure 19.16 Thin, fragile skin of the back of the hand due to osteoporosis.

Skin and the gastrointestinal tract

There are numerous interrelationships between the skin and the gastrointestinal tract, and only the more important ones fall within the scope of a book of this size.

DERMATITIS HERPETIFORMIS

This itchy, blistering disorder is strongly associated with an absorptive defect of the small bowel. Small-bowel mucosal biopsy demonstrates partial villous atrophy in some 70–80 per cent of patients with dermatitis herpetiformis. There are also some minor functional absorptive abnormalities in most patients. This gut disorder is, in fact, a form of gluten enteropathy (as is coeliac disease) and can be improved by a gluten-free diet.

PEUTZ–JEGHERS SYNDROME

This is a rare, autosomal dominant disorder in which perioral and labial pigmented macules occur in association with jejunal polyps. Pigmented macules also occur over the fingers.

GARDENER'S SYNDROME

In this dominant disorder, epidermoid cysts and benign epidermal tumours occur in association with colonic polyposis.

Hepatic disease

In severe chronic hepatocellular liver failure, hypoalbuminaemia occurs, which results in the curious sign of whitening of the fingernails (Fig. 19.17). Severe liver

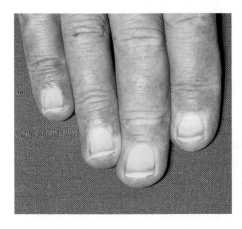

Figure 19.17 White fingernails due to liver disease.

failure may also cause multiple spider naevi to develop over the arms, upper trunk and face. These vascular anomalies consist of a central 'feeding' blood vessel ('the body') with numerous fine radiating 'legs'. Their cause is uncertain, but they may be related to the plasma levels of unconjugated oestrogens.

In biliary cirrhosis, severe pruritus develops, resulting in excoriations and prurigo papules. Jaundice and a generalized dusky pigmentation are seen in addition.

Systemic causes of pruritus

- End-stage renal failure (uraemia) often causes persistent severe itch. The itch is accompanied by a dusky, grey-brown pigmentation.
- Obstructive jaundice from any cause results in intolerable itching.
- Thyrotoxicosis sometimes causes itching, but does not seem to be due to the sweatiness or increased warmth of the skin experienced by such patients.
- Itching is sometimes a complaint of patients with hyperparathyroidism.
- The symptom of itch is occasionally a sign of Hodgkin's disease or, less often, of another type of lymphoma. Rarely, the itch is a presenting symptom of the neoplasm.
- Itch is a well-known disabling complaint of patients with polycythaemia rubra vera. For some curious reason, the itch may be a particular problem when these patients have a bath.
- It has often been claimed that patients with diabetes have pruritus, but if this is the case, it must be extremely rare. Diabetics are prone to candidiasis, which causes perigenital itch, and it is possible that this is how the idea began.

Summary

- Certain skin disorders are precipitated by an underlying malignancy. These include acanthosis nigricans, erythema gyratum repens, acquired ichthyosis and necrolytic migratory erythema.

- Necrolytic migratory erythema is a persistent, erosive, migratory rash associated with excess glucagon secretion from a pancreatic alpha cell tumour or hyperplasia.

- Acanthosis nigricans causes velvety thickening in the flexures, a generalized increase in pigmentation and an increase in skin tags and seborrhoeic warts. It is mainly seen in gastrointestinal malignancies, but also occurs in some endocrine disorders and obesity.
- Acquired ichthyosis occurs in lymphoma, but also in AIDS and leprosy.
- Dermatomyositis, bullous pemphigoid and the figurate erythemas are associated with malignant disease in some patients. Erythema gyratum repens is an odd erythematous rash with a 'wood-grain' pattern, which is specifically associated with visceral malignancy.
- In pretibial myxoedema, there are reddened plaques on the lower legs. It is seen in 5 per cent of thyrotoxic patients and is accompanied by exophthalmos.
- Necrobiosis lipoidica is strongly associated with diabetes. In this condition, persistent, irregular, yellowish plaques occur on the lower legs. Histologically, granulomatous inflammation surrounds areas of collagenous degeneration.
- Eruptive xanthomata (due to mixed hyperlipidaemia), ulceration (due to neuropathy causing perforating ulcers or due to ischaemia and infection) and generalized diffuse granuloma annulare are also associated with diabetes.
- Skin thinning, striae distensae, acne and susceptibility to skin infection are features of Cushing's syndrome and due to increased secretion of glucocorticoids from the adrenal cortex. Generalized hyperpigmentation is also a feature of Addison's disease, caused by destruction of the adrenal cortex.
- Polycystic ovaries or ovarian tumours cause androgenization (virilization), with increased limb and facial hair, seborrhoea and acne.
- The skin manifestations of vitamin deficiency include phrynoderma in retinol deficiency, pellagra in nicotinic acid deficiency and scurvy in ascorbic acid deficiency.
- Dermatitis herpetiformis is an autoimmune, itchy, blistering disease in which 70 per cent of patients show jejunal partial villous atrophy and a minor degree of malabsorption.
- White fingernails due to hypoalbuminaemia and multiple spider naevi are characteristic of severe liver disease.
- Generalized pruritus is a feature of renal failure, obstructive jaundice (especially biliary cirrhosis), thyrotoxicosis, lymphoma, polycythaemia rubra vera and hyperparathyroidism.

Disorders of pigmentation

Melanin pigment is produced in melanocytes in the basal layer of the epidermis. The degree of racial pigmentation does not depend on the number of melanocytes present, but on their metabolic activity and the size and shape of their melanin-producing organelles – the melanosomes. Melanocytes account for 5–10 per cent of the cells in the basal layer of the epidermis. They are dendritic (Fig. 20.1), but appear as 'clear cells' in formalin-fixed sections (Fig. 20.2).

Melanin synthesis is controlled by melanocyte-stimulating hormone and is influenced by oestrogens and androgens. Melanocytes are also stimulated by ultraviolet radiation (UVR) and by other irritative stimuli.

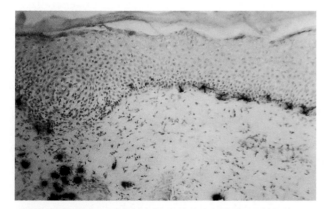

Figure 20.1 Dihydroxyphenylalanine (DOPA) oxidase reaction to reveal melanocytes in the basal layer of the epidermis as blackened cells with dendritic processes.

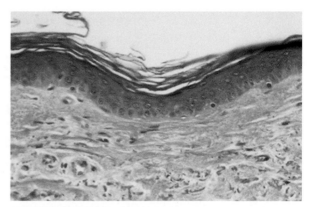

Figure 20.2 Formalin-fixed histological section of normal skin showing several 'clear cells' at the base representing melanocytes.

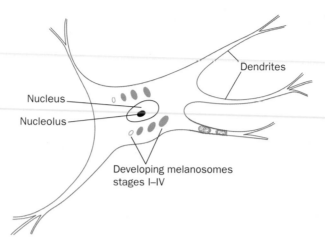

Figure 20.3 Diagram of a melanocyte showing dendrites and different stages of melanosomes.

Melanin is a complex, black-brown polymer synthesized from the amino acid dihydroxyphenylalanine (L-DOPA; Fig. 20.3). Two forms of melanin exist: 'ordinary' melanin, known as eumelanin, and a reddish melanin synthesized from cysteinyl DOPA, known as phaeomelanin.

Melanin synthesis is initially catalysed by a copper-containing enzyme known as tyrosinase, which also catalyses the transformation of L-DOPA to tyrosine.

Melanin is produced in melanocytes, but 'donated' via their dendrites to neighbouring keratinocytes. The melanin granules then ascend through the epidermis in the keratinocytes. Melanosomes go through several stages of melanin synthesis during their melaninization (stages I–IV). Mature melanosomes aggregate into melanin granules and it is these granular particles within keratinocytes that give protection against damage from UVR.

Melanin in keratinocytes is black and absorbs all visible light, UVR and infrared radiation. It is also a powerful electron acceptor and may have other uncharacterized protective functions.

Excessive pigmentation is known as hyperpigmentation, and decreased pigmentation is known as hypopigmentation. Both may be localized or generalized. Non-melanin pigments may also cause skin darkening.

Generalized hypopigmentation

OCULOCUTANEOUS ALBINISM

There are several varieties of genetically determined defects in melanin synthesis, the most common of which is recessively inherited oculocutaneous albinism.

Affected individuals have a very pale or even pinkish complexion with flaxen, white or slightly yellowish hair and very light-blue or even pink eyes. Albinos are also subject to nystagmus, either horizontal or rotatory. In addition, they are photophobic and often have serious refractive errors. They are extremely sensitive to the harmful effects of solar irradiation and in sunny climates often develop skin cancers.

Albinos have a normal number of melanocytes in the basal layer of the epidermis, but lack tyrosinase and are unable to synthesize melanin. If hair is plucked and incubated in a medium containing L-DOPA, the hair bulb does not turn black, as it does normally.

Management

Albino patients must learn to protect themselves against UVR with sunscreens and avoidance of sun wherever possible. Regular checking to detect early changes of skin cancer is also important.

OTHER FORMS OF ALBINISM

There are several other types of albinism, most of which are recessive. In Hermanski–Pudlak syndrome, there is an associated clotting defect due to a platelet abnormality. This is 'tyrosinase positive' and hair bulbs turn black after they are incubated with L-DOPA.

In several types of albinism, the abnormality of melanin synthesis is confined to the eyes.

Localized hypopigmentation

PIEBALDISM

In this condition, there is a white forelock and white patches on the skin surface. In Waardenburg's syndrome, the condition is associated with sensory deafness.

VITILIGO

Definition

This is a common skin disorder in which there is focal failure of pigmentation due to destruction of melanocytes that is thought to be mediated by immunological mechanisms.

Clinical features

Sharply defined areas of depigmentation appear (Fig. 20.4). The depigmented patches are often symmetrical, especially when they are over the limbs and face. Odd patterns sometimes occur, as when depigmented patches develop over the location of endocrine glands.

It is more noticeable in summer when the surrounding skin is sunburnt. It is a serious cosmetic problem for darkly pigmented people.

The condition often starts in childhood and either spreads, ultimately causing total depigmentation, or persists, with irregular remissions and relapses.

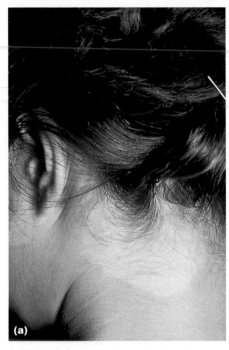
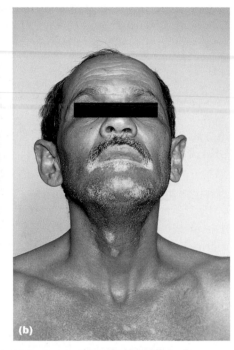

Figure 20.4 (a) A sharply defined patch of vitiligo on the neck. (b) Vitiligo in a dark-skinned patient.

In *halo naevus* (Sutton's naevus), the depigmentation of vitiligo begins around one or a few compound naevi.

Pathogenesis and epidemiology

Vitiligo occurs in 1–2 per cent of the population and is more common when it has occurred in other members of the family. It is also more common in diabetes, thyroid disease and alopecia areata, and appears to be due to an autoimmune attack on melanocytes.

Treatment

Treatments with topical corticosteroids or photochemotherapy with long-wave ultraviolet irradiation (PUVA) are sometimes effective in stimulating repigmentation, but the response is irregular. Reassurance and cosmetic camouflage are sufficient for most patients.

Case 21

Mohammed was aged 23 when he first developed a sharply defined, white area on his face. Over the following months, the patch enlarged and others appeared. His uncle had had vitiligo. Treatment for Mohammed's vitiligo did not seem to help a great deal, but, after several years, some of the patches repigmented spontaneously.

Table 20.1 Causes of localized hypopigmentation

Disorder	Comment
Vitiligo	Destruction of melanocytes; common; acquired; multiple, sharply defined, non-pigmented patches anywhere
Pityriasis versicolor	Superficial yeast infection (*Malassezia furfur*) leading to disturbance in pigment production; common; multiple, pale, scaling patches on trunk
Pityriasis alba	Mild, patchy eczema of the face in children causing a disturbance in pigment production
Leprosy	One or several paler macules on trunk or limbs that are hypoaesthetic
White macules of tuberous sclerosis	Uncommon developmental anomaly affecting central nervous system, connective tissue and skin; several 'maple leaf'-shaped, hypopigmented macules
Naevus anaemicus	Rare, developmental, solitary white patch, usually on trunk; thought to have a vascular basis
Chemical toxicity	May look like vitiligo; seen in workers in the rubber industry exposed to paratertiary benzyltoluene

OTHER CAUSES OF LOCALIZED DEPIGMENTATION OF SKIN

In many countries, the fear of leprosy makes the differential diagnosis of a 'white patch' an urgent and vitally important issue. The causes are summarized in Table 20.1. Examination in long-wave UVR distinguishes total depigmentation (as in vitiligo) and helps identify areas of depigmentation. It also detects the yellow-green fluorescence in some cases of pityriasis versicolor.

Hyperpigmentation

It has to be determined whether the pigmentation is due to melanin or some other pigment (Table 20.2).

Generalized melanin hyperpigmentation is seen in *Addison's disease* due to destruction of the adrenal cortex from tuberculosis, autoimmune influences, metastases or amyloidosis. Pigmentation is marked in the flexures and exposed areas, but the mucosae and nails are also hyperpigmented. The diagnosis is supported by hypotension, hyponatraemia and extreme weakness. The hyperpigmentation is due to an excess of pituitary peptides resulting from the lack of adrenal steroids. After bilateral adrenalectomy, pigmentation may be extreme (*Nelson's syndrome*).

Generalized hyperpigmentation may be part of *acanthosis nigricans* (see page 283), which is much more marked in the flexures and is accompanied by exaggerated skin markings and skin tags.

Table 20.2 Non-melanin causes of brown-black discoloration

Haemosiderin – from broken haem pigment in extravasated blood
Homogentisic acid – deposited in cartilage, in particular, in the inherited metabolic defect known as alkaptonuria
Unknown pigment in thickened stratum corneum of severe disorders of keratinization such as lamellar ichthyosis
Drugs and heavy-metal toxicity: dark pigmentation of skin and mucosae seen in silver, gold, mercury and arsenic poisoning; amiodarone and phenothiazines cause slate-grey, dusky skin pigmentation in exposed sites; minocycline may cause patchy pigmentation in exposed or other sites

A 'bronzed appearance' is seen in *primary haemochromatosis* (bronzed diabetes), in which iron is deposited in the viscera, including the pancreas (giving rise to diabetes) and the liver (causing cirrhosis). The increased pigmentation is caused by both iron and excess melaninization in the skin. Increased pigment is also evident in secondary haemosiderosis. Generalized hyperpigmentation is also seen in cirrhosis, particularly biliary cirrhosis, chronic renal failure, glycogen storage disease and Gaucher's disease. Biliary cirrhosis and renal failure are usually accompanied by severe pruritus.

Drugs can cause generalized diffuse hyperpigmentation, patchy generalized or localized hyperpigmentation. Classic examples are due to the rare heavy metal intoxications. Arsenic ingestion causes a generalized 'raindrop' pattern of hyperpigmentation, and topical silver preparations cause 'argyria', producing a dusky, greyish discoloration of the skin and mucosae.

Modern drugs can also produce darkening. Minoxycycline (Minocin) can cause darkening of the scars of acne; it can also produce dark patches on exposed areas. The pigment is a complex of iron, the drug and melanin and the condition is only partially reversible. Amiodarone, the antiarrhythmic drug, causes a characteristic greyish colour on exposed sites. The phenothiazines, in high doses over long periods, produce a purplish discoloration in the exposed areas due to the deposition of a drug–melanin complex in the skin. Chlorpromazine is particularly prone to doing this.

Carotenaemia produces an orange-yellow, golden hue due to the deposition of beta-carotene in the skin. It is seen in food faddists who eat large amounts of carrots and other red vegetables. Beta-carotene is also given for the condition of erythropoietic protoporphyria (see page 261).

Canthexanthin is another carotenoid that produces a similar skin colour and was sold for this purpose to simulate a 'bronzed' suntan. Pigment crystals were found in the retina of patients taking the drug and it has been withdrawn for this reason.

Transient skin discoloration is seen in methaemoglobinaemia and sulphaemoglobinaemia due to dapsone administration.

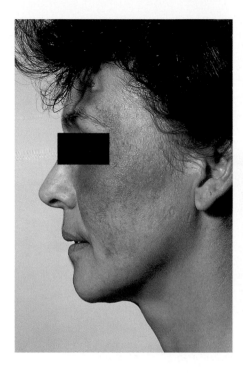

Figure 20.5 Macular grey-brown pigmentation in naevus of Ota.

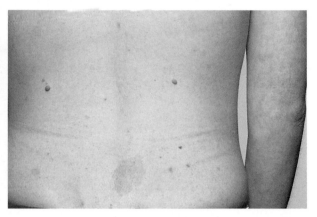

Figure 20.6 Light-brown macule (*café au lait*) due to Von Recklinghausen's disease.

LOCALIZED HYPERPIGMENTATION

Mongolian spots, the naevus of Ota and the naevus of Ito are large, flat, grey-brown patches and can be confused with bruising and other conditions (Fig. 20.5). *Café au lait* patches are part of neurofibromatosis (Von Recklinghausen's disease, see page 199). Numerous flat, light-brown macules, which vary from $0.5\,cm^2$ to $4\,cm^2$ are present all over the skin surface – and characteristically in the axillae alongside the neurofibromata (Fig. 20.6).

Not dissimilar brown macules are found on the lips and around the mouth and on the fingers in Peutz–Jeghers syndrome, accompanied by small-bowel polyps, and in Albright's syndrome, in which there are associated bone abnormalities.

A very common type of localized hyperpigmentation is chloasma. This facial pigmentation may be part of the increased pigmentation of pregnancy or may occur independently. The cheeks, periocular regions, forehead and neck may be affected in this so-called 'mask of pregnancy' (Fig. 20.7).

Post-inflammatory hyperpigmentation may be due to melanocytic hyperplasia occurring as part of epidermal thickening in chronic eczema, particularly atopic eczema. This is transient and of no real consequence.

It may also be due to the shedding of melanin from the damaged epidermis into the dermis, where it is engulfed by macrophages. This 'tattooing' may last many months. It is seen in lichen planus (Fig. 20.8; see also page 144) and in fixed drug eruption (see page 95).

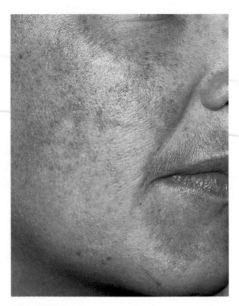

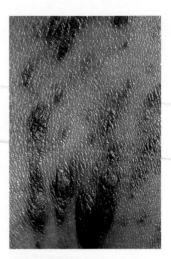

Figure 20.8 Dark patches following resolution of lichen planus.

Figure 20.7 Diffuse brown pigmentation of the cheek in chloasma.

Summary

- Melanin pigment is a complex, brown-black polymer, synthesized from dihydroxyphenylalanine by DOPA oxidase and tyrosinase in melanocytes in organelles known as melanosomes. These organelles are injected via dendrites into keratinocytes.

- Oculocutaneous albinism is a recessively inherited disorder in which there is a normal number of melanocytes but a tyrosinase deficiency. Albinos have fair skin, white/yellow hair and light-blue eyes. They are very sun sensitive and need careful protection from the sun. In piebaldism, there is a white forelock and white patches on the skin.

- In vitiligo, there are well-defined, multiple patches of depigmentation, which usually persist or spread but can remit. It affects 1–2 per cent of the population and appears to be autoimmune in origin. It may respond to corticosteroids or PUVA.

- Other causes of localized areas of depigmentation include leprosy, in which the patches are hypoaesthetic, pityriasis versicolor due to a superficial yeast infection and pityriasis alba, which is a kind of eczema in children.

- Generalized hyperpigmentation (including the mucosae and nails) due to excess pituitary melanocyte-stimulating hormone occurs in Addison's disease resulting from adrenal cortex disease or in Nelson's syndrome after bilateral adrenalectomy. It is also seen as part of acanthosis nigricans.

- Other causes of generalized pigmentation include primary haemochromatosis, hepatic cirrhosis, Gaucher's disease and renal failure.

- Dark pigmentation due to non-melanin pigments is seen in bruising (due to haemosiderin), in alkaptonuria (due to homogentisic acid) and after drug administration. Drugs that can cause pigmentation are minoxycline, amiodarone and agents containing silver, gold and mercury. Chlorpromazine can cause a dusky, purplish facial pigmentation; a golden-yellow colour is evident in carotenaemia.

- Mongolian spots, naevus of Ito and naevus of Ota are slate-grey, localized patches due to a particular kind of naevus.

- Other localized areas of hyperpigmentation may occur after skin inflammation. *Café au lait* patches are seen in neurofibromatosis. A more diffuse type of facial hyperpigmentation that is mostly seen in women is known as chloasma.

Management of skin disease

Psychological aspects of skin disorder

DOES SKIN DISORDER AFFECT THE PSYCHE?

The skin is vital to interpersonal relationships. It is a vital part of our communications system. If it is destroyed or deranged in any way, 'unfriendly messages' are transmitted. Instead of the message, 'Here is a healthy, harmless member of the human race', the signal from an abnormal skin is interpreted as announcing, 'Beware of the contagion'. There is a primitive dislike and distrust of individuals with skin disease or skin deformity. Skin problems seem to engender genuine fear and revulsion, perhaps as a hangover from primitive stages of human development when the avoidance of people with infected of infested skin had a survival advantage.

Interestingly, patients with obvious skin disease are also very disturbed by its appearance and tend to shun the company of others and become quite isolated. These attitudes are known collectively as 'the leper complex'. Reassurance and the use of prostheses, hairpieces and cosmetic camouflage should be encouraged rather than sneered at.

Patients with obvious disease of exposed areas, widespread skin disease and persistently itchy skin become depressed and need sympathy and general support, but some may need psychotropic drugs and psychiatric help.

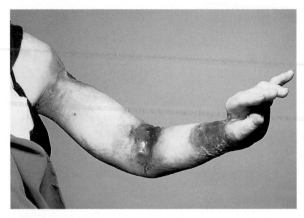

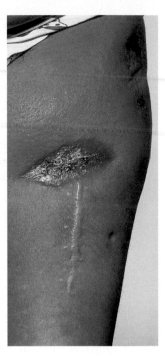

Figure 21.1 Dermatitis artefacta: an eroded area on the arm with scars due to self-mutilation.

Figure 21.2 Dermatitis artefacta: a scarred area on the thigh from self-induced injury.

DOES THE PSYCHE AFFECT THE SKIN?

A question frequently asked by patients is, 'Is it my nerves, doctor?' For the most part, there is no truth to this suggestion. 'Stress' of all kinds can precipitate or aggravate all kinds of disease, including cardiovascular, gastrointestinal and skin diseases, but there is very little evidence that psychological abnormality causes skin disorder.

The major exception is *dermatitis artefacta*, a skin disorder that is entirely self-induced. The degree of insight varies among patients: some admit scratching, picking or rubbing, but say they are unable to stop doing it; others hotly deny producing the injury to the skin.

The extent of the injury is itself varied. Clearly, in some patients the problem is hysterical in the psychiatric sense. At one end of the scale, nodular prurigo (see page 120) can be said to be a form of dermatitis artefacta. At the other end of the scale, there is a devastating injury resulting in serious permanent disability (Fig. 21.1).

In some cases, the artefactual injury is frank malingering for obvious gain (Fig. 21.2). Psychotherapy and psychotropic drugs appear to offer very little and the artefacts may persist for years.

DELUSIONS OF PARASITOSIS

This is a rare psychosis in which the individual believes that his or her skin is infested with insects or worms. Often, sufferers will bring to the doctor rolled up horn or other skin debris and point proudly to the 'infesting insect'. They may point to blemishes on the skin as evidence of their problem. These patients' beliefs are quite unshakeable, and beyond psychiatrists' help. The drug pimozide has been said to be helpful for patients with delusional parasitosis.

BODY IMAGE

We all have a particular 'view' of ourselves and a special 'concern' over our own visual worth. Curiously, some individuals have a distorted body image amounting to a delusional belief. Too much hair, too little hair, discolorations and minor blemishes can all become a major focal point of complaint. Dysmorphophobia is a term used to describe this, not uncommon, condition.

Skin disability

Skin disease can be as disabling as disease of other organ systems. Disability from skin disease consists of physical, emotional and social components. The physical disability derives from decreased mobility due to the abnormal stratum corneum present in eczema, psoriasis or the ichthyotic disorders. The abnormal horn lacks extensibility and cracks when stretched. The abnormally stiff dermis in scleroderma or scarring also affects mobility. The emotional disability stems from the psychological problems discussed above and can lead to serious depression and its consequences. The social disability stems from the 'isolation' imposed by both the patients themselves and society at large. It results in domestic and occupational problems.

Topical treatments for skin disease

Drugs for use topically are incorporated into vehicles, which include greasy single-phase ointments, creams, which are mostly oil in water, or water in oil emulsions or aqueous lotions. Pastes are thick substances containing a particulate solid phase; alcoholic lotions have some limited use, for example for scalp treatments; gels are semi-solid, translucent water-filled or alcohol-filled matrices, which are quite useful at times, for example for scalp disorders.

In general, ointments are prescribed for chronic scaling conditions, including psoriasis and persistent eczema; creams and lotions are prescribed for acute and exudative disorders. When the disorder is weeping and exudative, bathing and wet dressings are required. Gauze dressings kept moist with saline or dilute potassium permanganate solution (1:8000) or aluminium subacetate solution (8 per cent) should be used. Shampoos are helpful for psoriasis and seborrhoeic dermatitis of the scalp.

HOW MUCH TO PRESCRIBE?

It takes about 25 g to cover the body completely on one occasion with a cream or ointment; 50 g would be sufficient for a topical treatment for a bilateral hand dermatitis for a month. Clearly, 100 g would be needed for the hands and feet.

Emollients and cleansing preparations need to be prescribed in much larger quantities.

ADVERSE SIDE EFFECTS FROM TOPICAL PREPARATIONS
(Table 21.1)

If a patient does not improve with the topical medicine prescribed, it may be because:

- there is an adverse effect from use of the preparation (e.g. contact allergy)
- the condition has been wrongly diagnosed
- the patient has not used the medication
- the condition is resistant to the treatment prescribed.

EMOLLIENTS

Emollients (moisturizers) act by occluding the skin surface with a lipid film, which prevents evaporation of water from the surface, allowing it to accumulate within the stratum corneum. Emollients may be single-phase oils or greasy ointments, oil-in-water or water-in-oil emulsions, either as creams or lotions.

Emollients have important effects. They:

- make the stratum corneum swell and flatten so that the skin looks and feels smoother
- increase the extensibility of skin so that it cracks less
- decrease binding forces between the horn cells and decrease scaling
- decrease itch
- have some intrinsic anti-inflammatory properties, decrease epidermal mitotic activity and have anti-prostaglandin synthetase activity.

Table 21.1 Adverse side effects of topical medications

Effect	Significance
Allergic contact dermatitis (dermatitis medicamentosa) to the drug or a component of the vehicle	Eczematous rash at site of application, e.g. from neomycin
Irritation of the skin	Eczematous rash at site of application, e.g. from benzoyl peroxide
Photosensitivity	Erythematous or eczematous rash at exposed site of application, e.g. from a halogenated salicylanilide antimicrobial
Acneiform folliculitis	Acneiform rash at site of application, particularly in acne-prone areas
Absorption of drug or component of the preparation	Systemic toxicities, dependent on particular preparation

Uses of emollients

- Emollients may be all that is required for patients with mild ichthyotic disorders.
- They are also useful for patients with eczema, particularly atopic dermatitis.
- Emollients help patients with psoriasis and other chronic scaling dermatoses.

TOPICAL CORTICOSTEROIDS

There are numerous preparations containing topical corticosteroids, with different potencies (Table 21.2). Their predominant use is for eczematous dermatoses, but they are also useful in psoriasis. They have marked anti-inflammatory and antiproliferative effects. A major part of their action is in inducing lipocortin – the endogenous inhibitor of phospholipase A2 – which is important in the generation of eicosanoid compounds involved in the inflammatory process.

Adverse side effects from topical corticosteroids (Table 21.3)

If enough corticosteroid is absorbed, there is suppression of the pituitary–adrenal axis and adrenal atrophy. If even more is absorbed, a Cushingoid-like state can develop (Fig. 21.3). A general guideline is that not more than 50 g 0.1 per cent betamethasone 17-valerate ointment or cream should be used per week, or not more than 30 g 0.1 per cent clobetasol 17-propionate.

Table 21.2 Classification of corticosteroids according to potency

Category	Activity	Examples
1	Mild (weak)	Hydrocortisone Clobetasone butyrate
2	Moderately potent	Flurandrenolone Desoxymethasone
3	Potent	Betamethasone-17-valerate Fluocinolone acetonide
4	Very potent	Clobetasone-17-propionate Halcinonide Ulabetasol

Table 21.3 Side effects of topical corticosteroids

Absorption and pituitary–adrenal axis suppression and hypercortisonism

Skin-thinning effects causing telangiectasia, striae and fragility

Depressed wound healing

Masked infection, particularly ringworm (tinea incognito)

Miscellaneous, including acne, hirsutes and depigmentation

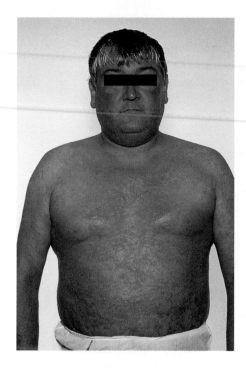

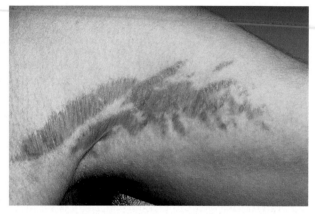

Figure 21.3 Iatrogenic Cushing's syndrome due to the use of large amounts of potent topical corticosteroid (fluocinolone acetonide) over a 3-year period.

Figure 21.4 Striae distensae from the use of potent topical corticosteroids over a 6-month period.

The effects on the skin include:

- skin thinning and striae (Fig. 21.4), resulting from the wasting action of corticosteroids on the dermal connective tissue
- masked infection, particularly ringworm, resulting in extensive and unusual-appearing ringworm (tinea incognito).

Note. Dilution of proprietary preparations is *not* advised because the formulations are complex and the important excipients are also diluted and may be ineffective when the dilution is made. Dilution does not necessarily decrease the effect proportionately.

Case 22

Jeremy, aged 9, had had eczema since he was a few weeks of age, but it had markedly worsened in the past 4 months, as had his asthma. Apart from the obvious severe eczema, he had marked xeroderma. He started to improve when he was treated regularly with emollients two or three times per day. He was also helped by the use of a weak corticosteroid (clobetasone butyrate) twice daily and a strong corticosteroid applied to the sites where there was severe eczema (mometasone furoate) once daily. Care was taken to ensure that he did not use excessive amounts of corticosteroids, in order to avoid the problems of skin thinning and pituitary–adrenal axis suppression.

TOPICAL ANTIMICROBIAL AGENTS

It should be remembered that:

- All that weeps and contains pus is not infected: many inflamed skin disorders are exudative but not infected.
- Some imidazole and older halogenated phenolic compounds may irritate; some antibiotics (e.g. neomycin) sensitize.
- It is quite easy to induce bacterial resistance, and agents that may be used systemically should not be used topically.

Amongst the safest and most useful compounds for bacterial and fungal infections are the imidazoles (e.g. econazole, miconazole, isoconazole), the triazoles (naftifine, terbinafine) and povidone iodine. The antibiotic mupirocin is very useful. Aciclovir, famiciclovir and idoxuridine are antiviral preparations used for herpes simplex, the first of these also being used for herpes zoster.

Surgical aspects of the management of skin disease

The surgical aspects of dermatology are increasingly important in dermatological practice.

- There is a growing demand for the removal of moles, seborrhoeic warts and similar benign lesions.
- The incidence of skin cancers of all types is increasing.
- There is increasing demand and ability to treat the skin changes of photodamage.

BIOPSY

The removal of a small fragment of skin tissue by trephine (punch biopsy) for routine histological preparation for electron microscopy, immunofluorescence or microbial culture is usually adequate. Sharp, disposable trephines are available of 2–6 mm in diameter. Sutures are not necessary for biopsies of less than 4 mm diameter taken this way, and only occasionally for 4 mm trephines. The following are useful tips for taking biopsies.

- Choose a new or typical lesion or the edge of an established lesion.
- It may be necessary to biopsy at different times or to sample different lesions.
- Handle the biopsy as gently as possible.
- Take care when biopsying human immunodeficiency virus (HIV)-positive and hepatitis B-positive patients – the laboratories need to be notified beforehand.
- Patients with bleeding diatheses and heart disease may need prophylactic treatment.

ABLATIVE PROCEDURES

These are mainly used to treat seborrhoeic and viral warts and solar keratoses, but also for minor, benign, localized lesions.

LASER TREATMENT

Lasers are high-intensity, coherent light sources of particular wavelengths, and are employed for their destructive capacity. The particular tissue effect is influenced by the energy, the wavelength and the pulse duration of the emission, as well as by the colour, thickness and depth of the tissue. Lasers are particularly useful for the destruction of vascular birthmarks, but other kinds of lesions can also be tackled.

CURETTAGE AND CAUTERY

Sharp, spoon-shaped curettes or disposable ring curettes are used. After curettage, the base is lightly touched with the tip of an electrocautery loop. Local anaesthesia is required beforehand. Curetted tissue should be examined histologically.

CRYOTHERAPY

This is used to treat viral warts and solar keratoses. A device supplying a fine spray of liquid nitrogen is often used. The frozen skin turns snow white and needs to stay this colour for 15–20 seconds before tissue destruction is complete.

Caution is required when treating lesions on the fingers, as the digital nerves can be damaged. Patients *must* be warned to expect pain and blistering at the frozen site and be told to keep the site covered.

SHAVE EXCISIONS

This procedure is only suitable for benign, raised, dome-shaped lesions, such as stable melanocytic naevi, as some abnormal tissue is left behind. After local anaesthesia, the lesion is shaved off flush with the skin surface with a sharp scalpel. The raw base is then lightly cauterized with an electrocautery loop. The tissue removed is sent for histological examination.

EXCISION OF SMALL TUMOURS

Benign moles, dermatofibromas and small basal cell carcinomas are examples of lesions that can be easily removed by elliptical incisions around the lesion. Margins of at least 3 mm need to be left at the sides of the lesion. The margins of the excision are then sutured *without tension*, using a silk or synthetic suture material. If the incision is parallel to Langer's lines on the limbs and trunk but in the 'crease' lines on the face, scarring should be minimal. Keloid scars sometimes develop in patients aged 12–30 years with excisions over the shoulders, upper arms and front of the chest.

Systemic therapy (see Table 21.4)

In many cases, topical treatments are also available and decisions as to whether to use a topical or a systemic agent need to be made. Some of the considerations are as follows.

- Systemic agents usually carry a greater risk of adverse side effects than topical agents.
- Systemic agents tend to have more potent therapeutic effects than topical agents.
- Many patients prefer a topical agent because they fear the side effects of systemic treatment.
- Some patients dislike using topical treatment and would prefer to take the risk of side effects.
- Topical treatment is impracticable in patients with widespread skin disease and in the elderly and infirm.

The options need to be discussed with the patient.

SYSTEMIC CORTICOSTEROIDS

If these are needed, both the risks and the benefits of such treatment should be understood by all. Their action is predominantly suppressive by virtue of their anti-inflammatory properties. Systemic (and very potent topical) corticosteroids can precipitate pustular psoriasis.

RETINOIDS

Although the usage of isotretinoin and acitretin differs, the precautions and side effects are quite similar. There is a serious danger of teratogenicity if the drug is given to a woman in the reproductive age group, and contraception is important. Acitretin is mostly excreted quite quickly, but in the presence of alcohol is 'back metabolized' to the, now withdrawn, etretinate, which is stored in the fat and detectable in the blood for 2–3 years. Contraception is required for this period. Particular care must be taken with isotretinoin, as this drug is given for severe acne and many young women are exposed to it. The mode of action of the retinoid drugs is uncertain, but there appear to be fundamental effects on cellular differentiation.

Patients on retinoids require monitoring for hepatotoxicity and elevation of serum lipids every 4–8 weeks, and for bone toxicity annually.

Table 21.4 Details of systemic drugs

Drug	Usual dose	Main indications	Main side effects	Comments
Corticosteroids	5–50 mg daily (prednisolone equivalent)	Severe eczema, severe drug reactions, severe autoimmune disease and hypersensitivity disorders, bullous diseases	Hypertension, diabetes, osteoporosis, psychosis, infections, gastrointestinal, bleeding skin thinning and striae, adrenocortical suppression	Lowest dose possible is needed; monitoring 4-weekly when 'stabilized', more frequently early in treatment; caution is needed on stopping treatment because of adrenocortical suppression – gradual reduction in dose is necessary; dose needs to increase during intercurrent illness
Retinoids				
Acitretin	0.5–1.0 mg/kg body weight daily	Severe psoriasis and disorders of keratinization, multiple non-melanoma skin cancers	*Minor:* cheilitis, drying of oral/ nasal/ocular mucosae, diffuse hair loss, paronychiae, pruritus *Major:* teratogenicity, hepatotoxicity, rise in serum lipids, bone toxicity – hyperostosis and ossification of ligaments	Effects start after 4 weeks; relapse is usual after stopping; careful monitoring is required every 4–8 weeks
Isotretinoin	0.5–1.0 mg/kg body weight daily	Severe acne	As above	Effects start after 4 weeks; initial aggravation is common; relapse after stopping is unusual; careful monitoring is required monthly over a 4-month course of treatment

Drug	Dose	Indications	Side effects	Comments
Methotrexate	5–25 mg weekly	Severe psoriasis (pustular erythrodermic, arthropathic and severe recalcitrant plaque type), pemphigus/pemphigoid	Hepatotoxicity with eventual fibrosis, myelotoxicity; nausea and mucositis may occur as acute effects	Regular monitoring is required (4–8-week intervals); liver biopsies are required after a cumulative dose of 1.5 g; may be given in combination with steroids for bullous disease
Azathioprine	50–150 mg daily	Lupus erythematosus and other autoimmune disorders, pemphigus/pemphigoid	Nausea, myelosuppression	Often used in combination with corticosteroids; monitoring is required to check on blood picture every 4–8 weeks
Cyclosporin	2–5 mg/kg body weight daily	Severe psoriasis (erythrodermic or recalcitrant plaque type), severe atopic dermatitis	Renal toxicity and hypertension; nausea and hirsutes are sometimes a problem; over the long term, development of neoplastic disease is a possibility	Potent immunosuppressive agent; interactions with ketoconazole may occur; monitoring 4–6 weekly is advised
Dapsone	25–150 mg daily	Leprosy, dermatitis herpetiformis	Haemolysis, methaemoglobinaemia, sulphaemoglobinaemia, fixed drug eruption; a granulocytosis is recorded	Monitoring every 4–8 weeks is advised

METHOTREXATE

This is an antimetabolite that effectively stops cell division by blocking DNA synthesis. It also has many other metabolic effects. It is used both for its antiproliferative actions and for its immunosuppressive effects. Patients require regular monitoring for myelotoxicity and hepatotoxicity every 4–8 weeks and may need liver biopsies after a cumulative dose of more than 1.5 g because of the frequency of serious liver toxicity, particularly in those who abuse alcohol.

AZATHIOPRINE

This is an antimetabolite that also blocks DNA synthesis, whose prime use in dermatology is for its immunosuppressive activity. As with methotrexate, patients on azathioprine require regular monitoring for myelotoxicity. Before use, the patient should be checked for an inherited enzyme defect (thiopurine methyl transferase) to avoid serious toxicity.

CYCLOSPORIN

This drug blocks lymphokine synthesis by lymphocytes. It is a very potent immunosuppressive agent. Patients on the drug should be monitored for renal toxicity and hypertension every 4–8 weeks.

DAPSONE (DIAMINOSULPHONE)

The mode of action of this drug is unclear. Its antimicrobial effects may be unrelated to its anti-inflammatory activity. It causes haemolysis and methaemoglobinaemia and is myelotoxic.

ANTIFUNGALS

Griseofulvin, terbinafine and itraconazole are effective against dermatophyte infections. Itraconazole, fluconazole and ketoconazole are effective against infections with yeast-like micro-organisms. The doses and side effects are given in Table 21.5.

Phototherapy for skin disease

Many patients with psoriasis and some with acne and atopic dermatitis improve in the summertime after being out in the sun. It is the ultraviolet portion of the solar spectrum (see page 27) that seems to aid these patients, and artificial sources

Table 21.5 Doses and side effects of antifungal agents

Drug	Dose	Indication	Side effects
Griseofulvin	0.5–1.0 g daily	Ringworm infection only	Headaches, photosensitivities
Ketoconazole	200 mg daily	Systemic mycoses, severe ringworm and yeast infections	Nausea, rashes, headaches, liver damage in the elderly
Amphotericin	250 mg/kg daily by i.v. infusion	Systemic candidiasis	Multiple toxicities including renal, neurological and hepatic
Fluconazole	50 mg daily	Candidiasis, especially in immunosuppressed patients	Nausea, rash
Itraconazole	100–200 mg daily	Ringworm and yeast infections	Nausea
Terbinafine	250 mg daily	Ringworm and onychomycosis	Nausea, rash

of ultraviolet radiation (UVR) are often used in treatment. Natural sunshine can also be used if the local weather conditions permit. Special 'spas' have been established at the Dead Sea in Israel, around the Black Sea and elsewhere.

Treatment with the 'sunburn' part of the UV spectrum (UVB: 280–320 nm) is sometimes used to treat patients with psoriasis. Caution is necessary to prevent burning in the short term and chronic photodamage and skin cancers in the long term by giving the minimum dose of UVR necessary to clear the patient's problems.

PUVA treatment

A more usual form of phototherapy in recent years is photochemotherapy with long-wave UVR (UVA) known as PUVA. In this treatment, the skin is photosensitized with psoralen drugs, given either orally 2 hours before irradiation or topically (in a bath) immediately before the UVR.

The oral drug used is mostly 8-methoxy psoralen, given in a dose of approximately 0.6 mg/kg body weight per day. Photochemotherapy with UVA has become a standard treatment for patients with severe and generalized psoriasis and is successful in 70–80 per cent of patients within 6–8 weeks. Usually, treatment is given two or three times per week, starting at a low dose and gradually increasing the dose until a good effect is obtained.

Patients with T-cell lymphoma of the skin (mycosis fungoides, Sézary syndrome) and some with atopic eczema also benefit.

Burning is a danger, and sun-sensitive patients must be treated very carefully with low doses. Nausea is common and due to the psoralen. Dry skin is also a side effect in the short term. Unfortunately, it has been found that some 8–10 years after 'high-dose' PUVA treatment, there is a greatly increased incidence of skin cancers – particularly squamous cell carcinoma. Other forms of skin cancer and chronic photodamage also seem to be increased after UVA.

Goggles or glasses that block UVA must be used during treatment and for 24 hours afterwards to prevent cataracts. Male patients need to cover their external genitalia because of the risk of neoplasia.

Summary

- The skin is important in communication and there is fear and dislike of skin disorders, causing social isolation and depression in patients.
- Stress may precipitate but not cause skin disorders. Patients may produce a variety of lesions (dermatitis artefacta). Rarely, patients may harbour a delusion that their skin is infested by insects.
- Dysmorphophobia describes the problem of people's distorted self-image (e.g. their nose is too big, they have too much hair).
- Skin disease may be both physically and emotionally disabling.
- In general, ointments are used for chronic scaling disorders, whereas creams and lotions are used for acute and exudative disorders.
- Emollients occlude the skin surface, prevent evaporation and cause a build up of water in the stratum corneum. They soothe, smooth and soften the skin. They have some anti-inflammatory actions and enhance desquamation. They are helpful for patients with eczema, psoriasis and ichthyosis.
- Topical corticosteroids are absorbed and may cause pituitary–adrenal axis suppression with adrenal cortical atrophy if appreciable amounts are applied (e.g. if more than 50 g of betamethasone valerate ointment or more than 30 g of clobetasol propionate ointment are used per week).
- Topical corticosteroids also cause skin thinning and marked infection.
- Imidazoles and povidone iodine preparations are amongst the safest and most useful of the topical antimicrobial agents.
- Skin surgery is a growing area of work for dermatologists because of a growing demand for the removal of moles, warts and other blemishes. In addition, surgical techniques, laser treatments and cryotherapy have become increasingly sophisticated.
- Potent systemic therapies are often available, but are more likely to cause significant adverse side effects. These include the systemic corticosteroids, the oral retinoids, methotrexate, azathioprine, cyclosporin and dapsone.
- Oral antifungal agents include terbinafine, griseofulvin and itraconazole.
- Phototherapy may be the most suitable form of treatment for generalized skin disease. This includes PUVA, UVB and spa treatments.

Bibliography

Books of interest

Adler, M.W. (ed.) 1990 *ABC of Sexually Transmitted Disease*. London: BMJ Publishing Group.

Ashton, R.E. (ed.) 1992 *Differential Diagnosis in Dermatology* (second edition). Oxford: Radcliffe Medical Press.

Darmon, M. and Blumenberg, M. (eds) 1993 *Molecular Biology of the Skin: the keratinocyte*. London: Academic Press.

Freinkel, R. and Woodley, D. (eds) 2001 *The Biology of Skin*. Carnforth: Parthenon.

Harper, J. (ed.) 1990 *Handbook of Paediatric Dermatology*. London: Butterworths.

Hawk, J.L.M. (ed.) 1999 *Photodermatology*. London: Arnold.

Levene, G.M. and Goolamali, S.K. (eds) 1986 *Diagnostic Picture Tests in Dermatology*. London: Wolfe.

Lowe, N. and Marks, R. 1998 *Retinoids. A Clinician's Guide* (second edition). London: Martin Dunitz.

McKee, P.H. 1999 *Essential Skin Pathology*. St Louis, MI: C.V. Mosby.

Marks, R. (ed.) 1981 *Coping with Psoriasis*. London: Sheldon Press.

Marks, R. (ed.) 1992 *Eczema*. London: Martin Dunitz.

Marks, R. (ed.) 1999 *Skin Disease in Old Age* (second edition). London: Martin Dunitz.

Marks, R. 2001 *Sophisticated Emollients*. Stuttgart: Thieme International.

Marks, R. and Leyden, J.J. (eds) 2002 *Dermatologic Therapy in Current Practice*. London: Martin Dunitz.

Marks, R. and Ortanne, J.P. 1999 *Photodamaged Skin: clinical signs, causes and management*. London: Martin Dunitz.

Marks, R., Dykes, P.J. and Motley, R. 1993. *Clinical Signs and Procedures in Dermatology*. London: Martin Dunitz.

Marks, R., Leveque, J.L. and Voegeli, R. (eds) 2002 *The Essential Stratum Corneum*. London: Martin Dunitz.

Reonigk, R.K. and Roegnik, H.H. (eds) 1993 *Surgical Dermatology*. London: Martin Dunitz.

Sharvill, D.E. (ed.) 1988 *Skin Signs of Systemic Disease*. London: Pocket Picture Guides.

Reference books

Braun-Falco, O., Plewig, G. et al. 2000. *Dermatology*. Berlin: Springer-Verlag.

Champion, R.H., Burton, J.L., Burns, D.A. and Breathnach, S.M. (eds) 1998 *Textbook of Dermatology* (sixth edition, in four volumes). Oxford: Blackwell Science.

Goldsmith, L.A. (ed.) 1991 *Physiology, Biochemistry and Molecular Biology of the Skin* (second edition). Oxford: Oxford University Press.

McKee, P.H. 1989 *Pathology of the Skin with Clinical Correlations*. Philadelphia, PA: J.B. Lippincott Co.

Selected articles and reviews

Barbargallo, J., Tager, P., Ingleton, R., Hirsch, R.J. and Weinberg, J.M. 2002: Cutaneous tuberculosis. Diagnosis and treatment. *American Journal of Clinical Dermatology* **3**, 319–328.

Chartier, M.B., Hoss, D.M. and Grant Kels, J.M. 2002: Approach to the adult female patient with diffuse non scarring alopecia. *Journal of the American Academy of Dermatology* **47**, 809–818.

English, J. 2001: Current concepts in contact dermatitis. *British Journal of Dermatology* **145**, 527–529.

Huang, C.L., Nordlund, J.J. and Boissy, R. 2002: Vitiligo. A manifestation of apoptosis? *American Journal of Clinical Dermatology* **5**, 301–308.

Kroumpouzos, G. and Cohen, L.M. 2001: Dermatoses of pregnancy. *Journal of the American Academy of Dermatology* **45**, 1–19.

Leung, D.Y.M. and Soter, N.A. 2001: Cellular and immunologic mechanisms in atopic dermatitis. *Journal of the American Academy of Dermatology* **44**(1), S1–S12.

Marks, R. 1999: The significance and measurement of scaling. *Journal of Dermatology* **26**, 713–717.

Nakagawa, S. and Bos, J.D. 2001: Role of Langerhans cells in the skin. What's new? *Journal of the European Academy of Dermatology and Venereology* **15**, 399–401.

Nickolff, B.J. 1999: The immunologic and genetic basis of psoriasis. *Archives of Dermatology* **135**, 1104–1110.

Takigawa, M. 2002: Histamine and cutaneous allergy: old friend, new player. *Journal of Dermatology* **20**, 263–266.

Index

Note: page numbers in **bold** refer to figures, page numbers in *italics* refer to information contained in tables